S. MELOCHE

MW01412821

DRUG FACTS

1998

FACTS AND COMPARISONS ®

A Wolters Kluwer Company

St. Louis

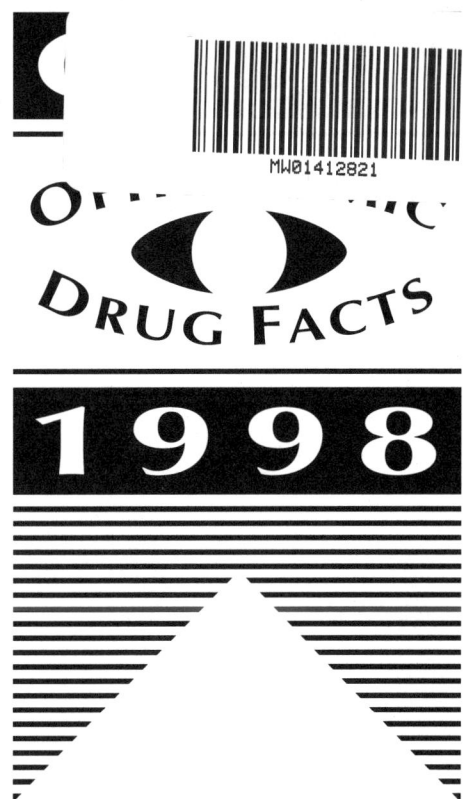

ODF

OPHTHALMIC DRUG FACTS

1998

Ophthalmic Drug Facts®

Copyright © 1998 by Facts and Comparisons®

All rights reserved. No part of this publication may be reproduced or transmitted in any form or by any means, electronic or mechanical, including photocopy, recording, or any information storage data base or retrieval system, or be put into a computer, without prior permission in writing from Facts and Comparisons®, the publisher.

Adapted from *Drug Facts and Comparisons®* loose-leaf drug information service.

ISBN 1-57439-008-2
ISSN 1043-1780

Printed in the United States of America

The information contained in this publication is intended to supplement the knowledge of healthcare professionals regarding ophthalmic drug information. This information is advisory only and is not intended to replace sound clinical judgment or individualized patient care in the delivery of healthcare services. Facts and Comparisons® disclaims all warranties, whether expressed or implied, including any warranty as to the quality, accuracy or suitability of this information for any particular purpose.

Published by
Facts and Comparisons®
A **Wolters Kluwer** Company
111 West Port Plaza, Suite 300
St. Louis, Missouri 63146-3098
314/216-2100
800/223-0554 Customer Service
314/878-5563 Fax

ODF

1998

Ophthalmic Drug Facts Editorial Panel:

Jimmy D. Bartlett, OD, DOS
Professor of Optometry,
School of Optometry
Professor of Pharmacology
School of Medicine
University of Alabama at Birmingham

Richard G. Fiscella, RPh, MPH
Clinical Associate Professor
Department of Pharmacy Practice
University of Illinois at Chicago

N. Rex Ghormley, OD, FAAO
Contact Lens and Vision Care Consultants
St. Louis, Missouri

Siret D. Jaanus, PhD
Professor of Pharmacology and Chairman
Department of Biological Sciences
State University of New York
State College of Optometry
New York, New York

J. James Rowsey, MD
Professor and Chairman
Department of Ophthalmology
University of South Florida
College of Medicine
Tampa, Florida

Thom J. Zimmerman, MD, PhD
Chairman of Department of
Ophthalmology and Visual Sciences
Professor of Pharmacology & Toxicology
University of Louisville

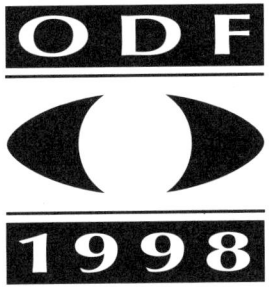

Facts and Comparisons Editorial Advisory Panel:

Dennis J. Cada, PharmD
Executive Editor, The Formulary

Timothy R. Covington, PharmD, MS
Anthony and Marianne Bruno Professor of Pharmacy
Director, Managed Care Institute
School of Pharmacy, Samford University

Daniel A. Hussar, PhD
Remington Professor of Pharmacy
Philadelphia College of Pharmacy and Science

Louis Lasagna, MD
Dean, Sackler School of Graduate Biomedical Sciences
Tufts University

James R. Selevan, BSEE, MD
CIO, Senior Vice President
Monarch Healthcare

Richard W. Sloan, MD, RPh
Chairman and Residency Program Director
Department of Family Practice
York Hospital
Clinical Associate Professor
Pennsylvania State University

David S. Tatro, PharmD
Drug Information Consultant
San Francisco, California

Thomas L. Whitsett, MD
Professor of Medicine and Pharmacology
Director, Clinical Pharmacology Program
University of Oklahoma Health Sciences Center

Facts and Comparisons Staff:

Vin Parker
president

Steven K. Hebel, BS Pharm
director, editorial/production

Bernie R. Olin, PharmD
director of drug information

Cathy H. Reilly
coordinating editor

Noël A. Shamleffer
special projects editor

Julie Scott
quality control editor

Beverly Donnell
Linda Jones
Bridget Sinclair
Orlando Thomas
assistant editors

TABLE OF CONTENTS

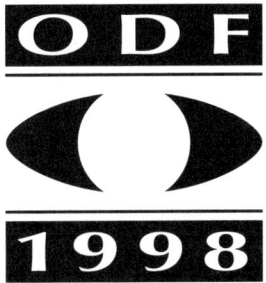

EDITOR'S PREFACE

The mission of *Ophthalmic Drug Facts* is to provide reliable and objective ophthalmic drug information and facilitate therapeutic decision making. This book is intended to promote efficient, quality eye health care. Although general information is available for ophthalmic drugs, there are very few sources that provide comparative drug and drug product information in a concise format; none is as comprehensive.

Ophthalmic Drug Facts was conceived and developed through a team approach and will be of value to both the student and eyecare practitioner. Ophthalmologists, optometrists and opticians should find this text particularly valuable in their daily practices.

Ophthalmic Drug Facts provides a broad range of information including pharmacologic and pharmacokinetic information on drug entities, commercial product information and specific formulation availability. The text is arranged in a pharmacotherapeutic format, with emphasis on drug action and current product availability rather than on pathophysiology of disease states.

Ophthalmic Drug Facts is a comprehensive ophthalmic drug information resource. Detailed information on specific entities is included as well as many drug combinations. There is also a comprehensive section of contact lens products and extemporaneous preparations. Selected bibliographies are provided for all chapters. In addition, *Ophthalmic Drug Facts* includes valuable information on:

- Systemic medications for ocular conditions
- Systemic drugs affecting the eye
- Unlabeled uses for FDA-approved drugs
- Orphan ophthalmic agents and investigational drugs
- Selected Clinical Practice Guidelines of the American Optometric Association
- Excipient glossary
- Ophthalmic product manufacturer index

New information of importance in the *1998 Edition* includes: Two new agents for glaucoma: brimonidine *(Alphagan)* and latanoprost *(Xalatan)*; a new anti-infective, cidofovir *(Vistide)*; a new ganciclovir implant *(Vitrasert)*; and a new H_1-receptor antagonist, olopatadine HCl *(Patanol)*; three new chapters: Extemporanous Preparations, Systemic Medications Used for Ocular Conditions and Selected American Optometric Association Clinical Practice Guidelines; new Chapter Summary tables; revised Excipient Glossary; and more administration and dosage illustrations.

We hope the reader finds this a valuable guide in ophthalmic drug product selection and use. As any practitioner is aware, ophthalmic practice is constantly adapting to incorporate the latest information. We intend to continue the effort with future editions; therefore, your comments, criticisms and suggestions are always welcome.

Jimmy D. Bartlett, OD, DOS
Richard G. Fiscella, RPh, MPH
N. Rex Ghormley, OD, FAAO
Siret D. Jaanus, PhD
J. James Rowsey, MD
Thom J. Zimmerman, MD, PhD

INTRODUCTION

Ophthalmic Drug Facts is a comprehensive ophthalmic drug information compendium. The unique format is designed to facilitate comparisons between drugs. To enable the reader to quickly locate needed information, it has been organized by:

- Therapeutic drug class
- Table of contents
- Chapter summary tables
- Comprehensive alphabetical index
- Extensive cross-referencing

The following pages explain the organization and contents of *Ophthalmic Drug Facts* in detail. All readers are urged to review this information to ensure efficient and effective use of *Ophthalmic Drug Facts.*

♦ Editorial Policy

Accurate, unbiased information; concise, standardized presentation; comparative, objective format; and timely delivery are the principal editorial guidelines governing *Ophthalmic Drug Facts*. Review of FDA-approved product labeling, hundreds of journal articles, textbooks, policies and recommendations from many authoritative and official groups form the base of evaluation of information for *Ophthalmic Drug Facts.* FDA-approved indications and dosage recommendations are included. In addition, other established or potential uses are discussed and are designated as *"Off-labeled Uses."*

Most of the products listed are protected by letters of patent and their names are trademarked and registered by the firm whose name appears with the product. Identification of the product distributor is given in parentheses next to the brand name. The distributor may or may not be the actual manufacturer or fabricator of the final dosage form. Listing of specific products is an indication only of availability on the market and does not constitute an endorsement or recommendation.

Products which contain identical amounts of active ingredients are listed together for comparison as an aid in product selection. Drug product interchange is regulated by state laws; listing of products together does not imply that they are therapeutically equivalent or legally interchangeable. Caution is particularly advised when comparing sustained release, timed release or repeat action dosage forms.

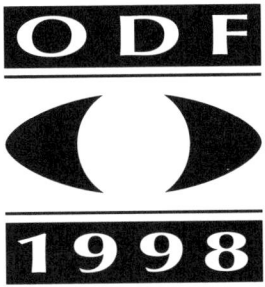

♦ Editorial Panel

The Editorial Panel for *Ophthalmic Drug Facts* is an interdisciplinary group of established, respected and renowned clinicians and researchers. The panel includes recognized experts in the fields of ocular pharmacology, therapeutics and drug information. These experts contribute the introductory material, review monographs and provide direction for *Ophthalmic Drug Facts.*

The *Drug Facts and Comparisons* Editorial Advisory Panel consists of a very distinguished group of physicians, pharmacologists and pharmacists. This panel reviews monographs and provides editorial direction for the entire Facts and Comparisons data base.

♦ Organization

Information in *Ophthalmic Drug Facts* is organized by therapeutic use. Twelve chapters are divided into groups and subgroups to facilitate comparisons of drugs and drug products with similar uses. The remaining chapters provide information on chapter summary tables, ophthalmic dosage forms and routes of administration, nonsurgical adjuncts, contact lens care, systemic drugs affecting the eye, extemporaneous preparations, systemic medications used for ocular conditions, drugs with unlabeled ophthalmic uses, investigational and orphan drugs, and selected American Optometric Association Clinical Practice Guidelines.

Products most similar in content or use are listed together. This format of presenting the facts makes it easy to make comparisons of identical, similar or related products. Because drugs are listed by use, some drugs may be listed in more than one section of the book.

♦ Index

The alphabetical index includes page references for drugs by their generic name, brand or trade name *(italics)* and therapeutic group names. Additionally, many synonyms, pharmacological actions and therapeutic uses for agents are included.

♦ Chapter Introductions

The chapter introduction provides information about the drugs in each therapeutic class. It also discusses general treatment guidelines. A selected bibliography located at the end of each chapter introduction provides additional sources of information.

♦ Drug Monographs

Prescribing information is presented in comprehensive drug monographs. General information on a group of closely related drugs may be presented in a group monograph. Specific information relating to a particular drug is presented in an individual monograph under the generic name of the drug. All monographs are divided into sections identified with bold titles for ease in locating the desired information.

Actions: This section gives a brief summary of the known pharmacologic and pharmacokinetic properties.

Indications: All FDA-approved indications or uses are listed. When available, drug monographs also include "Off-labeled Uses." These include investigational uses for drugs and uses not yet approved by the FDA.

Contraindications: This section specifies those conditions in which the drug should NOT be used.

Warnings and Precautions: These sections list conditions in which use of the drug may be hazardous, precautions to observe and parameters to monitor during therapy.

Drug Interactions: A brief summary of documented, clinically significant drug-drug, drug-food and drug-lab test interactions is provided.

Adverse Reactions: Reported adverse reactions are presented. Incidence data on adverse effects are included when available.

Overdosage: The clinical manifestations of toxicity and treatment of overdosage are given for most agents.

Patient Information: This section provides the essential information to be communicated to the patient by the health professional to allow the patient to safely and effectively administer the medication.

Administration and Dosage: Dosage ranges and methods of administration are presented.

♦ Charts and Tables

Charts and tables are included in many monographs to make drug-drug comparisons easier. Examples of tables include: Pharmacokinetics (onset, peak and duration of action), routes of administration, dosage ranges and adverse reactions.

♦ Special Features

Contact Lens Care Products: Chapter 13 provides guidelines and product information for hard, soft and rigid gas permeable contact lens care.

Extemporaneous Preparations: Chapter 14 provides guidelines for the use and preparation of extemporaneous compounding of ophthalmic solutions.

Systemic Drugs Affecting the Eye: Chapter 15 discusses the effects systemic drugs have on ocular structures and functions.

Systemic Medications Used for Ocular Conditions: Chapter 16 discusses systemic medications and their uses and dosing in ocular conditions.

Drugs with Unlabeled Ophthalmic Uses: Chapter 17 discusses FDA-approved drugs that are being used for unlabeled ophthalmic purposes.

Orphan Drugs: Chapter 18 briefly describes Orphan Drug legislation and includes a table that provides generic name, trade name, indication and manufacturer information on Orphan Drugs for ophthalmic conditions.

Investigational New Drugs: Chapter 18 also outlines the FDA drug approval process and includes a table that provides generic name, trade name (if available), therapeutic class or use, and manufacturer information for ophthalmic drugs on the horizon.

American Optometric Association Clinical Practice Guidelines: We have reprinted three of the most relevant guidelines for the practicing eye care professional and student.

Excipient Glossary: This glossary lists pharmaceutical excipients found in ophthalmic products. The functions and strengths of these adjuncts are briefly described.

Manufacturer Index: This index provides the unique manufacturer/labeler codes found in the National Drug Code (NDC) numbers, as well as the addresses and phone numbers of the manufacturers and distributors of ophthalmic products listed in *Ophthalmic Drug Facts.*

♦ Cost Index

The healthcare and pharmaceutical industries are undergoing rapid changes to improve the efficiency with which services can be offered and the economic productivity of various business relationships that have been formed in this new environment. A consequence of these developing business relationships has been the formulation of various drug pricing plans that are now in effect for managed care organizations, hospital and physician networks, wholesale distributors, and other pharmaceutical and endpoint users of medications. Since the complexity of these relationships precludes accurate prediction of medication cost, we have deleted the cost comparison data (Cost Index) from this edition of *Ophthalmic Drug Facts.*

♦ Product Listings

Individual products are listed following each monograph. The format and components of the product listings are discussed below and illustrated on the following page.

1. **Chapter title** is located at the top of the right-hand page.
2. **Generic titles** appear at the beginning of general drug monographs and individual drug monographs.
3. **Cross references** to the appropriate drug monograph appear for complete prescribing information.
4. **Distribution status** of products is indicated as *Rx* or *otc.*
5. **Products are grouped** by dosage form or strength.
6. **Identical brand name products** are listed in alphabetical order. Combination products are listed in tables to facilitate comparisons. Products most similar in formulation are listed next to each other.
7. **Package sizes** are given for all dosage forms and strengths of each product.
8. **Products available by their generic name** from multiple sources are indicated as available from (Various) distributors. Selected multiple-source distributors and manufacturers are provided. The list of distributors and manufacturers is intended to provide an example and is not an attempt to be comprehensive.
9. **Distributor's name** is given in parentheses next to the product name.

ATROPINE SULFATE (2)

For complete prescribing information, refer to the Cycloplegic Mydriatrics group (3)
monograph.

Indications:

Mydriasis/Cycloplegia: For cycloplegic refraction or pupil dilation in acute inflammatory conditions of iris and uveal tract.

Administration and Dosage:

Solution:

Adults – Uveitis: Instill 1 or 2 drops into the eye(s) up to 4 times daily.

Children – Uveitis: Instill 1 or 2 drops of 0.5% solution into the eye(s) up to 3 times daily.

Refraction: Instill 1 or 2 drops of 0.5% solution into the eye(s) twice daily for 1 to 3 days before examination.

Ointment: Apply a small amount in the conjunctival sac up to 3 times daily.

Compress the lacrimal sac by digital pressure during and for 2 to 3 minutes after instillation.

Individuals with heavily pigmented irides may require larger doses.

Storage: Keep away from heat.

Rx	**Atropine Sulfate Ophthalmic** (Various, eg, Bausch & Lomb, Fougera, Pharmafair, Zenith-Goldline) (4)	**Ointment**: 1%	In 3.5 and UD 1 g.
Rx	**Isopto Atropine** (Alcon)	**Solution**: 0.5%	In 5 ml Drop-Tainers.[1]
Rx	**Atropine Sulfate** (Various, eg, Alcon, Allergan, Bausch & Lomb, Optopics, Pharmafair, Rugby, Zenith-Goldline) (6)	(8) **Solution**: 1%	In 2, 5 and 15 ml and UD 1 ml. (7)
Rx	**Atropine Care** (Akorn)		In 2, 5 and 15 ml.[2]
Rx	**Atropine-1** (Optopics)		In 2, 5 and 15 ml.
Rx	**Atropisol** (Ciba Vision)		(5) In 1 ml Dropperettes.[3]
Rx	**Isopto Atropine** (Alcon)	(9)	In 5 and 15 ml Drop-Tainers.[1]
Rx	**Atropine Sulfate** (Alcon)	**Solution**: 2%	In 2 ml.

[1] With 0.01% benzalkonium chloride, 0.5% hydroxypropyl methylcellulose and boric acid.
[2] With 0.01% benzalkonium chloride, hydroxypropyl methylcellulose and boric acid.
[3] With benzalkonium chloride, EDTA and boric acid.

ODF

1

Dosage Forms And Routes Of Administration

For ophthalmic drugs to be effective, they must reach ocular tissues in relatively high concentrations. Depending on the specific diagnostic or therapeutic objective, ophthalmic drugs may be delivered to the eye through various routes of administration, including:

- Topical
- Oral
- Parenteral
- Periocular
- Intracameral
- Intravitreal

TOPICAL ADMINISTRATION

Topical application is the most common route of administration for ophthalmic drugs. Advantages include convenience, simplicity, noninvasive nature and the ability of the patient to self-administer. Because of blood and aqueous losses of drug, topical medications do not typically penetrate in useful concentrations to posterior ocular structures and usually are of no therapeutic benefit for diseases of the retina, optic nerve and other posterior segment structures.

Inactive Ingredients

The following inactive agents may be present in ophthalmic products:

Preservatives destroy or inhibit multiplication of microorganisms introduced into the product by accident.

benzalkonium chloride
benzethonium chloride
cetylpyridinium chloride
chlorobutanol
EDTA
mercurial preservatives
(phenylmercuric nitrate, phenylmercuric acetate, thimerosal)
methyl/propylparabens
phenylethyl alcohol
sodium benzoate
sodium propionate
sorbic acid

Viscosity-Increasing Agents slow drainage of the product from the eye, thus increasing retention time of the active drug. Increased bioavailability may result.

carboxymethylcellulose sodium
dextran 70
gelatin
glycerin
hydroxyethyl cellulose
hydroxypropyl methylcellulose
methylcellulose
PEG
poloxamer 407
polysorbate 80
propylene glycol
polyvinyl alcohol
polyvinylpyrrolidone (povidone)

Antioxidants prevent or delay deterioration of products by oxygen in the air.

EDTA
sodium bisulfite
sodium metabisulfite
sodium thiosulfate
thiourea

Wetting Agents reduce surface tension, allowing drug solution to spread.

polysorbate 20 and 80
poloxamer 282
tyloxapol

Buffers help maintain ophthalmic products in the range of pH 6 to 8, which is the comfortable range for ophthalmic instillation.

acetic acid
boric acid
hydrochloric acid
phosphoric acid
potassium bicarbonate
potassium borate
potassium carbonate
potassium citrate
potassium phosphate
potassium tetraborate
sodium acetate
sodium bicarbonate
sodium biphosphate
sodium borate
sodium carbonate
sodium citrate
sodium hydroxide
sodium phosphate

Tonicity Agents help the ophthalmic product solutions to be isotonic with the preocular tear film. Products in the sodium chloride equivalence range of 0.9% ± 0.2% are considered isotonic and will help prevent ocular irritation and tissue damage. A range of 0.6% to 1.8% is usually comfortable for ophthalmic use.

buffers
dextran 40 and 70
dextrose
glycerin
potassium chloride
propylene glycol
sodium Cl

Packaging Standards

To help reduce confusion in labeling and identification of various topical ocular medications, drug packaging standards have been proposed. When fully implemented by the ophthalmic drug industry, the standard colors for drug labels and bottle caps will include the following:

Topical Ophthalmic Drug Packaging Standards

Therapeutic class	Proposed color
Beta blockers	Yellow, blue or both
Mydriatics and cycloplegics	Red
Miotics	Green
Nonsteroidal anti-inflammatory drugs	Grey
Anti-infectives	Brown, tan
Carbonic anhydrase inhibitors	Orange

Medications

Solutions and Suspensions: Most topical ocular preparations are commercially available as solutions or suspensions that are applied directly to the eye from the bottle, which serves as the eye dropper. Avoid touching the dropper tip to the eye because this can lead to contamination of the medication and may also cause ocular injury. Resuspend suspensions (notably, many ocular steroids) by shaking to provide an accurate dosage of drug.

Betaxolol 0.25% (*Betoptic S*) and rimexolone (*Vexol*) are classified by the FDA as suspensions, but are much less viscous products suspended in carbonol gels than is pilocarpine (*Pilopine HS*). A drop can be administered with less concern for prolonged blurry vision. Although *Betoptic S* and *Vexol* are classified technically as suspensions, little shaking is required to suspend or resuspend these agents.

RECOMMENDED PROCEDURES FOR ADMINISTRATION OF SOLUTIONS AND SUSPENSIONS
1. Wash hands thoroughly before administration.
2. Tilt head backward or lie down and gaze upward.
3. Gently grasp lower eyelid below eyelashes and pull the eyelid away from the eye to form a pouch.
4. Place dropper directly over eye. Avoid contact of the dropper with the eye, finger or any surface.
5. Look upward just before applying a drop.
6. Release the lid slowly and close eyes gently.
7. With eyes closed, apply gentle pressure with fingers to the inside corner of eye for 2-3 minutes (see Figure 1). This retards drainage of the solution from the intended area.
8. Do not rinse the dropper.
9. Do not use eye drops that have changed color or contain a precipitate.
10. If more than one type of ophthalmic drop is used, wait ≥ 5 minutes before administering the second agent.

Solutions and Suspension - Drops

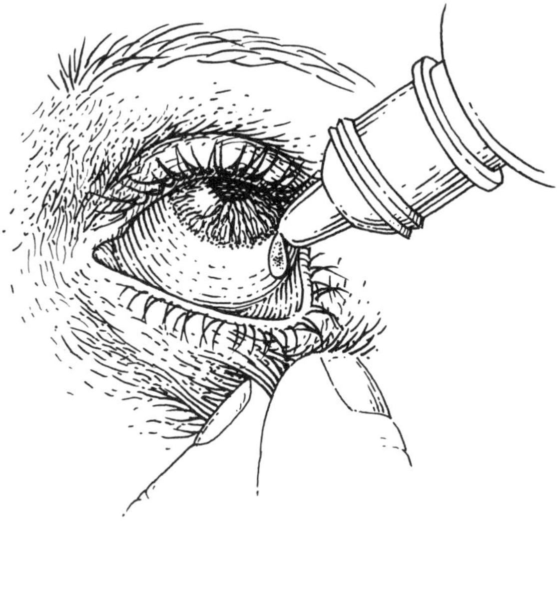

Nasolacrimal Occlusion

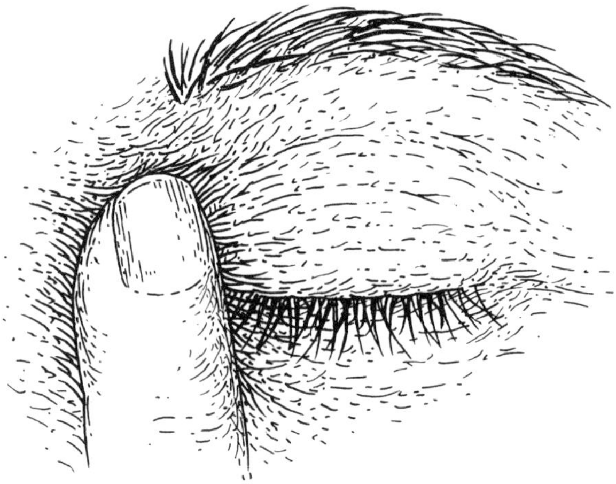

Ointments: The primary purpose for an ophthalmic ointment vehicle is to prolong drug contact time with the external ocular surface. This is particularly useful for treating children, who may "cry out" topically applied solutions, and for medicating ocular injuries, such as corneal abrasions, when the eye is to be patched. Administer solutions before ointments. Ointments preclude entry of subsequent drops.

RECOMMENDED PROCEDURES FOR ADMINISTRATION OF OINTMENTS
1. Wash hands thoroughly before administration. 2. Tilt head backward or lie down and gaze upward. 3. Gently pull down the lower lid to form a pouch. 4. Place 0.25 to 0.5 inch of ointment with a sweeping motion inside the lower lid by squeezing the tube gently and slowly release the eyelid. 5. Close the eye for 1 to 2 minutes. 6. Temporary blurring of vision may occur. Avoid activities requiring visual acuity until blurring clears. 7. Remove excessive ointment around the eye or ointment tube tip with a tissue. 8. If using more than one kind of ointment, wait about 10 minutes before applying the second agent.

See ointment administration illustrations on following page.

Ointments

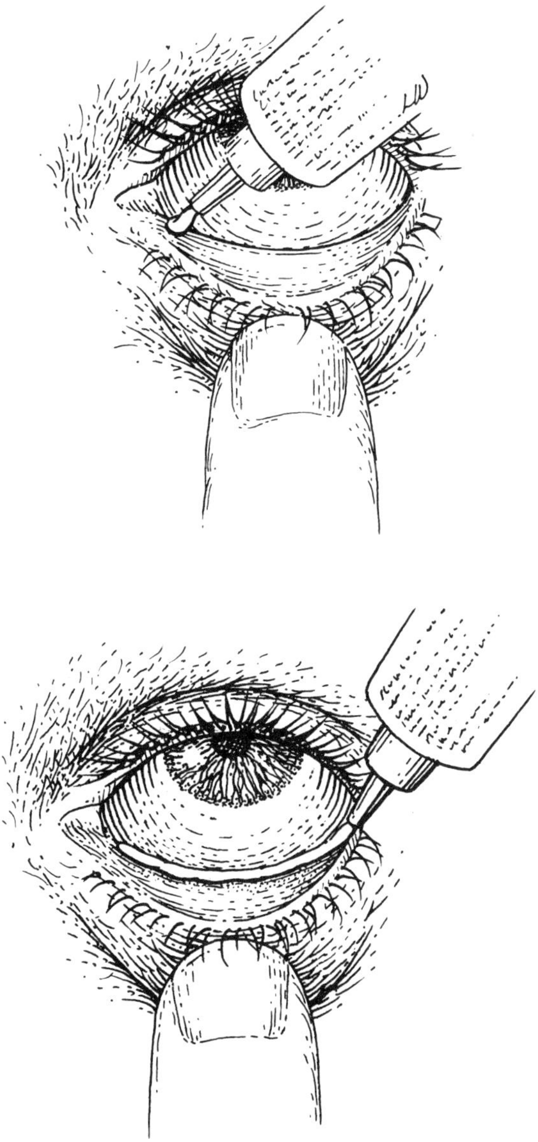

Gels: Ophthalmic gels are similar in viscosity and clinical usage to ophthalmic ointments. Pilocarpine (*Pilopine HS*), betaxolol 0.25% (*Betoptic S*), and rimexolone (*Vexol*) are three ophthalmic products formulated in carbopol gels. *Pilopine HS* is more viscous, like traditional gel, and is applied at bedtime to avoid blurred vision. Timolol maleate (*Timoptic XE*) is a slightly viscous solution that forms a gel when placed in contact with the cations in the preocular tear fluid. This formulation provides a prolonged contact time for the *Timoptic XE* within the precorneal tear film.

Sprays: Although not commercially available, some practitioners use mydriatics or cycloplegics, alone or in combination, administered as a spray to the eye to dilate the pupil or for cycloplegic examination. This is most often used for pediatric patients, and the solution is administered using a sterile perfume atomizer or plastic spray bottle.

Lid Scrubs: Commercially available eyelid cleansers or antibiotic solutions or ointments can be applied directly to the lid margin for the treatment of noninfectious blepharitis. This is best accomplished by applying the medication to the end of a cotton-tipped applicator and then scrubbing the eyelid margin several times daily. The gauze pads supplied with commercially available eyelid cleansers are also convenient.

Lid Scrub - Cotton-Tipped Applicator

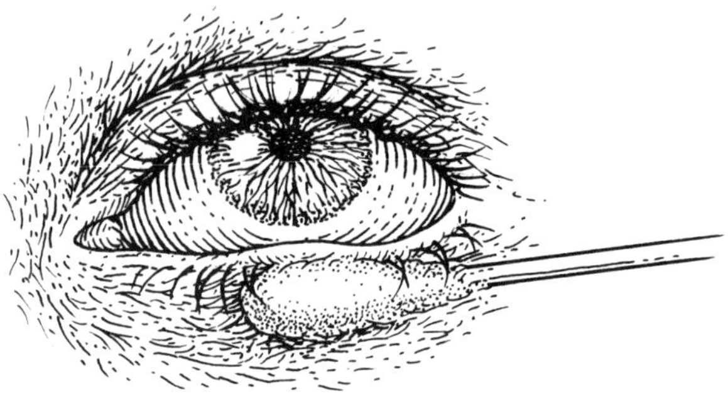

Lid Scrub - Gauze

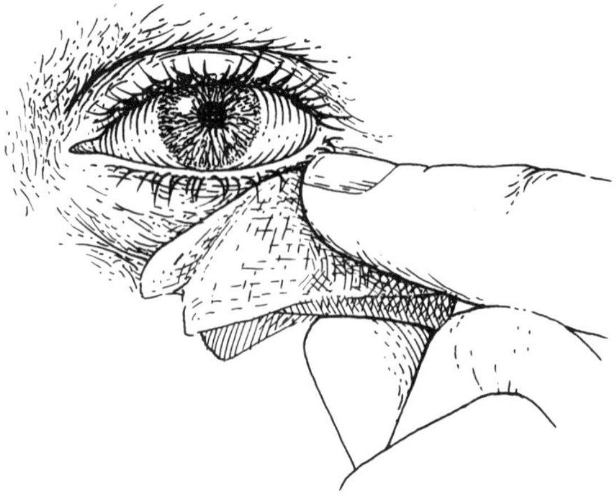

Devices

Contact Lenses: Soft contact lenses can absorb water-soluble drugs and release them to the eye over prolonged periods of time. This has the clinical advantage of promoting sustained release of solutions or suspensions that would otherwise be removed quickly from the external ocular tissues. Soft contact lenses as drug delivery devices are most often used in the management of dry eye disorders, but the technique is occasionally used for the treatment of ocular infections, including corneal ulcers.

Corneal Shields: Non-cross-linked, homogenized, porcine or bovine scleral collagen shields are available. These devices are placed as a bandage on the cornea following surgery or injury, protecting and lubricating the cornea. Topical antibiotics have been used in conjunction with the shield to promote healing of corneal ulcers.

Cotton Pledgets: Small pieces of cotton can be saturated with ophthalmic solutions and placed in the conjunctival sac. These devices allow a prolonged ocular contact time with solutions that are normally administered topically into the eye. The clinical use of pledgets is usually reserved for the administration of mydriatic solutions such as cocaine or phenylephrine. This drug delivery method promotes maximum mydriasis in an attempt to break posterior synechiae or to dilate sluggish pupils.

Filter Paper Strips: Sodium fluorescein and rose bengal dyes are commercially available as drug-impregnated filter paper strips. The strips help ensure sterility of sodium fluorescein which, when prepared in solution, can become easily contaminated with *Pseudomonas aeruginosa.* These dyes are used diagnostically to disclose corneal injuries, infections such as herpes simplex, and dry eye disorders.

Artificial Tear Inserts: A rod-shaped pellet of hydroxypropyl cellulose without preservative (*Lacrisert*) is inserted into the inferior conjunctival sac with a specially designed applicator. Following placement, the device absorbs fluid, swells, and then releases the nonmedicated polymer to the eye for up to 24 hours. The device is designed as a sustained-release artificial tear for the treatment of dry eye disorders.

Membrane-Bound Inserts: A membrane-controlled drug delivery system (*Ocusert*) delivers a constant quantity of pilocarpine to the eye for up to 1 week. Placed onto the bulbar conjunctiva under the upper or lower eyelid, it is a useful substitute for pilocarpine drops or gel in glaucoma patients who cannot comply with more frequent drug instillation or in those with ocular or visual side effects from pilocarpine solutions.

GENERAL CONSIDERATIONS IN TOPICAL OPHTHALMIC DRUG THERAPY

Proper administration is essential to optimal therapeutic response. In many instances, health professionals may be too casual when instructing patients on proper use of ophthalmics. The administration technique used often determines drug safety and efficacy.

- The normal eye retains ≈ 10 mcl of fluid (adjusted for blinking). The average dropper delivers 25 to 50 mcl/drop. There is no value in instilling more than one properly placed drop.
- Minimize systemic absorption of ophthalmic drops by compressing the canaliculus and lacrimal sacs for 3 to 5 minutes after instillation. This retards passage of drops via nasolacrimal duct into areas of potential absorption such as nasal and pharyngeal mucosa.
- Because of rapid lacrimal drainage and limited eye capacity, if multiple-drop therapy is indicated, the best interval between drops is 5 minutes. This ensures that the first drop is not flushed away by the second or that the second is not diluted by the first.
- Factors that may increase absorption from ophthalmic doseforms include lax eyelids of some patients, usually the elderly, which creates a greater reservoir for retention of drops, and hyperemic or diseased eyes.
- Eyecup use is discouraged due to risk of contamination and spreading disease.
- Ophthalmic suspensions mix with tears less rapidly and remain in the cul-de-sac longer than solutions.
- Ophthalmic ointments maintain contact between the drug and ocular tissues by slowing the clearance rate to as little as 0.5% per minute. Ophthalmic ointments provide maximum contact between drug and external ocular tissues.
- Ophthalmic ointments may impede delivery of other ophthalmic drugs to the affected side by serving as a barrier to contact.
- Ointments may blur vision during the waking hours. Use with caution in conditions where visual clarity is critical (eg, operating motor equipment, reading) or use at bedtime.
- Monitor expiration dates closely. Do not use outdated medication.
- Solutions and ointments are frequently misused. Do not assume that patients know how to maximize safe and effective use of these agents. Combine appropriate patient education and counseling with prescribing and dispensing of ophthalmics.

ORAL ADMINISTRATION

Although most ocular diseases respond to topical therapy, some disorders require systemic drug administration to achieve adequate therapeutic levels of drug in ocular tissue. Oral administration of certain drugs may be the most effective route of drug delivery. Examples of commonly used oral medications include: Carbonic anhydrase inhibitors for the treatment of glaucoma, corticosteroids for Graves' ophthalmopathy and optic neuritis, analgesics for the management of pain associated with ocular injury, antibiotic therapy of preseptal cellulitis and antihistamine therapy for acute allergic angioneurotic edema of the eyelids.

Some oral preparations for ocular use are available as sustained-release formulations, notably acetazolamide (eg, *Diamox Sequels*).

PARENTERAL ADMINISTRATION

Intramuscular (IM) and intravenous (IV) injections are occasionally used for the treatment of ocular disorders. Hydroxocobalamin (vitamin B_{12}; [eg, *Hydro Cobex*]) and some antibiotics (eg, penicillin) may be administered through the IM route. The continuous IV infusion of various antibiotics may be required for the treatment of endophthalmitis and other severe ocular infections.

PERIOCULAR/PERIBULBAR ADMINISTRATION

When higher concentrations of drugs are required than can be delivered to the eye by topical, oral or parenteral administration, drugs can be injected locally into the periocular tissues. Periocular drug administration includes injections under the bulbar conjunctiva (subconjunctival), under Tenon's capsule (sub-Tenon's) and behind the globe itself (retrobulbar). Drugs most often delivered in this manner include corticosteroids and antibiotics. Local anesthetics are commonly administered via retrobulbar or peribulbar injection prior to cataract extraction and other intraocular surgical procedures.

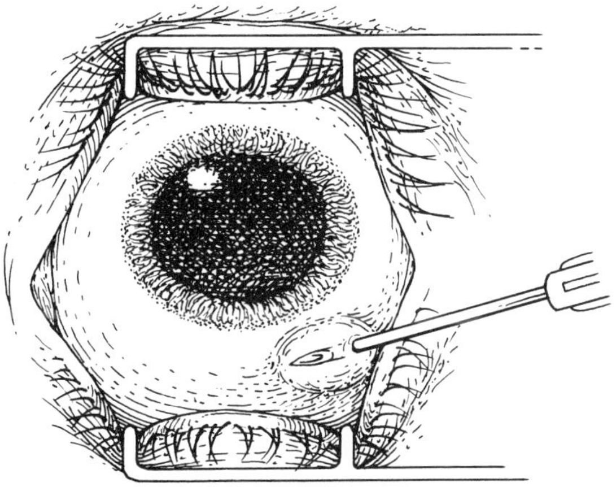

INTRACAMERAL ADMINISTRATION

Although the term "intracameral" technically denotes injection of drug into the globe, contemporary usage of the term implies administering the drug directly into the anterior chamber of the eye. This is most commonly associated with cataract extraction, during which a viscoelastic substance is injected into the anterior chamber to protect the corneal endothelium. Antibiotics are not routinely injected into the anterior chamber. This procedure is associated with a significant risk of complications as well as drug toxicity.

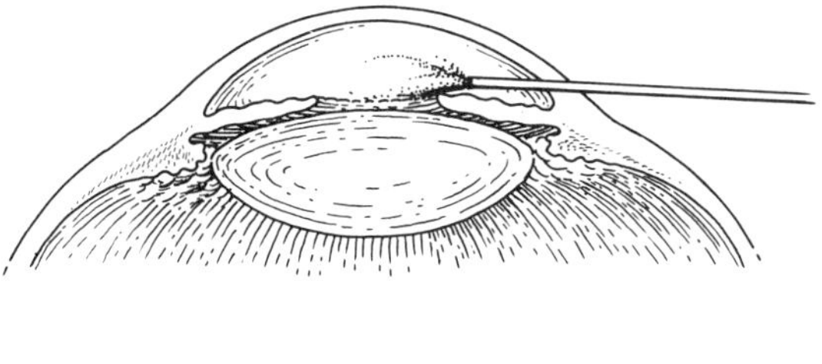

INTRAVITREAL ADMINISTRATION

The intravitreal injection of drugs is primarily reserved as a heroic effort to rescue eyes with severe acute intraocular inflammation or eyes that have failed to respond to more conservative therapy. Intravitreal antibiotics may be the treatment of choice for endophthalmitis. Intravitreal liquid silicone is used for the treatment of complicated retinal detachment. Recently, intravitreal ganciclovir has been used with some success in treating cytomegalovirus retinitis in patients with acquired immunodeficiency syndrome (AIDS).

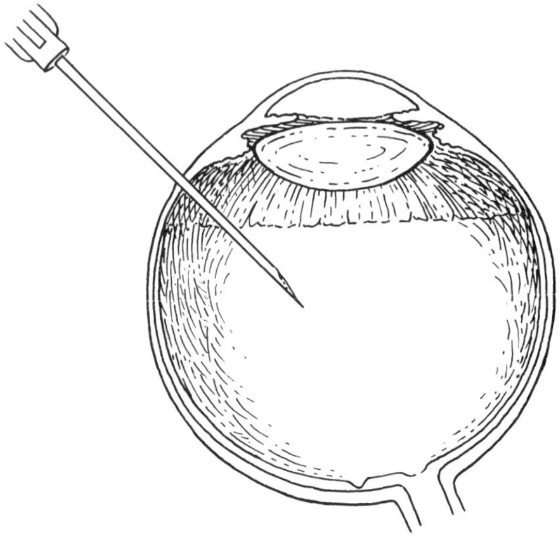

Jimmy D. Bartlett, OD, DOS
University of Alabama at Birmingham

For More Information

Bartlett JD, Jaanus SD, eds. Clinical Ocular Pharmacology, ed. 3. Boston: Butterworth-Heinemann, 1995.

Bartlett JD, Wesson MD, et al. Efficacy of a pediatric cycloplegic administered as a spray. *J Am Optom Assoc* 1993;64:617.

Feibel RM. Current concepts in retrobulbar anesthesia. *Surv Ophthalmol* 1985;30:102.

Fraunfelder FT. Drug-packaging standards for eye drop medications. *Arch Ophthalmol* 1988;106:1029.

Fraunfelder FT. Extraocular fluid dynamics: How best to apply topical ocular medication. *Trans Am Ophthalmol Soc* 1976;74:457.

Fraunfelder FT, Hanna C. Ophthalmic drug delivery systems. *Surv Ophthalmol* 1974;18:292.

Halberg GP, et al. Drug delivery systems for topical ophthalmic medication. *Ann Ophthalmol* 1975;7:1199.

Jain MR. Drug delivery through soft contact lenses. *Br J Ophthalmol* 1988;72:150.

Lamberts DW. Solid delivery devices. *Int Ophthalmol Clin* 1980;20:63.

MacKeen DL. Aqueous formulations and ointments. *Int Ophthalmol Clin* 1980;20:79.

Martin DF, Parks DJ, Mellow SD, et al. Treatment of cytomegalovirus retinitis with intraocular sustained-release ganciclovir implant. A randomized controlled clinical trial. *Arch Opthalmol* 1994;112:1531–39.

Reynolds LA, Closson RG. eds. Extemporaneous Ophthelmic Preparations. Vancouver, WA: Applied Therapeutics, 1993.

Robin JS, Ellis PP. Ophthalmic ointments. *Surv Ophthalmol* 1978;22:335.

Sharp J, Hanna C. Use of a spray to deliver drugs to the eye. *J Arkansas Med Soc* 1977;73:462.

Silbiger J, Stern GA. Evaluation of corneal collagen shields as a drug delivery device for the treatment of experimental *Pseudomonas* keratitis. *Ophthalmology* 1992;99:889.

Templeton WC, Eiferman RA, et al. *Serratia* keratitis by contaminated eyedroppers. *Am J Ophthalmol* 1982;93:723.

Wesson MD, Bartlett JD, Swiatocha J, et al. Efficacy of a cycloplegic administered as a spray. *J Am Optom Assoc* 1993;64:637.

Zimmerman TJ, et al. Improving the therapeutic index of topically applied ocular drugs. *Arch Ophthalmol* 1984;102:551.

Zimmerman TJ, Sharir M, et al. Therapeutic index of pilocarpine, carbachol and timolol with nasolacrimal occlusion. *Am J Ophthalmol* 1992;114:1.

ODF

2

Ophthalmic Dyes

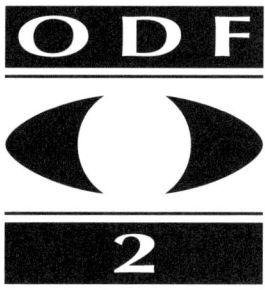

Dyes are used for a variety of diagnostic ocular procedures. Ophthalmic dyes in current use include sodium fluorescein, fluorexon, rose bengal and indocyanine green. Topical sodium fluorescein and rose bengal have proven valuable for assessment of ocular surface integrity, while intravenous and oral fluorescein have proven useful for evaluating anterior segment and retinal vascular function. More recently, indocyanine green has greatly enhanced observation of the choroidal circulation.

FLUORESCEIN SODIUM

Fluorescein sodium is a yellow water-soluble dibasic acid dye of the xanthine series that produces an intense green fluorescent color in alkaline (> pH 5) solution. Fluorescein is used to demonstrate defects of corneal epithelium. It does not actually stain tissues, but is useful as an indicator dye. The normal precorneal tear film appears yellow or orange with fluorescein. The intact corneal epithelium resists penetration of water-soluble fluorescein and is not colored by it. Any break in the epithelial barrier permits rapid fluorescein penetration. Whether resulting from trauma, infection or other causes, epithelial defects of the cornea appear bright green and are easily visualized. If epithelial loss is extensive, topical fluorescein will penetrate into the aqueous and is readily visible biomicroscopically as a green flare.

Fluorescein sodium exhibits a high degree of ionization at physiologic pH. Therefore, it does not penetrate the intact corneal epithelium or form a firm bond with vital tissue. When exposed to light, fluorescein absorbs certain wavelengths and emits fluorescent light of longer wavelength. Factors which can affect its fluorescence include its concentration, the pH of the solution, the presence of other substances and the intensity and wavelength of the absorbed light. At pH 8, fluorescein reaches its maximum intensity.

Ophthalmic uses of fluorescein include applanation tonometry, detection of foreign bodies, fitting of rigid contact lenses, determination of tear breakup time, Seidel's test, fluorescein angiography and vitreous fluorophotometry.

For topical ocular use, fluorescein may be administered as a solution or by fluorescein-impregnated filter paper strips (eg, *Fluorets*). Since fluorescein in solution is susceptible to bacterial contamination, multidose formulations are dispensed with a preservative such as chlorobutanol. For diagnostic purposes such as applanation tonometry, a local anesthetic is included in the formulation.

Fluorescein-impregnated filter paper strips are useful for routine office procedures such as contact lens fitting and lacrimal system evaluation. Bacterial contamination is minimized when the strips are stored in a dry state. When wetted with water or an irrigating solution, the dye is released from the strip and can be applied to the eye by gently touching the conjunctiva.

Intravenous fluorescein (fluorescein angiography) is used for detection of vascular abnormalities of the fundus. Following injection into the antecubital vein, the dye appears in the central retinal artery. Integrity of the retina and choroid may be determined.

Oral fluorescein can be administered by mixing fluorescein powder or several vials of 10% injectable fluorescein in a citrus drink over ice (see the Unlabeled Ophthalmic Uses chapter). Time of onset of maximal fluorescence is 45 to 60 minutes compared to seconds via the injectable route. Fasting enhances the serum concentration of the dye. Oral fluorescein can be used to study disorders characterized by late leakage of dye such as cystoid macular edema, to study retinal vascular abnormalities in young diabetic patients, and to document retinal pigment epithelial detachment, central serous choroidopathy and optic disc edema.

Topical application of fluorescein has been associated with minimum adverse effects. The most common side effect of intravenous use is nausea. The oral route appears to have the clinical advantage of less frequent side effects.

FLUOREXON

With a molecular size nearly twice that of fluorescein, fluorexon penetrates hydrophilic contact lenses at a much slower rate. Upon ocular instillation, it yields a pale, yellow-brown color. These properties make it useful as an adjunct in the fitting of soft contact lenses. However, the dye can stain hydrophilic lenses if significant amounts become trapped between lens and cornea or if the dye remains in contact with the soft lens for 10 minutes or more. Fluorexon is not recommended for use with high-water content soft lenses since the possibility of discoloration is much greater and more difficult to reverse than with lower-water content lenses.

Fluorexon has a lower fluorescent intensity than fluorescein. For optimum fluorescence, a special yellow filter is recommended. The dye generally causes little or no discomfort when instilled on the eye. Due to its larger molecular size, it is a less effective stain for epithelial defects, erosions and contact lens-induced effects than fluorescein. Like rose bengal, it will stain degenerated cells and mucus threads.

INDOCYANINE GREEN

Indocyanine green is a tricarbocyanine dye, available commercially under the trade name of *Cardio-Green*, and has been advocated for visualization of choroidal vessels with infrared absorption angiography. Toxic effects have not been associated with intravenous use of the dye when manufacturer's recommended dosage regimens have been followed. Data for routine diagnostic use are lacking since this dye is not in common clinical use.

ROSE BENGAL

An iodine derivative of fluorescein, rose bengal stains cells of the cornea and conjunctiva (including the nuclei and cell walls) a red color. More recent evidence indicates that this dye stains both normal and degenerated or dead cells. Staining will occur whenever there is poor protection of the surface epithelium by the preocular tear film. It appears that rose bengal is not a vital dye and that stained cells actually lose vitality upon exposure to the dye and undergo morphologic changes. It also will stain the mucus of the precorneal tear film. When applied as a solution or from a moistened filter paper strip, this dye can aid in the evaluation of keratoconjunctivitis sicca, corneal abrasions and detection of foreign bodies. A correlation may exist between intensity of staining and lack of a cellular barrier (preocular tear film) between the ocular surface and the dye.

Rose bengal can cause pronounced irritation and discomfort following instillation, particularly in more severely diseased eyes and with use of higher concentrations of dye. A topical anesthetic may be used to alleviate the discomfort, particularly if the solution formulation is employed. Application of dye using the commercially available filter paper strip usually results in less discomfort.

Rose bengal can stain eyelids, cheeks, fingers and clothing in a concentration-dependent manner. Keeping the amount of dye at a minimum and irrigating the eye can help circumvent this problem.

LISSAMINE GREEN

Lissamine green is suitable for vital staining of the cornea and conjunctiva. It stains degenerated cells, dead cells and precipitated mucus. The staining properties of the 1% solution are almost identical with 1% rose bengal, with rose bengal staining red and lissamine green a bluish-green color. The dye is also suitable for double staining with red dyes since it is possible to distinguish either component separately (red or green) and staining by both components (blue) by means of a green filter.

Lissamine green 1% has been compared with rose bengal 1% in assessment of keratoconjunctivitis sicca. The results are comparable, but lissamine green appears to be comparatively less irritating. The dye can also be helpful in detecting recurrent corneal erosions, dendritic ulcers and punctate or corneal staining from poorly fitting contact lenses.

The antiviral activity of the dye has also been investigated. In a rabbit model of herpetic epithelial keratitis, application of rose bengal significantly reduced viral replication and recovery, whereas lissamine green had no effect.

Lissamine green, unlike rose bengal, does not sting when applied to the eye and the dye is readily visible in red, inflamed eyes. No adverse effects have been observed with topical ocular use. Lissamine green will discolor the skin upon contact.

Siret D. Jaanus, PhD
State University of New York

For More Information

Bartlett JD, Jaanus SD, eds. Clinical Ocular Pharmacology, ed. 3. Boston: Butterworth-Heinemann, 1995.

Brooks SE, Kaza V, Nakanura T, et al. Photo inactivation of Herpes Simplex Virus by Rose Bengal and Fluorescein. *Cornea* 1994;13:43.

Chodosh J, Dix RD, Howell RC, et al. Staining characteristics and antiviral activity of sulforhodamine B and lissamine green B. *Invest Ophthalmol Vis Sci* 1994;35:1046.

Dakryon Pharmaceuticals. Lissamine green colored ophthalmic demulcent. Product information, 1997.

Feenstra RPG, Tseng SCG. Comparison of fluorescein and rose bengal staining. *Arch Ophthalmol* 1992;99:605.

Hayashi K, et al. Indocyanine green angiography of central serous chorioretinopathy. *Int Ophthalmol Clin* 1986;9:37.

Kelley JS, Kincaid M. Retinal fluorography using oral fluorescein. *Arch Ophthalmol* 1979;97:2331.

Khurana AK, Chaudhary R, Ahluwalia BK, et al. Tear film profile in dry eye. *Acta Ophthamol* 1991;69:79–86.

Norn MS. Lissamine green. Vital staining of the cornea and conjunctiva. *Acta Ophthalmol* 1973;51:483.

Refojo MF, et al. A new fluorescent stain for soft hydrophilic lens fitting. *Arch Ophthalmol* 1972;87:275.

Romanchuk KG. Fluorescein: Physiochemical factors affecting its fluorescence. *Surv Ophthalmol* 1982;26:269.

Yannuzzi LA, et al. Effective differences in the formulation of intravenous fluorescein and related side effects. *Am J Ophthalmol* 1974;78:217.

Yannuzzi LA, Slakter JS, Sorenson JA, et al. Digital indocyanine green videoangiography and choroidal neovascularization. *Retina* 1992;12:191.

Yannuzzi LA, Sorenson JA, Guyer DR, et al. Indocyanine green videoangiography: current status. *Eur J Opthalmol* 1994;4:69.

FLUORESCEIN SODIUM

Actions:

Pharmacology: Sodium fluorescein, a yellow water-soluble dibasic acid xanthine dye, produces an intense green fluorescent color in alkaline (pH > 5) solution. Fluorescein demonstrates defects of corneal epithelium. It does not stain tissues, but is a useful indicator dye. Normal precorneal tear film will appear yellow or orange. The intact corneal epithelium resists fluorescein penetration and is not colored. Any break in the epithelial barrier permits rapid penetration. Whether resulting from trauma, infection or other causes, epithelial corneal defects appear bright green and are easily seen. If epithelial loss is extensive, topical fluorescein penetrates into the aqueous humor and is readily visible biomicroscopically as a green flare.

Indications:

Topical: In fitting contact lenses; in applanation tonometry; diagnosis and detection of corneal stippling, abrasions, ulcerations, herpetic lesions, foreign bodies (not epithelialized), contact lens pressure points; making lacrimal drainage test; wound leakage tests (Seidel's Test).

Injection: Diagnostic aid in ophthalmic angiography, including examination of the fundus; evaluation of the iris vasculature; distinction between viable and nonviable tissue; observation of the aqueous flow; differential diagnosis of malignant and nonmalignant tumors; determination of circulation time and adequacy. *Off-labeled use:* Oral fluorography for diagnosis of retinal vascular diseases.

Contraindications:

Hypersensitivity to fluorescein or any other component of the product; do not use with soft contact lenses (lenses may become discolored).

Topical: Not for injection. Do not use in intraocular surgery.

Warnings:

Topical (drops): Discontinue if sensitivity develops. May stain soft contact lenses. Do not touch dropper tip to any surface, as this may contaminate the solution.

Extravasation: Avoid extravasation during injection. The high pH can result in severe local tissue damage. Complications have occurred from extravasation: Sloughing of skin, superficial phlebitis, SC granuloma and toxic neuritis along the median curve in the antecubital area. Extravasation can cause severe pain in the arm for several hours. When significant extravasation occurs, discontinue injection and use conservative measures to treat damaged tissue and relieve pain (see Warnings).

Hypersensitivity: Exercise caution when administering to patients with a history of hypersensitivity, allergies or asthma. If signs of sensitivity develop, discontinue use.

Pregnancy: Category C. Avoid parenteral fluorescein angiography during pregnancy, especially in the first trimester. There are no reports of fetal complications during pregnancy.

Lactation: Fluorescein is excreted in breast milk. Use caution when administering to a nursing woman.

Children: Safety and efficacy for use in children have not been established.

Adverse Reactions:

Injection: Nausea; headache; GI distress; vomiting; syncope; hypotension and other symptoms and signs of hypersensitivity; cardiac arrest; basilar artery ischemia; thrombophlebitis at injection site; severe shock; convulsions; death (rare); temporary yellowish skin discoloration. Hives, itching, bronchospasm, anaphylaxis, pyrexia, transient dyspnea, angioneurotic edema and slight dizziness may occur. A strong taste may develop with use. Urine becomes bright yellow. Skin discoloration fades in 6 to 12 hours, urine fluorescence in 24 to 36 hours. Extravasation at injection site causes intense pain at the site and dull aching pain in the injected arm (see Warnings).

Patient Information:

May cause strong taste with use.

May cause temporary yellowish discoloration of the skin. Urine will turn bright yellow. Discoloration of skin fades in 6 to 12 hours; urine fluorescence in 24 to 36 hours.

Soft contact lenses may become stained. Do not wear lenses while fluorescein is being used. Whenever fluorescein is used, flush the eyes with sterile normal saline solution and wait at least 1 hour before replacing the lenses.

Administration and Dosage:

Topical: To detect foreign bodies and corneal abrasions, instill 1 or 2 drops of 2% solution; allow a few seconds for staining. Wash out excess with sterile irrigating solution.

Strips: Moisten strip with sterile water. Place moistened strip at the fornix in the lower cul-de-sac close to the punctum. For best results, patient should close lid tightly over strip until desired amount of staining is obtained. The patient should blink several times after application.

> *Applanation tonometry strips* – Anesthetize the eyes. Retract upper lid and touch tip of strip moistened with saline or ocular irrigating solution (eg, *Blinx*) to the bulbar conjunctiva on the temporal side until an adequate amount of stain is available for a clearly defined endpoint reading.

Injection: Inject the contents of the ampule or pre-filled syringe rapidly into the antecubital vein *after taking precautions to avoid extravasation.* A syringe, filled with fluorescein, is attached to transparent tubing and a 25-gauge scalp vein needle for injection. Insert the needle and draw blood to the hub of the syringe so that a *small* air bubble separates the blood in the tubing from the fluorescein. With the room lights on, slowly inject the blood back into the vein while watching the skin over the needle tip. If the needle has extravasated, the patient's blood will bulge the skin, and the injection should be stopped before any fluorescein is injected. When assured that extravasation has not occurred, the room light may be turned off and the fluorescein injection completed. Luminescence appears in the retina and choroidal vessels in 9 to 15 seconds and can be observed by standard viewing equipment.

If potential allergy is suspected, an intradermal skin test may be performed prior to IV administration (ie, 0.05 ml injected intradermally to be evaluated 30 to 60 minutes following injection).

In patients with inaccessible veins where early phases of an angiogram are not necessary, such as cystoid macular edema, 1 g fluorescein has been given orally. Ten to 15 minutes are usually required before evidence of dye appears in the fundus.

Adults – 500 to 750 mg injected rapidly into the antecubital vein.

Children – 7.5 mg/kg (3.5 mg/lb) injected rapidly into the antecubital vein.

Have 0.1% epinephrine IM or IV, an antihistamine, soluble steroid, aminophylline IV and oxygen available.

Storage: Store at 8° to 30°C (46° to 86°F). Do not use if solution contains a precipitate. Discard any unused solution. Keep out of the reach of children.

Rx	**AK-Fluor** (Akorn)	**Injection**: 10%	In 5 ml amps and vials.
Rx	**Fluorescite** (Alcon)		In 5 ml amps with syringes.
Rx	**Funduscein-10** (Ciba Vision)		In 5 ml amps.
Rx	**Ophthifluor** (Deklerht)		In 5 ml amps.
Rx	**AK-Fluor** (Akorn)	**Injection**: 25%	In 2 ml amps and vials.
Rx	**Fluorescite** (Alcon)		In 2 ml amps.
Rx	**Funduscein-25** (Ciba Vision)		In 3 ml amps.
Rx	**Fluorescein Sodium** (Various, eg, Alcon)	**Solution**: 2%	In 1, 2 and 15 ml.
otc	**Ful-Glo** (PBH Wesley Jessen)	**Strips**: 0.6 mg	In 300s.
otc	**Fluorets** (Akorn)	**Strips**: 1 mg	In 100s.
Rx	**Fluor-I-Strip-A.T.** (Wyeth-Ayerst)		In 300s.[1]
Rx	**Fluor-I-Strip** (Wyeth-Ayerst)	**Strips**: 9 mg	In 300s.[1]

[1] With boric acid, polysorbate 80, 0.5% chlorobutanol.

FLUOREXON

Actions:

Pharmacology: Fluorexon is a large molecular weight fluorescent solution for use as a diagnostic and fitting aid for patients with hydrogel (soft) contact lenses. Used with or without lens in place, when fluorescein is contraindicated to avoid staining lenses. It may be used in both soft and hard lenses.

Indications:

Contact lens fitting aid: Assessment of proper fitting characteristics of hydrogel lenses. For quickly and accurately locating the optic zone in aphakic or low-plus lenses.

Evaluation of corneal integrity of patients wearing hydrogel contact lenses. In many instances, arcuate staining will show definite correlation with the edge of the optic zone, indicating improper bearing surfaces.

For use in place of sodium fluorescein when conducting the tear breakup time (B.U.T.) test.

For conducting the applanation tonometry procedure without removing the lens.

For locating the lathe-cut index markings (toric lenses). Use as directed for fitting contact lenses.

Contraindications:

Hypersensitivity to fluorescein sodium.

Warnings:

Contact lenses: When used with lenses with > 55% hydration, some color may remain on lens. Remove by washing repeatedly with washing solution approved for the lens. Rinse with saline or water. Any residual coloring will wash out with the tear flow when the lens is reinserted in the eye. With highly hydrated lenses, the amount of coloring picked up will vary with exposure. Avoid unnecessary delays in examination procedure.

Precautions:

Hydrogen peroxide: Do not use hydrogen peroxide solutions to clean or sterilize lenses until all traces of fluorexon are removed because fluorexon molecules may bind to the lens.

Administration and Dosage:

Place 1 drop on the concave surface of the lens and place the lens immediately on the eye. Alternately place 1 or 2 drops in the lower cul-de-sac and have the patient blink several times.

As the dye passes under the lens, observe a central dark zone of 6 to 9 mm in diameter (ie, a limbal fluorescent ring about 2 mm wide) which forms after each blink. If such staining pattern cannot be observed immediately, slide the lens upward by gently pushing it with a finger, causing the dye to penetrate under the lens as it slides back into normal position. Additional drops may be used if the fluorescence starts to dissipate after prolonged examination. When the examination is completed, rinse the eye and lens with saline. The lens may be reinserted immediately, as opposed to the long waiting period required after the use of fluorescein.

Begin the examination immediately after instillation of fluorexon drops. The material tends to dissipate readily with the tear flow, leading to a progressive reduction in fluorescence. Prolonged examination may require sequential application of drops.

Applanation tonometry (without removing lens): After seating the patient at the slit lamp and instilling a drop of fluorexon along with a drop of proparacaine or similar topical anesthetic, the contact lens is displaced to one side onto the sclera with the finger and the procedure begun.

otc	**Fluoresoft** (Various, eg, Akorn, Holles)	**Solution:** 0.35%	In 0.5 ml pipettes (12s).

INDOCYANINE GREEN

Actions:

Pharmacology: Sterile, water soluble, tricarbocyanine dye with a peak spectral absorption at 800 to 810 nm in blood or blood plasma. Indocyanine green contains ≤ 5% sodium iodide.

Indocyanine green permits recording of indicator-dilution curves for both diagnostic and research purposes independently of fluctuations in oxygen saturation. In the performance of dye dilution curves, a known amount of dye is usually injected as a single bolus as rapidly as possible via a cardiac catheter into selected sites in the vascular system. A recording instrument (oximeter or densitometer) is attached to a needle or catheter for sampling of the blood-dye mixture from a systemic arterial sampling site.

The peak absorption and emission of indocyanine green lie in a region (800 to 850 nm) where transmission of energy by the pigment epithelium is more efficient than in the region of visible light energy. Because indocyanine green is also nearly 98% bound to blood protein, excessive dye extravasation does not take place in the highly fenestrated choroidal vasculature. It is, therefore, useful in both absorption and fluorescence infrared angiography of the choroidal vasculature when using appropriate filters and film in a fundus camera.

Pharmacokinetics: Following IV injection, indocyanine green is rapidly bound to plasma protein, of which albumin is the principle carrier (95%). Indocyanine green undergoes no significant extrahepatic or enterohepatic circulation; simultaneous arterial and venous blood estimations have shown negligible renal, peripheral, lung or cerebrospinal uptake of the dye. Indocyanine green is taken up from the plasma almost exclusively by the hepatic parenchymal cells and is secreted entirely into the bile. After biliary obstruction, the dye appears in the hepatic lymph, independently of the bile, suggesting that the biliary mucosa is sufficiently intact to prevent diffusion of the dye, though allowing diffusion of bilirubin. These characteristics make indocyanine green a helpful index of hepatic function.

Indications:

Angiography: For ophthalmic angiography.

In vivo diagnostics: For determining cardiac output, hepatic function and liver blood flow.

Warnings:

Pregnancy: Category C. It is not known whether indocyanine green can cause fetal harm when administered to a pregnant woman or can affect reproduction capacity. Give to a pregnant woman only if clearly indicated.

Lactation: It is not known whether this drug is excreted in breast milk. Exercise caution when indocyanine green is administered to a nursing woman.

Precautions:

Plasma fractional disappearance rate at the recommended 0.5 mg/kg dose has been reported to be significantly greater in women than in men; however, there was no significant difference in the calculated value for clearance.

Radioactive iodine uptake studies: Do not perform for at least a week following the use of indocyanine green.

Iodide allergy: Contains sodium iodide. Use with caution in individuals who have a history of allergy to iodides.

Drug Interactions:

Drug/Lab test interactions: Heparin preparations containing sodium bisulfite reduce the absorption peak of indocyanine green in blood. Do not use heparin as an anticoagulant for the collection of samples for analysis.

Adverse Reactions:

Anaphylactic or urticarial reactions have also occurred in patients without history of allergy to iodides. If such reactions occur, treat with appropriate agents (eg, epinephrine, antihistamines, corticosteroids).

Administration and Dosage:

Use 40 mg dye in 2 ml of aqueous solvent. In some patients, half the volume has been found to produce angiograms of comparable resolution. Immediately follow the injected dye bolus with a 5 ml bolus of normal saline. This injection regimen is designed to provide delivery of a spatially limited dye bolus of optimal concentration to the choroidal vasculature following IV injection.

Compatibility: Use only the Aqueous Solvent (pH, 5.5 to 6.5) provided, which is specially prepared Sterile Water for Injection, to dissolve indocyanine green because there have been reports of incompatibility with some commercially available Water for Injection products.

Storage/Stability: Indocyanine green is unstable in aqueous solution and must be used within 10 hours. However, the dye is stable in plasma and whole blood so that samples obtained in discontinuous sampling techniques may be read hours later. Use sterile techniques in handling the dye solution and in the performance of the dilution curves.

Indocyanine green powder may cling to the vial or lump together because it is freeze-dried in the vials. *This is not due to the presence of water.*

Rx	**Cardio-Green (CG)** (Becton-Dickinson)	**Powder for Injection**: 25 mg	In 10 ml amps of aqueous solvent (2s).
		50 mg	In 10 ml amps of aqueous solvent (2s).

ROSE BENGAL

Actions:

Pharmacology: Stains dead or degenerated epithelial cells (corneal and conjunctival) and mucus.

Indications:

Suspected corneal/conjunctival damage: A diagnostic agent when superficial corneal or conjunctival tissue damage is suspected. Effective aid for diagnosis of keratitis, squamous cell carcinomas, keratoconjunctivitis sicca, corrosions or abrasions, and for the detection of foreign bodies.

Contraindications:

Hypersensitivity to rose bengal or any component of the formulation.

Precautions:

Irritation: The solution may be irritating.

Contact lenses: Whenever rose bengal is used in patients with soft contact lenses, flush the eyes thoroughly with sterile normal saline solution and wait at least 1 hour before replacing the lens.

Administration and Dosage:

Strips: Thoroughly saturate tip of strip with sterile irrigating solution. Touch bulbar conjunctiva or lower fornix with moistened strip. The patient should blink several times after application.

otc	**Rose Bengal** (PBH Wesley Jessen)	**Strips:** 1.3 mg per strip	In 100s.
Rx	**Rosets** (Akorn)		In 100s.

LISSAMINE GREEN

Actions:

Pharmacology: Stains dead or degenerated corneal and conjunctival cells and precipitated mucus.

Indications:

For the temporary relief of burning and irritation due to dryness of the eye. Coloring agent for food and drugs.

Off-labeled Uses: Diagnostic aid for dry eye conditions and squamous cell metaplasia.

Contraindications:

Hypersensitivity to lissamine green or any component of the formulation.

Patient Information:

Do not touch tip of container to any surface.

If eye pain, vision changes, continued redness or eye irritation occurs or if the condition worses or persists for more than 72 hours, the patient should be instructed to contact their healthcare provider.

Administration and Dosage:

Instill 1 or 2 drops in the affected eye(s) as needed.

Stability: Do not use if solution changes color or becomes cloudy.

Rx	**Lissamine Green** (Dakryon)	**Solution**: 0.1%, 0.5%, 1%	Bot. 5 ml. In 3s.

ODF

3

LOCAL ANESTHETICS

Although the exact mechanism of action is unknown, local anesthetics prevent the generation and conduction of nerve impulses by reducing sodium permeability, increasing the electrical excitation threshold, slowing the nerve impulse propagation and reducing the rate of rise of the action potential. Their action is reversible; complete recovery of nerve function occurs with no evidence of structural damage to nerve tissue. The progression of anesthesia is related to the diameter, myelination and conduction velocity of affected nerve fibers. The order of loss of nerve function is as follows: Pain, temperature, touch, proprioception and skeletal muscle tone.

With the exception of cocaine, local anesthetics are synthetic, aromatic or heterocyclic compounds. Nearly all local anesthetics in current use are weakly basic tertiary amines. The structural components consist of an aromatic lipophilic portion, an intermediate alkyl chain and a hydrophilic hydrocarbon chain containing nitrogen. The intermediate chain is linked to the aromatic group by either an ester or an amide, which determines certain pharmacologic properties of the molecule.

CLASSIFICATION

Local anesthetics are divided into two groups: *Esters,* which are derivatives of para-aminobenzoic acid and *amides,* which are derivatives of aniline. The "ester" local anesthetics are metabolized by hydrolysis of the ester linkage by plasma esterase, probably plasma cholinesterase. The "amide" local anesthetics are metabolized in the liver, then excreted primarily in the urine as metabolites with a small fraction of unchanged drug. Biliary excretion may contribute to the disposition of lidocaine (eg, *Xylocaine*) and mepivacaine (eg, *Carbocaine*). Allergic reactions to local anesthetics occur almost exclusively to anesthetics with ester linkage (see Precautions). All commonly used topical anesthetics are of the ester type (see Table 1: Classification of Local Anesthetics).

Table 1: CLASSIFICATION OF LOCAL ANESTHETICS

Ester Linkage	**Amide Linkage** (Amides of benzoic acid)
A. Esters of benzoic acid: Cocaine	A. Lidocaine
B. Esters of meta-aminobenzoic acid: Proparacaine	B. Mepivacaine
C. Esters of para-aminobenzoic acid	C. Bupivacaine
1. Procaine	D. Etidocaine
2. Chloroprocaine	
3. Tetracaine	
4. Benoxinate	

In the amine form, local anesthetics tend to be only slightly soluble in water and, therefore, are usually formulated in the form of their hydrochloride salt, which is water soluble. Since local anesthetics are weak bases, with a pK_a between 8 and 9, they ionize in solution, enhancing stability and shelf-life. Upon contact with more neutral or alkaline environments (eg, tears), the nonionized form is liberated. The nonionized drug can penetrate tissues, including the cornea.

PHARMACOKINETICS

Various pharmacokinetic parameters of the local anesthetics can be significantly altered by the presence of hepatic or renal disease, addition of epinephrine, factors affecting urinary pH, renal blood flow, the route of administration and patient age. Onset of local anesthesia is dependent on the dissociation constant (pK_a), lipid solubility, pH of the solution, protein binding and molecular size. In general, local anesthetics with high lipid solubility or low pK_a have a faster onset. The duration of action of local anesthetics is proportional to the drug's contact time with nerve tissue. To prolong contact time of injectable local anesthetics, vasoconstrictors may be added, but such adjuncts are of no benefit when used with topical anesthetics. The use of vasoconstrictors (eg, epinephrine) in conjunction with local anesthetics promotes local hemostasis, decreases systemic absorption and prolongs the duration of action.

Systemic absorption of local anesthetics affects the cardiovascular system and central nervous system. At blood concentrations achieved with normal therapeutic doses of injectable anesthetics, changes in cardiac conduction, excitability, refractoriness, contractility and peripheral vascular resistance are minimal. However, toxic blood concentrations depress cardiac conduction and excitability, which may lead to atrioventricular block and ultimately to cardiac arrest. In addition, with toxic blood concentrations, myocardial contractility may be depressed and peripheral vasodilation may occur, leading to decreased cardiac output and arterial blood pressure.

Following systemic absorption, toxic blood concentrations of local anesthetics can produce CNS stimulation, depression or both. Apparent central stimulation may be manifested as restlessness, tremors and shivering, which may progress to convulsions. Depression and coma may occur, possibly progressing ultimately to respiratory arrest. Local anesthetics have a primary depressant effect on the medulla and on higher centers. The depressed stage may occur without a prior stage of CNS stimulation.

Rate of systemic absorption depends on total dose and concentration of drug, vascularity of administration site and presence of vasoconstrictors. Depending on route of administration, local anesthetics are distributed to some extent to all body tissues. High concentrations are found in highly perfused organs (eg, liver, lungs, heart, brain). The rate and extent of placental diffusion is determined by plasma protein binding, ionization and lipid solubility. It is the nonionized form of the drug that crosses cellular membranes to the site of action. Fetal:maternal ratios are inversely related to degree of protein binding. Only the free, unbound drug is available for placental transfer. Drugs with the highest protein binding capacity may have the lowest fetal:maternal ratios. Lipid-soluble, nonionized drugs readily enter the fetal blood from the maternal circulation.

OPHTHALMIC USES

Anesthetics in current clinical use have relatively low systemic and ocular toxicity. They have a sufficiently long duration of action, are stable in solution and usually lack interference with the actions of other drugs. These advantages make local anesthetics useful for such ocular procedures as tonometry, foreign body and suture removal, gonioscopy, nasolacrimal irrigation and probing and surgical procedures (see Table 2: Ophthalmic Uses of Local Anesthetics).

Table 2: OPHTHALMIC USES OF LOCAL ANESTHETICS	
Injectable	1. Facial nerve block 2. Retrobulbar or peribulbar anesthesia 3. Eyelid infiltration
Topical	1. Gonioscopy 2. Tonometry 3. Fundus contact lens biomicroscopy 4. Evaluation of corneal abrasions 5. Forced duction testing 6. Schirmer tear testing 7. Electroretinography 8. Lacrimal dilation and irrigation 9. Contact lens fitting 10. Superficial foreign body removal 11. Minor surgery of conjunctiva 12. Suture removal 13. Corneal epithelial debridement

Jimmy D. Bartlett, OD, DOS
University of Alabama at Birmingham

For More Information

Bartlett JD, Jaanus SD, eds. Clinical Ocular Pharmacology, ed. 3. Boston: Butterworth-Heinemann, 1995.

Burns RP, et al. Chronic toxicity of local anesthetics on the cornea. In: Leopold IH, Burns RP, eds. *Symposium on Ocular Therapy*. New York: Wiley, 1977.

Bryant JA. Local and topical anesthetics in ophthalmology. *Surv Ophthalmol* 1969;13:263.

Chandler MJ, et al. Provocative challenge with local anesthetics in patients with a prior history of reaction. *J Allergy Clin Immunol* 1987;79:883.

Norden LC. Adverse reactions to topical ocular anesthetics. *J Am Optom Assoc* 1976;47:730.

Rosenwasser GOD. Complications of topical ocular anesthetics. *Int Ophthalmol Clin* 1989;29:153.

Smith RB, Everett WG. Physiology and pharmacology of local anesthetic agents. *Int Ophthalmol Clin* 1973;13: 35.

Sobol WM, McCrary JA. Ocular anesthetic properties and adverse reactions. *Int Ophthalmol Clin* 1989;29:195.

Vettesse T, Breslin CW. Retrobulbar anesthesia for cataract surgery: Comparison of bupivacaine and bupivacaine-lidocaine combinations. *Can J Ophthalmol* 1985;20:131.

Webster RB. Local anesthetics for ophthalmic use. *Aust J Optom* 1974;57:399.

LOCAL ANESTHETICS, INJECTABLE

Actions:

Pharmacology: These agents prevent generation and conduction of nerve impulses by inhibiting ionic fluxes, increasing electrical excitation threshold, slowing nerve impulse propagation and reducing rate of rise of action potential. Progression of anesthesia is related to the diameter, myelination and conduction velocity of affected nerve fibers.

The use of vasoconstrictors (eg, epinephrine) with local anesthetics promotes local hemostasis, decreases systemic absorption and prolongs duration of action.

Pharmacokinetics: Various pharmacokinetic parameters can be significantly altered by presence of hepatic or renal disease, addition of epinephrine, factors affecting urinary pH, renal blood flow, administration route and age of patient.

Injectable Local Anesthetics Pharmacokinetics

Anesthetic	Onset (minutes)	Duration (hours)	Equivalent anesthetic concentration (%)	pK_a	Partition[1] coefficient	Systemic protein binding (%)
ESTERS						
Procaine[2]	2-5	0.25-1	2	9.1	0.02	5.8[3]
(w/Epinephrine)	nd	0.5-1.5				
Chloroprocaine[2]	6-12	0.5	2	9	0.14	nd
(w/Epinephrine)	nd	0.5-1.5				
AMIDES						
Lidocaine[2]	< 2	0.5-1	1	7.9	2.9	64.3
(w/Epinephrine)	< 2	2-6				
Mepivacaine[2]	3-5	0.75-1.5	1	7.8	0.8	77.5[4]
(w/Epinephrine)	nd	2-6				
Bupivacaine[2]	5	2-4	0.25	8.2	27.5	95.6[4]
(w/Epinephrine)	nd	3-7				
Etidocaine[2]	3-5	5-10	0.5	7.7	141	94[4]
(w/Epinephrine)	nd	3-7				

[1] n-Heptane/Buffer, pH 7.4. nd – No data.
[2] Values in this line are for infiltrative anesthesia.
[3] Nerve homogenate binding.
[4] Plasma protein binding.

Local anesthetics are divided into two groups: *Esters,* which are derivatives of para-aminobenzoic acid, and *amides,* which are derivatives of aniline. The "ester" local anesthetics are metabolized by hydrolysis of the ester linkage by plasma esterase, probably plasma cholinesterase. The "amide" local anesthetics are metabolized primarily in the liver, then excreted primarily in the urine as metabolites, with a small fraction of unchanged drug. Hypersensitivity reactions may occur with local anesthetics of the ester type (see Warnings).

Indications:

Refer to individual product listings.

Ophthalmic Uses of Local Anesthetics

Route	Use
Injectable	Facial nerve block Retrobulbar anesthesia Eyelid infiltration

Contraindications:

Hypersensitivity to local anesthetics, para-aminobenzoic acid (amides only) or parabens.

Warnings:

Head and neck area: Small doses of local anesthetics injected into the head and neck area, including retrobulbar, dental and stellate ganglion blocks, may produce adverse reactions similar to systemic toxicity seen with unintentional intravascular injections of larger doses. The injection procedures require the utmost care. Confusion, convulsions, respiratory depression or arrest and cardiovascular stimulation or depression have occurred. These reactions may be due to intra-arterial injection of the local anesthetic with retrograde flow to cerebral circulation. They may also be due to puncture of the dural sheath of the optic nerve during retrobulbar block with diffusion of any local anesthetic along the subdural space to the midbrain. Observe patient carefully. Monitor respiration and circulation. Do not exceed dosage recommendations.

> *Ophthalmic* – When local anesthetic solutions are used for retrobulbar block, complete corneal anesthesia usually precedes onset of clinically acceptable external ocular muscle akinesia. Therefore, presence of akinesia rather than anesthesia alone should determine readiness of the patient for surgery.
>
> *Cardiovascular reactions* are depressants. They may be the result of direct drug effect, the result of vasovagal reaction, particularly if the patient is in the sitting position. Failure to recognize premonitory signs such as sweating, feeling of faintness, changes in pulse or sensorium may result in progressive cerebral hypoxia and seizure, or serious cardiovascular catastrophe. Place patient in recumbent position and administer oxygen. Vasoactive drugs such as ephedrine or methoxamine may be administered IV.

Hypersensitivity reactions, including anaphylaxis, may occur in a small segment of the population allergic to para-aminobenzoic acid derivatives (eg, procaine, tetracaine, benzocaine). The amide-type local anesthetics have not shown cross-sensitivity with the esters. Hypersensitivity reactions and anaphylaxis have occurred rarely with lidocaine. Administer ester-type local anesthetics cautiously to patients with abnormal or reduced levels of plasma esterases.

Renal function impairment: Use mepivacaine with caution in patients with renal disease.

Hepatic function impairment: Because amide-type local anesthetics are metabolized primarily in the liver, patients with hepatic disease, especially severe hepatic disease, may be more susceptible to potential toxicity. Use cautiously in such patients.

Elderly: Repeated doses may cause accumulation of the drug or its metabolites or slow metabolic degradation. Give reduced doses.

Pregnancy: Category B (etidocaine, lidocaine). *Category C* (bupivacaine, chloroprocaine, mepivacaine). Safety for use in pregnant women, other than those in labor, has not been established.

Lactation: Safety for use in the nursing mother has not been established. It is not known whether local anesthetic drugs are excreted in breast milk.

Children: Due to lack of clinical experience, the administration of bupivacaine to children < 12 years of age is not recommended. Dosages in children should be reduced, commensurate with age, body weight and physical condition.

Precautions:

Dosage: Use the lowest dosage that results in effective anesthesia to avoid high plasma levels and serious adverse effects. Inject slowly, with frequent aspirations before and during the injection, to avoid intravascular injection. Perform syringe aspirations before and during each supplemental injection in continuous (intermittent) catheter techniques.

Inflammation or sepsis: Use local anesthetic procedures with caution when there is inflammation or sepsis in the region of proposed injection.

CNS toxicity: Monitor cardiovascular and respiratory vital signs and state of consciousness after each injection. Restlessness, anxiety, incoherent speech, lightheadedness, numbness and tingling of the mouth and lips, metallic taste, tinnitus, dizziness, blurred vision, tremors, twitching, depression or drowsiness may be early signs of CNS toxicity.

Special risk patients: Debilitated patients, acutely ill patients, children, obstetric delivery patients and patients with increased intra-abdominal pressure: Repeated doses may cause accumulation of the drug or its metabolites or slow metabolic degradation. Give reduced doses. Use anesthetics with caution in patients with severe disturbances of cardiac rhythm, hypotension, shock or heart block. Local anesthetics should also be used with caution in patients with impaired cardiovascular function because they may be less able to compensate for functional changes associated with the prolongation of A-V conduction produced by these drugs.

Malignant hyperthermia: Many drugs used during anesthesia are considered potential triggering agents for familial malignant hyperthermia. It is not known whether amide-type local anesthetics may trigger this reaction and the need for supplemental general anesthesia cannot be predicted in advance; therefore, have a standard protocol for management available.

Vasoconstrictors: Use solutions containing a vasoconstrictor with caution and in carefully circumscribed quantities in areas of the body supplied by end arteries or having otherwise compromised blood supply. Use with extreme caution in patients whose medical history and physical evaluation suggest the existence of hypertension, peripheral vascular disease, arteriosclerotic heart disease, cerebral vascular insufficiency or heart block; these individuals may exhibit exaggerated vasoconstrictor response.

Sulfite sensitivity: Some of these products contain sulfites. Sulfites may cause allergic-type reactions (eg, hives, itching, wheezing, anaphylaxis) in certain susceptible persons. Although the overall prevalence of sulfite sensitivity in the general population is probably low, it is seen more frequently in asthmatics or in atopic nonasthmatic persons.

Drug Interactions:

Intercurrent use: Mixtures of local anesthetics are sometimes employed to compensate for the slower onset of one drug and the shorter duration of action of the second drug. Toxicity is probably additive with mixtures of local anesthetics, but some experiments suggest synergisms. Exercise caution regarding toxic equivalence when mixtures of local anesthetics are employed.

Prior use of chloroprocaine may interfere with subsequent use of bupivacaine. Because of this, and because safety of intercurrent use of bupivacaine and chloroprocaine has not been established, such use is not recommended.

Some preparations contain vasoconstrictors. Keep this in mind when using concurrently with other drugs that may interact with vasoconstrictors.

Injectable Local Anesthetic Drug Interactions			
Precipitant drug	Object drug*		Description
Local anesthetics	Sulfonamides	⬇	The para-aminobenzoic acid metabolite of procaine, chloroprocaine and tetracaine inhibits the action of sulfonamides. Therefore, do not use procaine, chloroprocaine or tetracaine in any condition in which a sulfonamide drug is employed.

* ⬇ = Object drug decreased.

Adverse Reactions:

The most common acute adverse reactions are related to the CNS and cardiovascular systems. These are generally dose-related and may result from rapid absorption from the injection site, from diminished tolerance or from unintentional intravascular injection.

Dermatologic: Cutaneous lesions, urticaria, pruritus, erythema, angioneurotic edema (including laryngeal edema), sneezing, syncope, excessive sweating, elevated temperature and anaphylactoid symptoms (including severe hypotension). Skin testing is of limited value.

CNS: Restlessness, anxiety, dizziness, tinnitus, blurred vision, nausea, vomiting, chills, pupil constriction or tremors may occur, possibly proceeding to convulsions ($\approx$ 0.1% of local anesthetic epidural administrations). Excitement may be transient or absent, with depression being the first manifestation. This may quickly be followed by drowsiness merging into unconsciousness and respiratory arrest.

Postspinal headache; meningismus; arachnoiditis; palsies; apprehension; double vision; euphoria; sensation of heat, cold, numbness; and spinal nerve paralysis (spinal anesthesia) have also occurred.

Cardiovascular: Myocardial depression, hypotension (with spinal anesthesia due to vasomotor paralysis and pooling of blood in the venous bed), decreased cardiac output, heart block, syncope, bradycardia, ventricular arrhythmias (including tachycardia and fibrillation), cardiac arrest and fetal bradycardia (see Warnings).

Overdosage:

Acute emergencies from local anesthetics are generally related to high plasma levels encountered during therapeutic use or due to unintended subarachnoid injection.

Management: The first consideration is prevention.

Convulsions, as well as underventilation or apnea, are due to unintentional subarachnoid injection; maintain patent airway and assist or control ventilation with oxygen and a delivery system capable of permitting immediate positive airway pressure by mask. Evaluate circulation. If convulsions persist despite respiratory support, and if the status of the circulation permits, give small increments of an ultra short-acting barbiturate (eg, thiopental) or a benzodiazepine (eg, diazepam) IV. Circulatory depression may require administration of IV fluids and a vasopressor. If not treated immediately, convulsions and cardiovascular depression can result in hypoxia, acidosis, bradycardia, arrhythmias and cardiac arrest. Underventilation or apnea may produce these same signs and also lead to cardiac arrest if ventilatory support is not instituted. If cardiac arrest occurs, institute standard cardiopulmonary resuscitative measures.

Endotracheal intubation may be indicated.

Administration and Dosage:

The dose of local anesthetic administered varies with the procedure, vascularity of the tissues, depth of anesthesia, degree of required muscle relaxation, duration of anesthesia desired and the physical condition of the patient. Reduce dosages for children, elderly and debilitated patients and patients with cardiac or liver disease.

Infiltration or regional block anesthesia: Always inject slowly, with frequent aspirations, to prevent intravascular injection.

For detailed administration and dosage, refer to specific manufacturers' labeling.

Individual drug monographs are on the following pages.

LIDOCAINE HYDROCHLORIDE and LIDOCAINE COMBINATIONS

For complete prescribing information, refer to the Injectable Local Anesthetics group monograph.

Indications:

Retrobulbar or transtracheal injection: 4% solution.

Rx	**Xylocaine MPF** (Astra)	**Injection:** 4%	In 5 ml amps and 5 ml disp. syringe with laryngotracheal cannula.
Rx	**Duo-Trach Kit** (Astra)		In 5 ml pre-filled syringe with cannula.

MEPIVACAINE HYDROCHLORIDE

For complete prescribing information, refer to the Injectable Local Anesthetics group monograph.

Indications:

Peripheral nerve block: 1% or 2% solution.

Infiltration: 0.5% (via dilution) or 1% solution

Rx	**Carbocaine** (Sanofi Winthrop)	**Injection:** 1%	In 30 and 50 ml vials.[1]
Rx	**Mepivacaine HCl** (Various, eg, Schein, Zentih-Goldline)		In 50 ml vials.
Rx	**Polocaine** (Astra)		In 50 ml vials.
Rx	**Polocaine MPF** (Astra)		In 30 ml vials.
Rx	**Carbocaine** (Sanofi Winthrop)	**Injection:** 1.5%	In 30 ml vials.
Rx	**Polocaine MPF** (Astra)		In 30 ml vials.
Rx	**Carbocaine** (Sanofi Winthrop)	**Injection:** 2%	In 20 and 50 ml vials.[1]
Rx	**Polocaine** (Astra)		In 50 ml vials.
Rx	**Polocaine MPF** (Astra)		In 20 ml vials.
Rx	**Mepivacaine** (Various, eg, IDE, Moore, Schein, Zenith-Goldline)		In 50 ml vials.

[1] With methylparaben.

BUPIVACAINE HYDROCHLORIDE and BUPIVACAINE COMBINATIONS

For complete prescribing information, refer to the Injectable Local Anesthetics group monograph.

Indications:

Retrobulbar block: 0.75% solution.

Rx	**Bupivacaine HCl** (Abbott)	**Injection:**0.75%	In 20 ml amps and 20 ml *Abboject.*
Rx	**Marcaine HCl** (Sanofi Winthrop)		In 30 ml amps and 10 and 30 ml vials.
Rx	**Marcaine Spinal** (Sanofi Winthrop)		In 2 ml single dose amps.[1]
Rx	**Sensorcaine** (Astra)		In 30 ml amps.
Rx	**Sensorcaine MPF** (Astra)		In 30 ml amps and 10 and 30 ml vials.
Rx	**Sensorcaine MPF Spinal** (Astra)		In 2 ml amps.[1]
Rx	**Marcaine HCl** (Sanofi Winthrop)	0.75% with 1:200,000 epinephrine	In 30 ml amps.[2]
Rx	**Sensorcaine MPF** (Astra)		In 30 ml amps and 10 and 30 ml vials.[3]

[1] With 8.25% dextrose.
[2] With sodium metabisulfite and EDTA.
[3] With sodium metabisulfite.

ETIDOCAINE HYDROCHLORIDE

For complete prescribing information, refer to the Injectable Local Anesthetics group monograph.

Indications:

Retrobulbar: 1% or 1.5% solution.

Rx	**Duranest MPF** (Astra)	**Injection:** 1%	In 30 ml single dose vials.
		1% with 1:200,000 epinephrine	In 30 ml single dose vials.[1]
		1.5% with 1:200,000 epinephrine	In 20 ml amps.[1]

[1] With sodium metabisulfite.

LOCAL ANESTHETICS, TOPICAL

Actions:

Pharmacology: Local anesthetics stabilize the neuronal membrane so the neuron is less permeable to ions. This prevents the initiation and transmission of nerve impulses, thereby producing the local anesthetic action.

Studies indicate that local anesthetics influence permeability of the nerve cell membrane by limiting sodium ion permeability by closing the pores through which the ions migrate in the lipid layer of the nerve cell membrane. This limitation prevents the fundamental change necessary for the generation of the action potential.

Pharmacokinetics: Tetracaine and proparacaine are approximately equally potent. They have a rapid onset of anesthesia beginning within 13 to 30 seconds following instillation; the duration of action is 15 to 20 minutes.

Indications:

Corneal anesthesia of short duration (eg, tonometry, gonioscopy, removal of corneal foreign bodies and sutures); short corneal and conjunctival procedures; cataract surgery; conjunctival and corneal scraping for diagnostic purposes; paracentesis of the anterior chamber.

Ophthalmic Uses of Local Anesthetics

Route	Use
Topical	Gonioscopy
	Tonometry
	Fundus contact lens biomicroscopy
	Evaluation of corneal abrasions
	Forced duction testing
	Schirmer tear testing
	Electroretinography
	Lacrimal dilation and irrigation
	Contact lens fitting
	Superficial foreign body removal
	Minor surgery of conjunctiva
	Suture removal
	Corneal epithelial debridement

Contraindications:

Hypersensitivity to similar drugs (ester-type local anesthetics), para-aminobenzoic acid or its derivatives or to any other ingredient in these preparations; prolonged use, especially for self-medication (not recommended).

Warnings:

For topical ophthalmic use only. Prolonged use may diminish duration of anesthesia, retard wound healing and cause corneal epithelial erosions (see Adverse Reactions).

Systemic toxicity is rare with topical ophthalmic application of local anesthetics. It usually occurs as CNS stimulation followed by CNS and cardiovascular depression.

Protection of the eye from irritating chemicals, foreign bodies and rubbing during the period of anesthesia is very important. Advise the patient to avoid touching the eye until anesthesia has worn off.

Pregnancy: Category C. Safety for use during pregnancy has not been established. Use only when clearly needed and when potential benefits outweigh potential hazards to the fetus.

Lactation: Safety for use during lactation has not been established. Use only when clearly needed and when potential benefits outweigh potential hazards to the infant.

Children: Safety and efficacy for use in children have been well established through clinical experience although no studies exist.

Precautions:

Reduced plasma esterase: Use caution in patients with abnormal or reduced levels of plasma esterases.

Special risk patients: Use cautiously and sparingly in patients with known allergies, cardiac disease or hyperthyroidism.

Adverse Reactions:

Prolonged ophthalmic use of topical anesthetics has been associated with corneal epithelial erosions, retardation or prevention of healing of corneal erosions and reports of severe keratitis and permanent corneal opacification with accompanying visual loss and scarring or corneal perforation. Inadvertent damage may be done to the anesthetized cornea and conjunctiva by rubbing an eye to which topical anesthetics have been applied.

Tetracaine:

Transient stinging, burning and conjunctival redness may occur. A rare, severe, immediate-type allergic corneal reaction has been reported characterized by acute diffuse epithelial keratitis with filament formation and sloughing of large areas of necrotic epithelium, diffuse stromal edema, descemetitis and iritis.

Rarely, local reactions including lacrimation, photophobia and chemosis have occurred.

Proparacaine:

Local or systemic sensitivity occurs occasionally. At recommended concentration and dosage, proparacaine usually produces little or no initial irritation, stinging, burning, conjunctival redness, lacrimation or increased winking. However, some local irritation and stinging may occur several hours after instillation.

Rarely, a severe, immediate-type, hyperallergic corneal reaction may occur, which includes acute, intense and diffuse epithelial keratitis, a gray, ground-glass appearance, sloughing of large areas of necrotic epithelium, corneal filaments and, sometimes, iritis with descemetitis. Pupillary dilation or cycloplegic effects have been observed rarely.

Allergic contact dermatitis with drying and fissuring of the fingertips and softening and erosion of the corneal epithelium and conjunctival congestion and hemorrhage have been reported.

Patient Information:

Avoid continuous or prolonged use.

Avoid touching or rubbing the eye until the anesthesia has worn off because inadvertent damage may be done to the anesthetized cornea and conjunctiva.

To avoid contamination, do not touch dropper tip to any surface. Replace cap after using.

Do not use if discolored, cloudy or if it contains a precipitate. Protect from light.

Individual drug monographs are on the following pages.

TETRACAINE HYDROCHLORIDE

For complete prescribing information, refer to the Topical Local Anesthetics group monograph.

Administration and Dosage:

Solution: Instill 1 or 2 drops. Not for prolonged use.

Storage: Store at 8° to 27°C (46° to 80°F). Protect from light.

Rx	**Tetracaine HCl** (Various, eg, Alcon, Ciba Vision, Optopics, Schein)	**Solution:** 0.5%	In 1, 2 and 15 ml.
Rx	**AK-T-Caine PF** (Akorn)		In 15 ml.
Rx	**Pontocaine HCl** (Sanofi Winthrop)		In 15 ml Mono-drop and 59 ml.[1]

[1] With 0.4% chlorobutanol and 0.75% sodium chloride.

PROPARACAINE HYDROCHLORIDE

For complete prescribing information, refer to the Topical Local Anesthetics group monograph.

Administration and Dosage:

Deep anesthesia as in cataract extraction: 1 drop every 5 to 10 minutes for 5 to 7 doses.

Removal of sutures: Instill 1 or 2 drops 2 or 3 minutes before removal of sutures.

Removal of foreign bodies: Instill 1 or 2 drops prior to operating.

Tonometry: Instill 1 or 2 drops immediately before measurement.

Storage: Store at 8° to 24°C (46° to 75°F). Protect from light.

Rx	**Proparacaine HCl** (Various, eg, Moore, Raway, Rugby)	**Solution:** 0.5%	In 2, 15 ml and UD 1 ml.
Rx	**Alcaine** (Alcon)		In 15 ml Drop-Tainers.[1, 2]
Rx	**Ophthaine** (Apothecon)		In 15 ml.[3, 4]
Rx	**Ophthetic** (Allergan)		In 15 ml.[4, 5]

[1] With glycerin and 0.01% benzalkonium Cl.
[2] Refrigerate after opening.
[3] With glycerin, 0.2% chlorobutanol and benzalkonium Cl.
[4] Refrigerate.
[5] With 0.01% benzalkonium Cl, glycerin and sodium Cl.

MISCELLANEOUS LOCAL ANESTHETIC COMBINATIONS

For complete prescribing information, refer to the Topical Local Anesthetics group monograph.

Indications:

For procedures in which a topical ophthalmic anesthetic agent in conjunction with a disclosing agent is indicated: Corneal anesthesia of short duration (eg, tonometry, gonioscopy, removal of corneal foreign bodies); short corneal and conjunctival procedures.

Administration and Dosage:

Removal of foreign bodies or sutures; tonometry: 1 to 2 drops (in single instillations) in each eye before operating.

Deep ophthalmic anesthesia:

Proparacaine/fluorescein – Instill 1 drop in each eye every 5 to 10 minutes for 5 to 7 doses. Use of an eye patch is recommended.

Benoxinate/fluorescein – Instill 2 drops into each eye at 90 second intervals for 3 instillations.

Storage: Protect from light.

Rx	**Fluoracaine** (Akorn)	**Solution**: 0.5% proparacaine HCl and 0.25% fluorescein sodium	In 5 ml.[1, 2]
Rx	**Fluorescein Sodium with Proparacaine HCl** (Taylor Pharmaceuticals)		In 5 ml.[3]
Rx	**Fluress** (PBH Wesley Jessen)	**Solution**: 0.4% benoxinate HCl and 0.25% fluorescein sodium	In 5 ml with dropper.[4]
Rx	**Flurate** (Bausch & Lomb)		In 5 ml.
Rx	**Flu-Oxinate** (Taylor Pharmaceuticals)		In 5 ml.[5]

[1] Refrigerate.
[2] With glycerin, povidone, polysorbate 80 and 0.01% thimerosal.
[3] With povidone, glycerin, EDTA and 0.01% thimerosal.
[4] With povidone, boric acid and 1% chlorobutanol.
[5] With povidone, glycerin, EDTA and 1% chlorobutanol.

ODF

4

Mydriatics And Cycloplegics

Mydriatics are drugs that dilate the pupil. Adrenergic agonists are used for routine dilation of the pupil. Phenylephrine (eg, *Neo-Synephrine*) and epinephrine (eg, *Epifrin*) are the only direct-acting adrenergic agents available that produce mydriasis without cycloplegia. Epinephrine, however, is not used clinically for its mydriatic effects.

Anticholinergic agents administered topically to the eye for purposes of inhibiting accommodation are termed *cycloplegics*. Their primary use is for cycloplegic refraction and in the treatment of uveitis. Since these agents also inhibit action of the iris sphincter muscle, they are effective mydriatics. Of the cholinergic blocking agents, only tropicamide (eg, *Tropicacyl*) is used routinely for mydriasis. For most dilation procedures, the adrenergic or anticholinergic agents can be used either alone or in combination for maximum mydriasis.

MYDRIATICS

Phenylephrine Hydrochloride

Phenylephrine is a synthetic alpha-receptor agonist that is structurally similar to epinephrine. Following topical application on the eye, it contracts the iris dilator muscle and smooth muscle of the conjunctival arterioles, causing pupillary dilation and "blanching" of the conjunctiva. Mueller's muscle of the upper eyelid may be stimulated, widening the palpebral fissure.

For pupillary dilation, concentrations of 2.5% and 10% are commercially available. Maximum dilation occurs within 45 to 60 minutes, depending on the concentration used or number of drops instilled. The pupil size usually returns to pre-drug levels within 4 to 6 hours. Since phenylephrine has little or no effect on the ciliary muscle, mydriasis occurs without cycloplegia.

Phenylephrine 1% solution can be used in diagnosis of Horner's syndrome. Significant mydriasis can occur in the eye with a postganglionic lesion as compared to one with a normal innervation.

The mydriatic response to phenylephrine may be affected in situations that alter corneal epithelial integrity. Corneal abrasions or trauma from such procedures as tonometry or gonioscopy, as well as prior instillation of a topical anesthetic, can enhance its pharmacologic effect. Concentrations as small as 0.125%, as present in over-the-counter decongestants, can cause mydriasis if the corneal epithelium is damaged.

Since the topical instillation of phenylephrine can be accompanied by clinically significant ocular and systemic side effects, cardiovascular effects in particular, use of the 10% concentration should be avoided if possible. The 2.5% concentration is generally recommended for routine dilation, especially in infants and the elderly. The drug should be used with caution in patients with cardiac disease, hypertension, arteriosclerosis and diabetes. It is contraindicated in patients taking tricyclic antidepressants (eg, amitriptyline [eg, *Elavil*]), MAO inhibitors (eg, phenelzine [*Nardil*]), reserpine, guanethidine (eg, *Ismelin*) and methyldopa (eg, *Aldomet*).

CYCLOPLEGIC MYDRIATICS

Commonly used cycloplegic mydriatics include: Atropine (eg, *Isopto Atropine*), homatropine (eg, *Isopto Homatropine*), scopolamine (eg, *Isopto Hyoscine*), cyclopentolate (eg, *Cyclogyl*) and tropicamide (eg, *Tropicacyl*).

Both objective and subjective refractive procedures are employed to determine the nature of the refractive error. Under normal circumstances, this is best accomplished without interference from topically applied drugs that might adversely affect examination results. Under some circumstances, however, the instillation of cycloplegics may enable a more accurate refractive examination.

Use in Esotropia

Children with strabismus, especially esotropia, should receive a cycloplegic examination. It is important to uncover the full amount of hyperopia in young patients with suspected accommodative esotropia so that plus lenses can relieve the effort placed on the accommodative-convergence system. Some clinicians use cycloplegics in children who exhibit myopia for the first time to rule out accommodative spasm (pseudomyopia) as the underlying etiology. Patients who are unresponsive or inconsistent in their responses to subjective refraction will often benefit from cycloplegia. Cycloplegic refraction is also indicated to confirm the refractive amount in patients who exhibit symptoms of malingering or conversion reaction. Refraction of young children and infants is usually more accurate and easier with cycloplegics, since these patients may fixate any distance during the examination. Patients with suspected latent hyperopia will also benefit from cycloplegic refraction.

Contraindications: Since cycloplegics cause pupillary dilation, they are contraindicated in patients with extremely narrow anterior chamber angles or a history of angle-closure glaucoma. Use atropine with caution in patients with Down's syndrome and in patients receiving systemic anticholinergic drugs. Patients allergic to atropine can usually be given scopolamine, which will enable similar examination results.

Drug selection: Atropine provides the most effective cycloplegia of any currently available anticholinergic drug, and is indicated for the cycloplegic retinoscopy of infants and children up to 4 years of age with suspected accommodative esotropia. The use of atropine allows determination of the maximum amount of hyperopia.

Cyclopentolate has become the drug of choice for the cycloplegic refraction of strabismic patients over 4 years of age and nonstrabismic patients of any age. Although atropine is still preferred for patients under 4 years of age with suspected accommodative esotropia, there is a trend toward the use of cyclopentolate in these patients.

Clinical Procedures: The use of atropine for the refractive examination of patients with suspected accommodative esotropia requires that the medication be instilled at home for 1 to 3 days prior to the office visit. This allows time for maximum cycloplegia to occur.

Cyclopentolate is used in the practitioner's office and is instilled 30 to 60 minutes prior to refractive examination. Once maximum cycloplegia has occurred, retinoscopy or subjective refraction is performed. Considerable skill and judgment are required to interpret the findings and prescribe a useful refractive correction.

Use in Uveitis

Uveitis is an inflammation of the iris, ciliary body or choroid of the eye. The inflammation can be limited to the anterior structures or the posterior structures of the eye, or both; the clinical features depend on the site of involvement. Uveitis can be classified based on the anatomic site of inflammation. For example, uveitis involving the iris only is termed iritis. Another method to classify the uveal inflammation is based on whether it affects the anterior or posterior structures of the eye. Uveitis can also be classified as either granulomatous or nongranulomatous. Any clinical classification system has considerable overlap, but these classifications provide the opportunity to differentiate various clinical presentations and predict the natural course of the uveal inflammation.

Etiology: Uveitis is thought to be an immune-complex disease with T-cell antigen dysfunction playing a major role. Idiopathic anterior uveitis is the most common clinical presentation. Human leukocyte antigen (HLA) studies are being undertaken to identify individuals who might be predisposed to recurrent episodes of uveitis or whose uveitis might be associated with other conditions. Systemic disorders are often associated with uveitis and include collagen diseases such as rheumatoid arthritis, ankylosing spondylitis and systemic lupus erythematosus. Other systemic causes include metabolic diseases, granulomatous diseases and infectious diseases such as herpes zoster and herpes simplex.

Diagnosis: The signs and symptoms of uveitis depend largely on the anatomic site of inflammation. Anterior uveitis is characterized by conjunctival hyperemia, the distribution of which often follows a circumcorneal pattern. The pupil is frequently miotic, and there is almost always an anterior chamber reaction manifested by cells and flare. The intraocular pressure may be reduced, and there are often keratic precipitates on the corneal endothelium as seen with the slit lamp. Symptoms include ocular pain, photophobia and blurred vision. Cases of anterior uveitis that are bilateral, recurrent or resistant to treatment should be considered for more extensive diagnostic evaluation for the presence of underlying systemic disease.

Posterior uveitis is characterized by little or no pain, and although there can be some anterior chamber reaction, inflammation of the vitreous (vitritis) is most prominent. If the macula is involved or if the vitreous is sufficiently hazy to diminish vision, visual acuity will be affected.

Drug Selection: Cycloplegics are useful in the treatment of anterior uveitis because they often prevent posterior synechiae. Cycloplegia places the ciliary body and iris at rest, reducing many of the associated symptoms, and cycloplegics also reduce the anterior chamber reaction. Cyclopentolate, homatropine and atropine are the most commonly used cycloplegic agents for the treatment of uveitis.

Topical corticosteroids are usually administered in conjunction with cycloplegic therapy. In severe cases, periocular or oral steroids may also be considered; immunosuppressive agents can be used in cases where corticosteroids may not be effective. If uveitic glaucoma ensues, antiglaucoma therapy is usually initiated.

Jimmy D. Bartlett, OD, DOS
University of Alabama at Birmingham

Siret D. Jaanus, PhD
State University of New York

Thom Zimmerman, MD, PhD
University of Louisville

For More Information

Bartlett JD. Administration of and adverse reactions to cycloplegic agents. *Am J Optom Physiol Optics* 1978;55:227.

Bartlett JD, Jaanus SD, eds. Clinical Ocular Pharmacology, ed. 3. Boston: Butterworth-Heinemann, 1995.

Cremer SA, et al. Hydroxyamphetamine mydriasis in Horner's Syndrome. *Am J Ophthalmol* 1990;110:71.

Fraunfelder FT, Scafidi AF. Possible adverse effects from topical ocular 10% phenylephrine. *Am J Ophthalmol* 1978;85:862.

Gambill HD, et al. Mydriatic effect of four drugs determined by pupillograph. *Arch Ophthalmol* 1967;77:740.

Hendly DE, et al. Changing patterns of uveitis. *Am J Ophthalmol* 1987;103:131.

Larkin KM, Charap A, Cheetham JK, et al. Ideal concentration of tropicamide with hydroxyamphetamine 1% for routine pupillary dilation. *Ann Ophthalmol* 1989;21:340.

Manny RE, Fern KD, Zervas HJ, et al. 1% cyclopentolate hydrochloride: Another look at the time course of cycloplegia using an objective measure of the accommodative response. *Optom Vis Sci* 1993;70:651–65.

Montgomery DMI, Macewan CS. Pupil dilation with tropicamide. The effects on acuity, accommodation and refraction. *Eye* 1989;3:845.

Moore BD. Cycloplegic refraction of young children. *N Engl J Optom* 1988;41:10.

Paggiarino DA, Brancato LJ, Newton RE. The effect on pupil size and accommodation of sympathetic and parasympatholytic agents. *Ann Ophthalmol* 1993;25:244–53.

PHENYLEPHRINE HYDROCHLORIDE

Actions:

Pharmacology: Phenylephrine ophthalmic solution possesses predominantly α-adrenergic effects. In the eye, phenylephrine acts locally as a potent vasoconstrictor and mydriatic by constricting ophthalmic blood vessels and the radial muscle of the iris. The ophthalmic usefulness of phenylephrine is due to its rapid effect and moderately prolonged action.

Actions of different concentrations of phenylephrine are shown in the following table:

Phenylephrine Hydrochloride			
	Mydriasis/Vasoconstriction		
Strength of solution (%)	Maximal (min)	Recovery time (hrs)	Paralysis of accommodation
0.12	30 to 90	–	–
2.5	15 to 60	3	trace
10	10 to 60	6	slight

Although rare, systemic absorption of sufficient quantities of phenylephrine may lead to systemic α-adrenergic effects, such as rise in blood pressure, which may be accompanied by a reflex atropine-sensitive bradycardia.

Indications:

2.5% and 10%: Decongestant and vasoconstrictor and for pupil dilation in uveitis (posterior synechiae), open-angle glaucoma, refraction without cycloplegia, prior to surgery, ophthalmoscopic examination (funduscopy).

Contraindications:

Hypersensitivity to any component of the formulation; narrow-angle glaucoma or individuals with a narrow (occludable) angle who do not have glaucoma; in low birth weight infants and in some elderly adults with severe arteriosclerotic cardiovascular or cerebrovascular disease; during intraocular operative procedures when the corneal epithelial barrier has been disturbed.

Phenylephrine 10%: In infants, small children with low body weights, debilitated or elderly patients and in patients with aneurysms. The administration of phenylephrine is contraindicated in patients with long-standing insulin-dependent diabetes, hypertensive patients receiving reserpine or guanethidine, advanced arteriosclerotic changes, idiopathic orthostatic hypotension and in those patients with a known history of organic cardiac disease.

In individuals with an intraocular lens implant, the administration of 10% phenylephrine is contraindicated due to the possibility of dislodging the lens.

Warnings:

Phenylephrine 10%: There have been rare reports of the development of serious cardiovascular reactions, including ventricular arrhythmias and myocardial infarctions. These episodes, some fatal, have usually occurred in elderly patients with preexisting cardiovascular diseases.

Elderly: Use with caution. Due to the strong action of phenylephrine 2.5% to 10% on the dilator muscle, older individuals may also develop transient pigment floaters in the aqueous humor 30 to 45 minutes following administration. The appearance may be similar to anterior uveitis or microscopic hyphema.

Rebound miosis occurs in some elderly patients. Subsequent instillation of phenylephrine may produce less mydriasis than the initial instillation. This may be of clinical importance when dilating pupils prior to retinal detachment or cataract surgery. Exercise caution not to overdose these patients.

Pregnancy: Category C. Safety for use has not been established. Use only if clearly needed and potential benefits outweigh potential hazards to the fetus.

Lactation: It is not known whether this drug is excreted in breast milk. Use caution when phenylephrine HCl is administered to a nursing woman.

Children: Safety and efficacy for use in children have not been established. Phenylephrine 2.5% has been used for a "one application method" in combination with a preferred rapid-acting cycloplegic (see Administration and Dosage). Phenylephrine 10% is contraindicated in infants.

Precautions:

Systemic absorption: Exceeding recommended dosages or applying phenylephrine 2.5% to 10% to an instrumented, traumatized, diseased or postsurgical eye or adnexa, or to patients with suppressed lacrimation, as during anesthesia, may result in the absorption of sufficient quantities to produce a systemic vasopressor response.

A significant elevation in blood pressure is rare but has been reported following conjunctival instillation of recommended doses of phenylephrine 10%. Use with caution in children of low body weight, the elderly and patients with insulin-dependent diabetes, hypertension, hyperthyroidism, generalized arteriosclerosis or cardiovascular disease. Carefully monitor the posttreatment blood pressure of these patients and any patients who develop symptoms (see Contraindications).

The hypertensive effects of phenylephrine may be treated with an α-adrenergic blocking agent such as phentolamine mesylate, 5 mg to 10 mg IV, repeated as necessary.

Narrow-angle glaucoma: Ordinarily, mydriatics are contraindicated in glaucoma patients. However, when temporary pupil dilation may free adhesions, or when intrinsic vessel vasoconstriction may lower IOP, this may temporarily outweigh danger from coincident dilation.

Corneal effects: If the corneal epithelium has been denuded or damaged, corneal clouding may occur if phenylephrine 10% is instilled. This may be especially serious following corneal epithelium removal during retinal detachment surgery or vitrectomy. The corneas of diabetic patients may manifiest epithelial ulcerations as well as a slow rate of reepithelialization. Use of phenylephrine in such corneas may be especially hazardous.

Rebound congestion may occur with extended use of ophthalmic vasoconstrictors.

Sulfite sensitivity: Some of these products contain sulfites. Sulfites may cause allergic-type reactions (eg, hives, itching, wheezing, anaphylaxis) in certain susceptible persons. Although the overall prevalence of sulfite sensitivity in the general population is low, it is seen more frequently in asthmatics or in atopic nonasthmatic persons. Specific products containing sulfites are identified in the product listings.

Drug Interactions:

Anesthetics: Use anesthetics that sensitize the myocardium to sympathomimetics (eg, cyclopropane or halothane) cautiously. Local anesthetics can increase ocular absorption of topical drugs. Exercise caution when applying prior to use of phenylephrine.

β-adrenergic blocking agents: Systemic side effects may occur more readily in patients taking these drugs. A severe hypertensive episode and fatal intracranial hemorrhage possibly associated with ophthalmic use of phenylephrine was reported in one patient taking propranolol for hypertension.

MAOIs: When given with, or up to 21 days after MAOIs, exaggerated adrenergic effects may result. Supervise and adjust dosage carefully. The pressor response of adrenergic agents may also be potentiated by tricyclic antidepressants, propranolol, reserpine, guanethidine, methyldopa and anticholinergics (see Adverse Reactions).

Adverse Reactions:

Ophthalmic: Transitory stinging on initial instillation; blurring of vision; mydriasis; increased redness; irritation; discomfort; punctate keratitis; lacrimation; increased IOP. May cause rebound miosis and decreased mydriatic response to therapy in older persons.

Cardiovascular: Palpitations; tachycardia; cardiac arrhythmia; hypertension; collapse; extrasystoles; ventricular arrhythmias (ie, premature ventricular contractions); reflex bradycardia; coronary occlusion; subarachnoid hemorrhage; myocardial infarction; stroke; death associated with cardiac reactions. Headache or browache may occur.

> *Phenylephrine 10%* – Significant elevation of blood pressure is rare but can occur after conjunctival instillation. Exercise caution with elderly patients and children of low body weight. Carefully monitor the blood pressure of these patients. (See Warnings and Contraindications.) There have been rare reports of the development of serious cardiovascular reactions, including ventricular arrhythmias and myocardial infarctions. These episodes, some fatal, have usually occurred in elderly patients with preexisting cardiovascular diseases.

Miscellaneous: Headache; blanching; sweating; dizziness; nausea; nervousness; drowsiness; weakness; hyperglycemia.

Patient Information:

Potentially hazardous tasks: May cause temporary blurred vision. Observe caution while driving or performing other hazardous tasks.

If severe eye pain, headache, vision changes, acute eye redness or pain with light exposure occur, discontinue use and consult a physician.

To avoid contamination, do not touch dropper tip to any surface. Replace cap after using.

Do not use if solution changes color or becomes cloudy.

Administration and Dosage:

Vasoconstrictors and pupil dilation: Instill a drop of topical anesthetic. Follow in a few minutes by 1 drop of the 2.5% or 10% phenylephrine. The anesthetic prevents stinging and consequent dilution of solution by lacrimation. It may be necessary to repeat the instillation after 1 hour, again preceded by a topical anesthetic.

Uveitis: The formation of synechiae may be prevented by using the 2.5% or 10% solution and atropine to produce wide dilation of the pupil. However, the vasoconstrictor effect of phenylephrine may be antagonistic to the increase of local blood flow in uveal infection.

To free recently formed posterior synechiae, instill 1 drop of the 2.5% or 10% solution to the upper surface of the cornea. Continue treatment the following day, if necessary. In the interim, apply hot compresses for 5 or 10 minutes, 3 times daily using 1 drop of 1% or 2% solution of atropine sulfate before and after each series of compresses.

Glaucoma: Instill 1 drop of 10% solution on the upper surface of the cornea as often as necessary. The 2.5% and 10% solutions have been used in conjunction with miotics in patients with open-angle glaucoma. Phenylephrine reduces the difficulties experienced by the patient because of the small field produced by miosis. Hence, there may be marked improvement in visual acuity after using phenylephrine with miotic drugs.

Surgery: When a short-acting mydriatic is needed for wide dilation of the pupil before intraocular surgery, the 2.5% or 10% solution may be instilled from 30 to 60 minutes before the operation.

Refraction: Prior to determination of refractive errors, the 2.5% solution may be used effectively with homatropine HBr, atropine sulfate, cyclopentolate, tropicamide HCl or a combination of homatropine and cocaine HCl.

> *Adults* – Instill 1 drop of the preferred cycloplegic in each eye; follow in 5 minutes with 1 drop phenylephrine 2.5% solution and in 10 minutes with another drop of the cycloplegic. In 50 to 60 minutes, the eyes are ready for refraction.
>
> Since adequate cycloplegia is achieved at different time intervals after the necessary number of drops, different cycloplegics will require different waiting periods.
>
> *Children* – Instill 1 drop of atropine sulfate 1% in each eye; follow in 10 to 15 minutes with 1 drop of phenylephrine 2.5% solution and in 5 to 10 minutes with a second drop of atropine sulfate 1%. In 1 to 2 hours, the eyes are ready for refraction.
>
> For a "one application method", combine 2.5% phenylephrine solution with a cycloplegic, such as cyclopentolate, to elicit synergistic action. The additive effect varies depending on the patient. Therefore, when using a "one application method", it may be desirable to increase the concentration of the cycloplegic.

Ophthalmoscopic examination: Phenylephrine is rarely used alone for mydriasis. Maximum dilation is achieved in 45 to 60 minutes.

Diagnostic procedures: Heavily pigmented irides may require larger doses in all the following procedures:

Retinoscopy – When dilation of the pupil without cycloplegic action is desired, the 2.5% solution may be used alone.

Blanching test – Instill 1 to 2 drops of the 2.5% solution in the injected eye. After 5 minutes, examine for perilimbal blanching. If blanching occurs, the congestion is superficial and probably does not indicate iritis.

Stability: Prolonged exposure to air or strong light may cause oxidation and discoloration. Do not use if solution changes color, becomes cloudy or contains a precipitate.

Rx	**Phenylephrine HCl** (Various, eg, Steris)	**Solution**: 2.5%	In 15 ml.
Rx	**AK-Dilate** (Akorn)		In 2 and 15 ml.[1]
Rx	**Mydfrin 2.5%** (Alcon)		In 3 and 5 ml Drop-Tainers.[2]
Rx	**Neo-Synephrine** (Sanofi Winthrop)		In 15 ml.[3]
Rx	**Phenoptic** (Optopics)		In 2, 5 and 15 ml.
Rx	**Phenylephrine HCl** (Various, eg, Ciba Vision, Steris)	**Solution**: 10%	In 2 and 5 ml.
Rx	**AK-Dilate** (Akorn)		In 2 and 5 ml.[1]
Rx	**Neo-Synephrine** (Sanofi Winthrop)		In 5 ml.[4]
Rx	**Neo-Synephrine Viscous** (Sanofi Winthrop)		In 5 ml.[5]

[1] With benzalkonium chloride.
[2] With 0.01% benzalkonium chloride, EDTA and sodium bisulfite.
[3] With 1:7500 benzalkonium chloride.
[4] With 1:10,000 benzalkonium chloride.
[5] With 1:10,000 benzalkonium chloride and methylcellulose.

CYCLOPLEGIC MYDRIATICS

Actions:

Pharmacology: Anticholinergic agents (cholinergic antagonists) block the responses of the sphincter muscle of the iris and the muscle of the ciliary body to cholinergic stimulation, producing pupillary dilation (mydriasis) and paralysis of accommodation (cycloplegia).

Cycloplegic Mydriatics

Drug	Mydriasis Peak (minutes)	Mydriasis Recovery (days)	Cycloplegia Peak (minutes)	Cycloplegia Recovery (days)	Solution available
Atropine	30-40	7-10	60-180	6-12	0.5%-2%
Homatropine	40-60	1-3	30-60	1-3	2%-5%
Scopolamine	20-30	3-7	30-60	3-7	0.25%
Cyclopentolate	30-60	1	25-75	0.25-1	0.5%-2%
Tropicamide	20-40	0.25	20-35	< 0.25	0.25%-1%

Indications:

Mydriasis/Cycloplegia: For cycloplegic refraction and for dilating the pupil in inflammatory conditions of the iris and uveal tract. See individual monographs for specific indications.

Contraindications:

Primary glaucoma or a tendency toward glaucoma (eg, narrow anterior chamber angle); hypersensitivity to belladonna alkaloids or any component of the products; adhesions (synechiae) between the iris and the lens; children who have previously had a severe systemic reaction to atropine.

Warnings:

For topical ophthalmic use only: Not for injection.

Glaucoma: Determine the intraocular tension and the depth of the angle of the anterior chamber before and during use to avoid glaucoma attacks.

Elderly: Use these products with caution in the elderly and others where increased IOP may be encountered.

Pregnancy: Category C (atropine, cyclopentolate, homatropine). Safety for use during pregnancy has not been established. Give to a pregnant woman only if clearly needed.

Lactation: Atropine and homatropine may be detectable, in very small amounts, in breast milk. Although this is controversial, according to the American Academy of Pediatrics, these agents are compatible with breastfeeding. It is not known if cyclopentolate is excreted in breast milk. Exercise caution when administering to a nursing woman.

Children: Excessive use in children and in certain susceptible individuals may produce systemic toxic symptoms. Use with extreme caution in infants and small children.

> *Tropicamide and cyclopentolate* – May cause CNS disturbances, which may be dangerous in infants and children. Keep in mind the possibility of psychotic reaction and behavioral disturbance due to hypersensitivity to anticholinergic drugs. Use with extreme caution. Increased susceptibility to cyclopentolate has been reported in infants, young children and in children with spastic paralysis or brain damage. Feeding intolerance may follow ophthalmic use of this product in neonates. It is recommended that feeding be withheld for 4 hours after examination. Do not use in concentrations > 0.5% in small infants.

Precautions:

Systemic effects: Avoid excessive systemic absorption by compressing the lacrimal sac by digital pressure during and for 2 to 3 minutes after instillation.

Down's syndrome/children with brain damage: Use cycloplegics with caution. These patients may demonstrate a hyperreactive response to topical atropine.

Hazardous tasks: May produce drowsiness, blurred vision or sensitivity to light (due to dilated pupils); observe caution while driving or performing other tasks requiring alertness, coordination or physical dexterity.

Sulfite sensitivity: Some of these products contain sulfites which may cause allergic-type reactions (eg, hives, itching, wheezing, anaphylaxis) in certain susceptible persons. Although the overall prevalence of sulfite sensitivity in the general population is probably low, it is seen more frequently in asthmatics or in atopic nonasthmatic persons. Specific products containing sulfites are identified in the product listings.

Adverse Reactions:

Local: Increased intraocular pressure; transient stinging/burning; irritation with prolonged use (eg, allergic lid reactions, hyperemia, follicular conjunctivitis, blepharoconjunctivitis, vascular congestion, edema, exudate, eczematoid dermatitis).

Systemic: Dryness of the mouth and skin; blurred vision; photophobia with or without corneal staining; tachycardia; headache; parasympathetic stimulation; somnolence; visual hallucinations.

Other toxic manifestations of anticholinergic drugs include: Skin rash; abdominal distention in infants; unusual drowsiness; hyperpyrexia; vasodilation; urinary retention; diminished GI motility; decreased secretion in salivary and sweat glands, pharynx, bronchi and nasal passages. Severe manifestations of toxicity include: Coma; medullary paralysis; death. Severe reactions are manifested by hypotension with progressive respiratory depression.

Cyclopentolate and tropicamide have been associated with psychotic reactions and behavioral disturbances in children. Ataxia, incoherent speech, restlessness, hallucinations, hyperactivity, seizures, disorientation as to time and place, and failure to recognize people have occurred with cyclopentolate. CNS disturbances have also occurred in children with tropicamide.

Overdosage:

Ocular: If ocular overdosage occurs, flush eye(s) with water or normal saline. Use of a topical miotic may be required. If accidentally ingested, induce emesis or gastric lavage.

Systemic: If symptoms develop (see Adverse Reactions), patients usually recover spontaneously when the drug is discontinued. In cases of severe toxicity, give physostigmine salicylate (see individual monograph in the Agents for Glaucoma chapter). Have atropine (1 mg) available for immediate injection if physostigmine causes bradycardia, convulsions or bronchoconstriction.

Cyclopentolate toxicity may produce exaggerated symptoms (see Adverse Reactions). When administration of the drug product is discontinued, the patient usually recovers spontaneously. In case of severe manifestations of toxicity, the antidote of choice is physostigmine salicylate.

Children – Slowly inject 0.5 mg physostigmine salicylate IV. If toxic symptoms persist and no cholinergic symptoms are produced, repeat at 5 minute intervals to a maximum cumulative dose of 2 mg.

Adults and adolescents – Slowly inject 2 mg physostigmine salicylate IV. A second dose of 1 to 2 mg may be given after 20 minutes if no reversal of toxic manifestations has occurred.

Patient Information:

To avoid contamination, do not touch dropper tip to any surface. Replace cap after using.

May cause blurred vision. Do not drive or engage in any hazardous activities while the pupils are dilated.

May cause sensitivity to light. Protect eyes in bright illumination during dilation.

Keep out of the reach of children. These drugs should not be taken orally. Wash your own hands and the child's following administration.

If eye pain occurs, discontinue use and consult physician immediately.

Individual drug monographs are on the following pages.

ATROPINE SULFATE

For complete prescribing information, refer to the Cycloplegic Mydriatrics group monograph.

Indications:

Mydriasis/Cycloplegia: For cycloplegic refraction or pupil dilation in acute inflammatory conditions of iris and uveal tract.

Administration and Dosage:

Solution:

Adults – Uveitis: Instill 1 or 2 drops into the eye(s) up to 4 times daily.

Children – Uveitis: Instill 1 or 2 drops of 0.5% solution into the eye(s) up to 3 times daily.

Refraction: Instill 1 or 2 drops of 0.5% solution into the eye(s) twice daily for 1 to 3 days before examination.

Ointment: Apply a small amount in the conjunctival sac up to 3 times daily.

Compress the lacrimal sac by digital pressure during and for 2 to 3 minutes after instillation.

Individuals with heavily pigmented irides may require larger doses.

Storage: Keep away from heat.

Rx	**Atropine Sulfate Ophthalmic** (Various, eg, Bausch & Lomb, Fougera, Pharmafair, Zenith-Goldline)	**Ointment:** 1%	In 3.5 and UD 1 g.
Rx	**Isopto Atropine** (Alcon)	**Solution:** 0.5%	In 5 ml Drop-Tainers.[1]
Rx	**Atropine Sulfate** (Various, eg, Alcon, Allergan, Bausch & Lomb, Optopics, Pharmafair, Rugby, Zenith-Goldline)	**Solution:** 1%	In 2, 5 and 15 ml and UD 1 ml.
Rx	**Atropine Care** (Akorn)		In 2, 5 and 15 ml.[2]
Rx	**Atropine-1** (Optopics)		In 2, 5 and 15 ml.
Rx	**Atropisol** (Ciba Vision)		In 1 ml Dropperettes.[3]
Rx	**Isopto Atropine** (Alcon)		In 5 and 15 ml Drop-Tainers.[1]
Rx	**Atropine Sulfate** (Alcon)	**Solution:** 2%	In 2 ml.

[1] With 0.01% benzalkonium chloride, 0.5% hydroxypropyl methylcellulose and boric acid.
[2] With 0.01% benzalkonium chloride, hydroxypropyl methylcellulose and boric acid.
[3] With benzalkonium chloride, EDTA and boric acid.

HOMATROPINE HYDROBROMIDE

For complete prescribing information, refer to the Cycloplegic Mydriatics group monograph.

Indications:

Mydriasis/Cycloplegia: A moderately long-acting mydriatic and cycloplegic for refraction, and in the treatment of inflammatory conditions of the uveal tract. For preoperative and postoperative states when mydriasis is required.

Lens opacity: As an optical aid in some cases of axial lens opacities.

Administration and Dosage:

Uveitis: Instill 1 or 2 drops into the eye(s) up to every 3 to 4 hours.

Refraction: Instill 1 or 2 drops into the eye(s); repeat in 5 to 10 minutes if necessary.

Individuals with heavily pigmented irides may require larger doses.

Children: Use only the 2% strength.

Compress the lacrimal sac by digital pressure during and for 2 to 3 minutes after instillation.

Storage: Store at 8° to 24°C (46° to 75°F).

Rx	**Isopto Homatropine** (Alcon)	**Solution**: 2%	In 5 and 15 ml Drop-Tainers.[1]
Rx	**Homatropine HBr** (Various, eg, Alcon, Ciba Vision)	**Solution**: 5%	In 1, 2 and 5 ml.
Rx	**AK-Homatropine** (Akorn)		In 5 ml.
Rx	**Isopto Homatropine** (Alcon)		In 5 and 15 ml Drop-Tainers.[2]

[1] With 0.01% benzalkonium chloride, 0.5% hydroxypropyl methylcellulose and polysorbate 80.
[2] With 0.005% benzethonium chloride and 0.5% hydroxypropyl methylcellulose.

SCOPOLAMINE HYDROBROMIDE (Hyoscine Hydrobromide)

For complete prescribing information, refer to the Cycloplegic Mydriatics group monograph.

Indications:

Mydriasis/Cycloplegia: For cycloplegia and mydriasis in diagnostic procedures.

Iridocyclitis: For preoperative and postoperative states in the treatment of iridocyclitis.

Administration and Dosage:

Uveitis: Instill 1 or 2 drops into the eye(s) up to 4 times daily.

Refraction: Instill 1 or 2 drops into the eye(s) 1 hour before refracting.

Compress the lacrimal sac by digital pressure during and for 2 to 3 minutes after instillation.

Storage: Protect from light. Store at 8° to 27°C (46° to 80°F).

Rx	**Isopto Hyoscine** (Alcon)	**Solution:** 0.25%	In 5 and 15 ml Drop-Tainers.[1]

[1] With 0.01% benzalkonium chloride and 0.5% hydroxypropyl methylcellulose.

CYCLOPENTOLATE HYDROCHLORIDE

For complete prescribing information, refer to the Cycloplegic Mydriatics group monograph.

Indications:

Mydriasis/Cycloplegia: For mydriasis and cycloplegia in diagnostic procedures.

Administration and Dosage:

Adults: Instill 1 or 2 drops of 0.5%, 1% or 2% solution into eye(s). Repeat in 5 to 10 minutes, if necessary. Complete recovery usually occurs in 24 hours.

Children: Instill 1 or 2 drops of 0.5%, 1% or 2% solution into each eye. Follow in 5 to 10 minutes with a second application of 0.5% or 1% solution, if necessary.

Small infants: Instill 1 drop of 0.5% solution into each eye. Observe patient closely for at least 30 minutes following instillation.

Compress the lacrimal sac by digital pressure during and for 2 to 3 minutes after instillation.

Individuals with heavily pigmented irides may require higher strengths.

Storage: Store at 8° to 27°C (46° to 80°F).

Rx	**Cyclogyl** (Alcon)	**Solution**: 0.5%	In 2, 5 and 15 ml Drop-Tainers.[1]
Rx	**Cyclopentolate HCl** (Various, eg, Bausch & Lomb, Schein, Steris)	**Solution**: 1%	In 2, 5 and 15 ml.
Rx	**AK-Pentolate** (Akorn)		In 2 and 15 ml.[1]
Rx	**Cyclogyl** (Alcon)		In 2, 5 and 15 ml.[1]
Rx	**Cyclogyl** (Alcon)	**Solution**: 2%	In 2, 5 and 15 ml Drop-Tainers.[1]
Rx	**Pentolair** (Bausch & Lomb)	**Solution**: 1%	In 2 and 15 ml squeeze bottles.[2]

[1] With 0.01% benzalkonium chloride, EDTA and boric acid.
[2] With 0.01% benzalkonium chloride and EDTA.

TROPICAMIDE

For complete prescribing information, refer to the Cycloplegic Mydriatics group monograph.

Indications:

Mydriasis/Cycloplegia: For mydriasis and cycloplegia for diagnostic purposes.

Administration and Dosage:

Refraction: Instill 1 or 2 drops of 1% solution into the eye(s); repeat in 5 minutes. If patient is not seen within 20 to 30 minutes, instill an additional drop to prolong mydriatic effect.

Examination of fundus: Instill 1 or 2 drops of 0.5% solution 15 to 20 minutes prior to examination. Compress the lacrimal sac by digital pressure during and for 2 to 3 minutes after instillation to avoid excessive absorption.

Individuals with heavily pigmented irides may require larger doses.

Storage: Store away from heat. Do not refrigerate.

Rx	**Tropicamide** (Various, eg, Bausch & Lomb)	**Solution**:0.5%	In 2 and 15 ml.
Rx	**Mydriacyl** (Alcon)		In 15 ml Drop-Tainers.[1]
Rx	**Opticyl** (Optopics)		In 2 and 15 ml.
Rx	**Tropicacyl** (Akorn)		In 2 and 15 ml.
Rx	**Tropicamide** (Various, eg, Bausch & Lomb)	**Solution**: 1%	In 15 ml.
Rx	**Mydriacyl** (Alcon)		In 3 and 15 ml Drop-Tainers.[1]
Rx	**Opticyl** (Optopics)		In 2 and 15 ml.
Rx	**Tropicacyl** (Akorn)		In 2 and 15 ml.[2]

[1] With 0.01% benzalkonium chloride and EDTA.
[2] With 0.1% benzalkonium chloride and EDTA.

MYDRIATIC COMBINATIONS

These combinations induce mydriasis that is greater than that of either drug used alone at the concentrations present in these combination formulations. See individual monographs for complete prescribing information.

Indications:

Cyclomydril: Production of mydriasis.

Murocoll-2: For mydriasis, cycloplegia and to break posterior synechiae in iritis.

Administration and Dosage:

Cyclomydril: Instill 1 drop into each eye every 5 to 10 minutes, not to exceed 3 times.

Murocoll-2:

Mydriasis – Instill 1 or 2 drops into eye(s); repeat in 5 minutes, if necessary.

Postoperatively – Instill 1 or 2 drops into the eye(s) 3 or 4 times daily.

Rx	**Cyclomydril** (Alcon)	**Solution**: 0.2% cyclopentolate HCl and 1% phenylephrine HCl.	In 2 and 5 ml Drop-Tainers.[1]
Rx	**Murocoll-2** (Bausch & Lomb)	**Drops**: 0.3% scopolamine HBr and 10% phenylephrine HCl.	In 5 ml.[2]

[1] With 0.01% benzalkonium chloride, EDTA and boric acid.
[2] With 0.01% benzalkonium chloride, sodium metabisulfite and EDTA.

ODF

5

ANTIALLERGY AND DECONGESTANT AGENTS

Release of histamine, prostaglandins, leukotrienes and other less well-defined mediators from the mast cell during an allergic reaction can cause a variety of uncomfortable symptoms and sometimes life-threatening complications. Drug therapy is often successful in satisfactorily relieving associated signs and symptoms, especially when ocular tissues are affected.

Type I hypersensitivity reactions, also known as anaphylactic, immediate or IgE-mediated reactions, occur when an antigen such as a drug or pollen is reintroduced into an individual who has been previously exposed to the antigen. Upon initial exposure to the antigen, IgE antibodies are produced which attach to mast cells and make the cells susceptible to rupture when the patient is again exposed to the same antigen. Disruption (degranulation) of mast cells causes a release of large quantities of inflammatory mediators, including histamine, prostaglandins, leukotrienes and eosinophil chemotatic factor. Histamine activates H_1 receptors on blood vessels, causing vasodilation. These dilated blood vessels leak fluid, causing tissues to swell. Common symptoms and signs of local Type I reactions include redness, swelling and itching. Such reactions occur in hay fever, allergic conjunctivitis, asthma, bee stings and other chemical and toxin sensitivities (eg, penicillin). The following ocular diseases are characterized by Type I hypersensitivity reactions and may be treated with antihistamines or mast cell stabilizers.

ALLERGIC CONDITIONS

Seasonal Allergic Conjunctivitis

Allergic conjunctivitis can result from a variety of exogenous antigens and is often a component of more widespread allergic states. Airborne pollens, dust and other environmental contaminants constitute the largest single group of agents responsible for the disorder. Ophthalmic drugs and their preservatives/excipients which may cause allergic conjunctivitis include neomycin, sulfonamides, atropine and thimerosal. A careful patient history along with the typical appearance of conjunctival chemosis and hyperemia, together with itching and tearing, are necessary for the proper etiologic diagnosis.

Vernal Conjunctivitis

Affecting primarily adolescent males, vernal conjunctivitis is a bilateral inflammation involving the upper tarsal conjunctiva and sometimes the limbal conjunctiva. The disease is seasonal and has peak activity during the warm months of the year. It is characterized by the formation of large papillae having the appearance of cobblestones on the upper tarsal conjunctiva. Papillary hypertrophy can occur at the limbus and is characterized by a gelatinous thickening of the superior limbus. Tear histamine levels are significantly higher than in normal patients. Symptoms include intense itching during warm months and often a thick, ropy discharge. If the cornea becomes involved, photophobia may be marked. Significant papillary involvement of the upper lids may result in ptosis.

Atopic Keratoconjunctivitis

Atopic keratoconjunctivitis represents a hypersensitivity state caused by predispositional, constitutional or hereditary factors rather than by acquired hypersensitivity to specific antigens. Patients usually have a personal or family history of allergy, especially asthma or hay fever. Atopic dermatitis is characterized by patches of thickened, excoriated, lichenified skin which is usually dry and itchy. Ocular findings are characterized by conjunctival hyperemia and chemosis. Corneal involvement is not uncommon and may be evident as a classic shield ulcer or pannus.

Giant Papillary Conjunctivitis

Giant papillary conjunctivitis (GPC) is a specific conjunctival inflammatory reaction to materials on contact lenses (eg, protein), but has also been reported in patients wearing methylmethacrylate ocular prostheses. The condition is characterized by papillary hypertrophy and primarily affects the upper tarsal conjunctiva. Although the condition is similar in appearance to that of vernal conjunctivitis, it probably represents a chronic conjunctival inflammatory reaction to denatured proteins that are adherent to the anterior lens surface. Lens bulk (thickness and diameter) may also play a part. Once the conjunctival changes reach a certain point, itching, lens instability, mucoid discharge and contact lens intolerance occur.

DECONGESTANTS

The vasoconstrictor effect of the adrenergic agonists (ie, phenylephrine and the imidazole derivatives) makes them useful as topical ocular decongestants. Following instillation, conjunctival vessels constrict within minutes, causing the eye to whiten. Minor ocular irritation can be temporarily relieved.

Due to the relatively low concentrations required for ocular decongestion, phenylephrine and the imidazole derivatives generally do not cause systemic side effects. These products are designed for short-term use since they may mask symptoms of more serious ocular problems such as bacterial or other infections. If the condition does not respond to use of these products within 48 hours, a more serious condition should be suspected.

Phenylephrine

Phenylephrine (eg, *Neo-Synephrine*), a synthetic amine structurally similar to epinephrine has been used in over-the-counter products at concentrations of 0.12% or 0.125% which cause vasoconstriction with little or no pupillary dilation in eyes with intact corneal epithelium. Since a potential for mydriasis does exist at low concentrations, phenylephrine is contraindicated in eyes predisposed to angle-closure glaucoma. Prolonged or excessive use can result in rebound conjunctival hyperemia. The eye may become more congested and red as the effect of the drug begins to subside.

Phenylephrine can exhibit variable effectiveness since it is subject to oxidation on exposure to air, light or heat. The solution may show no evidence of discoloration. To prolong shelf-life, antioxidants such as sodium bisulfite may be added to the formulation.

Imidazole Derivatives

The imidazole derivatives, naphazoline (eg, *Naphcon*), tetrahydrozoline (eg, *Visine*) and oxymetazoline (eg, *Visine L.R.*), differ structurally from phenylephrine by replacement of the benzene ring with an unsaturated ring. Concentrations used for ocular vasoconstriction do not alter pupil size or raise intraocular pressure in the normal eye.

The imidazole derivatives do not differ significantly in their ability to relieve conjunctival congestion. After instillation, the blanching effect occurs within minutes and may last up to several hours. These agents are generally more stable in solution than phenylephrine, and have a longer shelf-life and duration of action. Imidazole derivatives are buffered to a pH of 6.2 and may sting upon initial instillation.

ANTIHISTAMINES, MAST CELL STABILIZERS AND NSAIDS

Since many of the signs and symptoms associated with Type I hypersensitivity reactions are due to release of histamine from mast cells, antihistamines can be effective in relieving at least some patient discomfort. Levocabastine, an H_1-receptor antagonist, has been formulated for topical ocular use without the presence of a decongestant. Ocular challenge studies have indicated that it can be effective and well tolerated for both prophylaxis and therapy of seasonal allergic conjunctivitis.

Ketorolac tromethamine (*Acular*) is the first NSAID approved for topical ocular use in seasonal allergic conjunctivitis (see the Anti-inflammatory Agents chapter). It can alleviate the ocular itching as well as other signs and symptoms that accompany the reaction.

Mast cell stabilizers can also be useful for certain ocular allergic signs and symptoms. Cromolyn sodium (*Crolom*) is formulated for ophthalmic use in the U.S. and lodoxamide tromethamine *(Alomide),* a recently developed mast cell stabilizer, is currently FDA-approved for the management of vernal keratoconjunctivitis.

COMBINATION PRODUCTS

In addition to vasoconstrictor substances, ocular decongestants may also contain preservatives, antihistamines, viscosity-increasing agents, buffers and astringents. Since preservatives may induce allergic reactions in some patients, unit-dose preservative-free products are being formulated.

PHARMACOLOGIC MANAGEMENT

Antihistamines can be given with or without decongestants, and are administered topically or orally, depending on the degree of involvement. Mast cell stabilizers such as cromolyn sodium (*Crolom*) and lodoxamide tromethamine (*Alomide*) are also effective and can even be used prophylactically. For severe reactions or when rapid relief of symptoms is warranted, topical or oral corticosteroids may be justified. In addition, ketorolac tromethamine (*Acular*), a nonsteroidal anti-inflammatory drug, is indicated for the relief of ocular itching due to seasonal allergic conjunctivitis (see the Anti-inflammatory Agents chapter).

Jimmy D. Bartlett, OD, DOS
University of Alabama at Birmingham

Siret D. Jaanus, PhD
State University of New York

For More Information

Abelson MB, Schaefer K. Conjunctivitis of allergic origin. *Surv Ophthalmol* 1993;38:115.

Bartlett JD, Jaanus SD, eds. Clinical Ocular Pharmacology, ed. 3. Boston: Butterworth-Heinemann, 1995.

Bartlett JD, Ross RN. Primary care of ocular allergy. *J Am Optom Assoc* 1990;61(6)(Suppl):S3–S46.

Bartlett JD, Swanson MW. Ophthalmic products. In: Covington T, ed. Handbook of Non-Prescription Drugs, ed. 10. Washington, DC: American Pharmaceutical Association, 1993:351.

Ciprandi G, Buscaglia S, et al. Drug treatment of allergic conjunctivitis. *Drugs* 1992;43:154.

Caldwell DR, Verin P, Hartwich-Young R, et al. Efficacy and safety of lodoxamide 0.1% vs cromolyn sodium 4% in patients with vernal keratoconjunctivitis. *Am J Ophthamol* 1992;113:632–37.

Donshik PC, et al. Treatment of contact lens-induced giant papillary conjunctivitis. *CLAO J* 1984;10:346.

DECONGESTANTS

Actions:

Pharmacology: The effects of sympathomimetic agents on the eye are concentration-dependent and include: Pupil dilation, increase in outflow of aqueous humor and vasoconstriction (alpha-adrenergic effects).

Higher concentrations of drug (ie, phenylephrine 2.5% and 10%) cause vasoconstriction and pupillary dilation for diagnostic eye exams, during surgery and to prevent synechiae formation in uveitis. Weak concentrations of phenylephrine (0.12%) and other alpha-adrenergic agonists (naphazoline; tetrahydrozoline) are used as ophthalmic decongestants (vasoconstriction of conjunctival blood vessels) and for symptomatic relief of minor eye irritations. Epinephrine is used for open-angle glaucoma and is not included in this monograph (see monograph in Agents for Glaucoma chapter).

Ophthalmic Vasoconstrictors

Vasoconstrictor	Duration of action (hr)	Available concentration	Prescription status
Naphazoline	3 to 4	0.012%	otc
		0.02%	otc
		0.03%	otc
		0.1%	Rx
Oxymetazoline	4 to 6	0.025%	otc
Phenylephrine	0.5 to 1.5	0.12%	otc
	—	2.5%	Rx
	—	10%	Rx
Tetrahydrozoline	1 to 4	0.05%	otc

Indications:

Refer to individual product listings for specific indications.

Contraindications:

Hypersensitivity to any of these agents; narrow-angle glaucoma or anatomically narrow (occludable) angle and no glaucoma; prior to peripheral iridectomy in eyes capable of angle closure because mydriatic action may precipitate angle closure.

Phenylephrine 10%: Infants and patients with aneurysms.

Warnings:

Anesthetics: Discontinue prior to use of anesthetics which sensitize the myocardium to sympathomimetics (eg, cyclopropane, halothane).

Local anesthetics can increase absorption of topically applied drugs; exercise caution when applying prior to use of phenylephrine. However, use of a local anesthetic prior to phenylephrine 2.5% or 10% may prevent stinging and enhance ocular drug penetration.

Overuse may produce rebound vasodilation and increased redness of the eye.

Phenylephrine 10%: There have been rare reports of the development of serious cardiovascular reactions, including ventricular arrhythmias and myocardial infarctions. These episodes, some fatal, have usually occurred in elderly patients with preexisting cardiovascular diseases.

Pregnancy: Category C. Safety for use in pregnancy is not established. Use only if clearly needed and if the potential benefits outweigh potential hazards to the fetus.

Lactation: Safety for use during breastfeeding has not been established. Use caution when administering to a nursing woman.

Children: Safety and efficacy have not been established. Phenylephrine 10% is contraindicated in infants.

Precautions:

Special risk patients: Use with caution in children of low body weight, the elderly and in the presence of hypertension, diabetes, hyperthyroidism, cardiovascular abnormalities, arteriosclerosis.

Narrow-angle glaucoma: Ordinarily, any mydriatic is contraindicated in patients with angle-closure glaucoma. However, when temporary pupil dilation may free adhesions, these advantages may temporarily outweigh danger from coincident pupil dilation.

Rebound congestion may occur with frequent or extended use of ophthalmic vasoconstrictors. Rebound miosis has occurred in older persons 1 day after receiving phenylephrine; reinstillation produced a reduction in mydriasis.

Systemic absorption: Exceeding recommended dosages of these agents or applying phenylephrine 2.5% to 10% solutions to the instrumented, traumatized, diseased or postsurgical eye or adnexa, or to patients with suppressed lacrimation, as during anesthesia, may result in the absorption of sufficient quantities to produce a systemic vasopressor response.

Pigment floaters: Older individuals may develop transient pigment floaters in the aqueous humor 30 to 45 minutes after instillation of phenylephrine. The appearance may be similar to anterior uveitis or to a microscopic hyphema.

Hazardous tasks: Phenylephrine may cause temporary blurred or unstable vision; observe caution while driving or performing other hazardous tasks.

Sulfite sensitivity: Some of these products contain sulfites that may cause allergic-type reactions (eg, hives, itching, wheezing, anaphylaxis) in certain susceptible persons. Although the overall prevalence of sulfite sensitivity in the general population is low, it is seen more frequently in asthmatics or in atopic nonasthmatic persons.

Drug Interactions:

Ophthalmic Sympathomimetic Drug Interactions			
Precipitant drug	Object drug*		Description
Anesthetics	Ophthalmic sympatho-mimetics	↑	Cautiously use anesthetics that sensitize the myocardium to sympathomimetics (eg, cyclopropane, halothane). Local anesthetics can increase absorption of topical drugs; exercise caution when applying prior to use of phenylephrine.
Beta blockers	Ophthalmic sympatho-mimetics	↑	Systemic side effects may occur more readily in patients taking these drugs.
MAOIs	Ophthalmic sympatho-mimetics	↑	When given with, or up to 21 days after MAOIs, exaggerated adrenergic effects may result. Supervise and adjust dosage carefully.

* ↑ = Object drug increased.

Also consider drug interactions that may occur with systemic use of the sympathomimetics.

Adverse Reactions:

Ophthalmic: Transitory stinging on initial instillation; blurring of vision; mydriasis; increased redness; irritation; discomfort; punctate keratitis; lacrimation; increased IOP.

Phenylephrine may cause rebound miosis and decreased mydriatic response to therapy in older persons.

Cardiovascular: Palpitation; tachycardia; cardiac arrhythmia; hypertension; collapse; extrasystoles; ventricular arrhythmias (ie, premature ventricular contractions); reflex bradycardia; coronary occlusion; subarachnoid hemorrhage; myocardial infarction; stroke; death associated with cardiac reactions. Headache or browache may occur.

Phenylephrine 10% – Significant elevation of blood pressure is rare but can occur after conjunctival instillation. Exercise caution with elderly patients and children of low body weight. Carefully monitor the blood pressure of these patients. (See Warnings and Precautions.) There have been rare reports of the development of serious cardiovascular reactions, including ventricular arrhythmias and myocardial infarctions. These episodes, some fatal, have usually occurred in elderly patients with preexisting cardiovascular diseases.

Miscellaneous: Blanching; sweating; dizziness; nausea; nervousness; drowsiness; weakness; hyperglycemia.

Patient Information:

Do not use beyond 48 to 72 hours without consulting a physician.

If irritation, blurring or redness persists, or if severe eye pain, headache, vision changes, floating spots, dizziness, decrease in body temperature, drowsiness, acute eye redness or pain with light exposure occur, discontinue use and consult a physician.

Do not use if you have glaucoma except under the advice of a physician.

Refer to the Dosage Forms and Administration chapter for more complete information.

Hazardous tasks: Phenylephrine may cause temporary blurred or unstable vision; observe caution while driving or performing other hazardous tasks.

Individual drug monographs are on the following pages.

PHENYLEPHRINE HYDROCHLORIDE

For complete prescribing information, refer to the Decongestants group monograph. The following section is included here for completeness to show all of the clinical uses of this drug.

Indications:

0.12%: A decongestant to provide relief of minor eye irritations.

Administration and Dosage:

Minor eye irritations: Instill 1 or 2 drops of the 0.12% solution in eye(s) up to 4 times daily as needed.

Stability: Prolonged exposure to air or strong light may cause oxidation and discoloration. Do not use if solution changes color, becomes cloudy or contains a precipitate.

otc	**AK-Nefrin** (Akorn)	**Solution:** 0.12%	In 15 ml.[1]
otc	**Prefrin Liquifilm** (Allergan)		In 20 ml.[2]
otc	**Relief** (Allergan)		Preservative free. In UD 0.3 ml.[3]
otc	**Zincfrin Solution** (Alcon)		In 15 and 30 ml Drop-Tainers.[3]

[1] With 0.005% benzalkonium chloride, 1.4% polyvinyl alcohol and EDTA.
[2] With 1.4% polyvinyl alcohol, 0.004% benzalkonium chloride and EDTA.
[3] With 0.01% benzalkonium Cl, polysorbate 80, 0.25% zinc sulfate.

NAPHAZOLINE HYDROCHLORIDE

For complete prescribing information, refer to the Decongestants group monograph.

Indications:

Redness: To soothe, refresh and remove redness due to minor eye irritation such as smoke, smog, sun glare, allergies or swimming.

Administration and Dosage:

Instill 1 or 2 drops into the conjunctival sac of affected eye(s) every 3 to 4 hours, up to 4 times daily.

Storage/Stability: Do not use if solution changes color or becomes cloudy.

otc	**Allerest Eye Drops** (Ciba Vision)	**Solution**: 0.012%	In 15 ml.[1]
otc	**Clear Eyes** (Ross)		In 15 and 30 ml.[2]
otc	**Clear Eyes ACR** (Ross)		In 15 and 30 ml.[3]
otc	**Degest 2** (Akorn)		In 15 ml.[4]
otc	**Naphcon** (Alcon)		In 15 ml.[5]
otc	**Allergy Drops** (Bausch & Lomb)		In 15 ml.[6]
otc	**Vaso Clear** (Ciba Vision)	**Solution**: 0.02%	In 15 ml.[7]
otc	**Vaso Clear A** (Ciba Vision)		In 15 ml.[8]
otc	**Comfort Eye Drops** (PBH Wesley Jessen)	**Solution**: 0.03%	In 15 ml.[9]
otc	**Maximum Strength Allergy Drops** (Bausch & Lomb)		In 15 ml.[10]
Rx	**Naphazoline HCl** (Various, eg, Rugby, Zenith-Goldline)	**Solution**: 0.1%	In 15 ml.
Rx	**AK-Con** (Akorn)		In 15 ml.[5]
Rx	**Albalon** (Allergan)		In 15 ml.[11]
Rx	**Nafazair** (Bausch & Lomb)		In 15 ml.[5]
Rx	**Naphcon Forte** (Alcon)		In 15 ml Drop-Tainers.[5]
Rx	**Vasocon Regular** (Ciba Vision)		In 15 ml.[12]

[1] With benzalkonium chloride, EDTA.
[2] With benzalkonium chloride, EDTA, 0.2% glycerin, boric acid.
[3] With benzalkonium chloride, EDTA, 0.25% zinc sulfate, 0.2% glycerin.
[4] With 0.0067% benzalkonium chloride, 0.02% EDTA, hydroxyethylcellulose, povidone.
[5] With 0.01% benzalkonium chloride, EDTA.
[6] With 0.2% PEG-300, 0.01% benzalkonium chloride.
[7] With 0.01% benzalkonium chloride, 0.25% polyvinyl alcohol, 1% PEG-400, EDTA.
[8] With 0.005% benzalkonium chloride, EDTA, 0.25% zinc sulfate, 0.25% polyvinyl alcohol, 1% PEG-400 .
[9] With 0.005% benzalkonium chloride and 0.02% EDTA.
[10] With 0.01% benzalkonium chloride, 0.5% hydroxypropyl methylcellulose and EDTA.
[11] With 0.004% benzalkonium chloride, EDTA, 1.4% polyvinyl alcohol.
[12] With benzalkonium chloride, polyvinyl alcohol, EDTA, PEG-8000.

TETRAHYDROZOLINE HYDROCHLORIDE

For complete prescribing information, refer to the Decongestants group monograph.

Indications:

Redness: For relief of redness of the eye due to minor irritations.

Burning/Irritation: For temporary relief of burning and irritation due to dryness of the eye or discomfort due to minor irritations or to exposure to wind or sun.

Administration and Dosage:

Instill 1 or 2 drops into eye(s) up to 4 times a day.

Stability: Do not use if solution changes color or becomes cloudy.

otc	**Tetrahydrozoline HCl** (Various, eg, Moore, Rugby, Steris)	**Solution:** 0.05%	In 15 and 30 ml.
otc	**AR Eye Drops - Astringent Redness Reliever** (Bausch & Lomb)		In 15 ml.[1]
otc	**Collyrium Fresh** (Wyeth-Ayerst)		In 15 ml.[2]
otc	**Eye Drops** (Bausch & Lomb)		In 15 ml.[3]
otc	**Eye Drops Extra** (Bausch & Lomb)		In 15 ml.[4]
otc	**Eyesine** (Akorn)		In 15 ml.[3]
otc	**Geneye** (Zenith Goldline)		In 15 ml.[5]
otc	**Geneye Extra** (Zenith Goldline)		In 15 ml.[6]
otc	**Mallazine Eye Drops** (Roberts Hauck)		In 15 ml.[3]
otc	**Murine Plus** (Ross)		In 15 and 30 ml.[7]
otc	**Optigene 3** (Pfeiffer)		In 15 ml.[5]
otc	**Tetrasine** (Optopics)		In 15 and 22.5 ml.[8]
otc	**Tetrasine Extra** (Optopics)		In 15 ml.[6]
otc	**Visine** (Pfizer)		In 15, 22.5 and 30 ml.[5]
otc	**Visine Allergy Relief** (Pfizer)		In 15 and 30 ml.[9]
otc	**Visine Moisturizing** (Pfizer)		In 15 and 30 ml.[10]

[1] With 0.25% zinc sulfate.
[2] With 0.01% benzalkonium chloride, 0.1% EDTA and 1% glycerin.
[3] With 0.01% benzalkonium chloride and EDTA.
[4] With 1% polyethylene glycol 400.
[5] With 0.01% benzalkonium chloride and 0.1% EDTA.
[6] With 1% polyethylene glycol 400, benzalkonium chloride and EDTA.
[7] With benzalkonium chloride, EDTA, 1.4% polyvinyl alcohol and 0.6% povidone.
[8] With benzalkonium chloride and EDTA.
[9] With 0.01% benzalkonium Cl, 0.1% EDTA and 0.25% zinc sulfate.
[10] With 0.013% benzalkonium chloride, 0.1% EDTA and 1% PEG-400.

OXYMETAZOLINE HYDROCHLORIDE

For complete prescribing information, refer to the Decongestants group monograph.

Indications:

Redness: For the relief of redness of the eye due to minor eye irritations.

Administration and Dosage:

Adults and children ≥ 6 years: Instill 1 or 2 drops in the affected eye(s) every 6 hours.

Stability: Do not use if solution changes color or becomes cloudy.

otc	**OcuClear** (Schering-Plough)	**Solution:** 0.025%	In 30 ml.[1]
otc	**Visine L.R.** (Pfizer)		In 15 and 30 ml.[1]

[1] With 0.01% benzalkonium chloride and 0.1% EDTA.

ANTIHISTAMINES

Actions:

Pharmacology: Antihistamines can be used alone or in combination with decongestants to provide relief of ocular irritation or congestion for the treatment of allergic or inflammatory ocular conditions. Antihistamines counteract the effects of histamine, a chemical released in the body in response to an antigen-antibody reaction that causes redness, itching and irritation of tissues, and can cause watery eyes, runny nose and sneezing.

Indications:

To provide relief of symptoms of allergic conjunctivitis (watering, itching eyes).

Contraindications:

Hypersensitivity to any component of the formulation; with monoamine oxidase (MAO) inhibitor use.

Warnings:

Elderly: The elderly may require lower doses. Antihistamines are more likely to cause dizziness, sedation, confusion and decreased blood pressure in the elderly.

Pregnancy: Category C. Safety for use has not been established. Use only if clearly needed and if the potential benefits outweigh the potential hazards to the fetus.

Lactation: Antihistamines appear in breast milk. Breastfeeding should be discouraged while using these medications.

Children: Antihistamine overdosage in children may cause hallucinations, convulsions and death. Antihistamines may decrease mental alertness. They produce hyperactivity in children. Caution should be used in children under 12 years of age.

Precautions:

Use with caution in the presence of asthma, coronary artery disease, digestive tract obstruction, enlarged prostate, glaucoma (narrow-angle), heart disease, hypertension, hyperthyroidism, irregular heartbeat, liver disease, peptic ulcer, pregnancy, urinary bladder obstruction.

Glaucoma: Because they produce angle closure, use with caution in persons with narrow angle or a history of glaucoma.

Topical antihistamines are potential sensitizers and may produce a local sensitivity reaction.

Drug Interactions:

Alcohol, sedatives (sleeping pills), tranquilizers, antianxiety medications and narcotic pain relievers all are known to react with antihistamines. The following drug and drug classes also interact with antihistamines: Anticoagulants, epinephrine, fluconazole, isocarboxazid, itraconazole, ketoconazole, macrolides, metronidazole, miconazole, phenelzine, procarbazine, selegiline, tranylcypromine.

Adverse Reactions:

Ophthalmic: Blurred and double vision; eye pain; dryness; sensitivity to light.

Systemic: Stomach ache; constipation; appetite changes; nausea; vomiting; diarrhea; drowsiness; dizziness; mental confusion; decreased coordination; fatigue; headache; sleeplessness; sleepiness; sore throat; pharyngitis; cough; dry nose, throat and mouth; thickening of mucus in respiratory tract; wheezing; stuffiness.

Cardiovascular: Irregular heartbeat; palpitations; hypotension.

Miscellaneous: Difficult urination; urine retention; ringing in the ears; rash; hives; excessive perspiration; chills.

Patient Information:

May cause drowsiness or dizziness. Use caution while driving or performing tasks requiring mental alertness. Avoid alcohol and other sedatives, hypnotics, tranquilizers, etc.

Elderly patients are more likely to experience dizziness, sedation, decreased coordination, mental confusion and fainting when they take antihistamines.

May produce unexpected excitation, restlessness, irritability and insomnia in rare instances. This is most likely in children and elderly patients.

Do not use for several days before allergy skin testing.

To avoid contamination, do not touch tip of the container to any surface. Replace cap after using.

Individual drug monographs are on the following pages.

LEVOCABASTINE HYDROCHLORIDE

Actions:

Pharmacology: Levocabastine is a potent, selective histamine H_1-receptor antagonist for topical ophthalmic use. Antigen challenge studies performed 2 and 4 hours after initial drug instillation indicated activity was maintained for at least 2 hours.

Pharmacokinetics: After instillation in the eye, levocabastine is systemically absorbed. However, the amount of systemically absorbed levocabastine after therapeutic ocular doses is low (mean plasma concentrations in the range of 1 to 2 ng/ml).

Clinical trials: Levocabastine instilled 4 times daily was significantly more effective than its vehicle in reducing ocular itching associated with seasonal allergic conjunctivitis.

Indications:

Allergic conjunctivitis: For the temporary relief of the signs and symptoms of seasonal allergic conjunctivitis.

Contraindications:

Hypersensitivity to any component of the product; while wearing soft contact lenses.

Warnings:

For ophthalmic use only: Not for injection.

Carcinogenesis/Mutagenesis/Fertility impairment: In female mice, levocabastine doses of 5000 and 21,500 times the maximum recommended ocular human use level resulted in an increased incidence of pituitary gland adenoma and mammary gland adenocarcinoma possibly produced by increased prolactin levels. The clinical relevance of this finding is unknown with regard to the interspecies differences in prolactin physiology and the very low plasma concentrations of levocabastine following ocular administration.

Pregnancy: Category C. Levocabastine is teratogenic (polydactyly) in rats when given in doses 16,500 times the maximum recommended human ocular dose. Teratogenicity (polydactyly, hydrocephaly, brachygnathia), embryotoxicity and maternal toxicity were observed in rats at 66,000 times the maximum recommended ocular human dose. There are no adequate and well controlled studies in pregnant women. Use during pregnancy only if the potential benefit justifies the potential risk to the fetus.

Lactation: Based on determinations of levocabastine in breast milk after ophthalmic administration of the drug to one nursing woman, it was calculated that the daily dose of levocabastine in the infant was about 0.5 mcg.

Children: Safety and efficacy in children < 12 years of age have not been established.

Adverse Reactions:

Mild, transient stinging and burning (15%); headache (5%); visual disturbances, dry mouth, fatigue, pharyngitis, eye pain/dryness, somnolence, red eyes, lacrimation/discharge, cough, nausea, rash/erythema, eyelid edema, dyspnea (1% to 3%).

Patient Information:

Shake well before using.

To prevent contaminating the dropper tip and suspension, take care not to touch the eyelid or surrounding area with the dropper tip of the bottle.

Keep bottle tightly closed when not in use. Do not use if the suspension has discolored. Store at controlled room temperature. Protect from freezing.

Administration and Dosage:

Shake well before using.

The usual dose is 1 drop instilled in the affected eye(s) 4 times daily. Treatment may be continued for up to 2 weeks.

Storage/Stability: Keep tightly closed when not in use. Do not use if the suspension has discolored. Store at controlled room temperature of 15° to 30°C (59° to 86°F). Protect from freezing.

Rx	**Livostin** (Ciba Vision)	**Ophthalmic suspension:** 0.05%	In 2.5, 5 and 10 ml dropper bottles.[1]

[1] With 0.15 mg benzalkonium chloride, propylene glycol, EDTA.

CROMOLYN SODIUM

Actions:

Pharmacology: In vitro and in vivo animal studies have shown that cromolyn inhibits the degranulation of sensitized mast cells that occurs after exposure to specific antigens. Cromolyn acts by inhibiting the release of histamine and other mediators from the mast cell.

Another activity demonstrated in vitro is the capacity of cromolyn to inhibit the degranulation of non-sensitized rat mast cells by phospholipase A and the subsequent release of chemical mediators. In another study, cromolyn did not inhibit the enzymatic activity of released phospholipase A on its specific substrate.

Cromolyn has no intrinsic vasoconstrictor, antihistaminic or anti-inflammatory activity.

Pharmacokinetics: Cromolyn is poorly absorbed. When multiple doses of cromolyn ophthalmic solution are instilled into normal rabbit eyes, < 0.07% of the dose is absorbed into the systemic circulation (presumably by way of the eye, nasal passages, buccal cavity and GI tract). Trace amounts (< 0.01%) of the dose penetrate into the aqueous humor, and clearance from this chamber is virtually complete within 24 hours after treatment is stopped.

In healthy volunteers, analysis of drug excretion indicates that approximately 0.03% of cromolyn is absorbed following administration to the eye.

Indications:

Conjunctivitis: Treatment of vernal keratoconjunctivitis, vernal conjunctivitis and vernal keratitis.

Contraindications:

Hypersensitivity to cromolyn or to any of the other ingredients.

Warnings:

Stinging/Burning: Patients may experience a transient stinging or burning sensation following instillation of cromolyn.

Duration/Frequency of therapy: The recommended frequency of administration should not be exceeded. Symptomatic response to therapy (decreased itching, tearing, redness and discharge) is usually evident within a few days, but longer treatment for up to 6 weeks is sometimes required. Once symptomatic improvement has been established, continue therapy for as long as needed to sustain improvement.

Contact lens use: As with all ophthalmic preparations containing benzalkonium chloride, users of soft (hydrophilic) contact lenses should refrain from wearing lenses while under treatment with cromolyn ophthalmic solution. Wear can be resumed within a few hours after discontinuation of the drug.

Concomitant therapy: If required, corticosteroids may be used concomitantly with cromolyn ophthalmic solution.

Pregnancy: Category B. In animals receiving parenteral cromolyn, adverse fetal effects (increased resorption and decreased fetal weight) were noted only at the very high parenteral doses that produced maternal toxicity. There are no adequate and well controlled studies in pregnant women. Use during pregnancy only if clearly needed.

Lactation: It is not known whether this drug is excreted in breast milk. Exercise caution when cromolyn is administered to a nursing woman.

Children: Safety and efficacy in children < 4 years of age have not been established.

Adverse Reactions:

The most frequently reported adverse reaction is transient ocular stinging or burning upon instillation. Other adverse reactions (infrequent) include: Conjunctival infection; wateriness; itchiness; dryness around the eye; puffiness; irritation; styes.

Patient Information:

Advise patients that the effect of cromolyn therapy is dependent on its administration at regular intervals, as directed.

Do not wear soft contact lenses while using cromolyn.

Administration and Dosage:

Instill 1 or 2 drops in each eye 4 to 6 times a day at regular intervals. One drop contains approximately 1.6 mg cromolyn sodium.

Rx	**Crolom** (Bausch & Lomb)	**Solution:** 4%	In 2.5 and 10 ml bottles with controlled drop tip.

LODOXAMIDE TROMETHAMINE

Actions:

Pharmacology: Lodoxamide is a mast cell stabilizer that inhibits, in vivo, the Type I immediate hypersensitivity reaction. Lodoxamide therapy inhibits the increases in cutaneous vascular permeability that are associated with reagin or IgE and antigen-mediated reactions. In vitro, lodoxamide stabilizes rodent mast cells and prevents release of mast cell inflammatory mediators and inhibits eosinophil chemotaxis. Although lodoxamide's precise mechanism of action is unknown, the drug may prevent calcium influx into mast cells upon antigen stimulation.

Lodoxamide has no intrinsic vasoconstrictor, antihistaminic, cyclooxygenase inhibition or other anti-inflammatory activity.

Pharmacokinetics: The disposition of lodoxamide was studied in six healthy adult volunteers receiving a 3 mg oral dose. Urinary excretion was the major route of elimination. The elimination half-life was 8.5 hours in urine. In a study in 12 healthy adult volunteers, topical administration of one drop in each eye 4 times per day for 10 days did not result in any measurable lodoxamide plasma levels at a detection limit of 2.5 ng/ml.

Indications:

Treatment of the ocular disorders referred to by the terms vernal keratoconjunctivitis, vernal conjunctivitis and vernal keratitis. *Off-labeled use:* Treatment of seasonal allergic conjunctivitis.

Contraindications:

Hypersensitivity to any component of this product.

Warnings:

For ophthalmic use only. Not for injection.

Contact lenses: As with all ophthalmic preparations containing benzalkonium chloride, instruct patients not to wear soft contact lenses during treatment with lodoxamide.

Pregnancy: Category B. There are no adequate and well controlled studies in pregnant women. Use during pregnancy only if clearly needed.

Lactation: It is not known whether lodoxamide is excreted in breast milk. Exercise caution when administering to a nursing woman.

Children: Safety and efficacy in children < 2 years of age have not been established.

Precautions:

Burning/Stinging: Patients may experience a transient burning or stinging upon instillation of lodoxamide. Should these symptoms persist, advise the patient to contact their physician.

Adverse Reactions:

Ophthalmic: Transient burning, stinging or discomfort upon instillation (≈ 15%); ocular itching/pruritus, blurred vision, dry eye, tearing/discharge, hyperemia, crystalline deposits, foreign body sensation (1% to 5%); corneal erosion/ulcer, scales on lid/lash, eye pain, ocular edema/swelling, ocular warming sensation, ocular fatigue, chemosis, corneal abrasion, anterior chamber cells, keratopathy/keratitis, blepharitis, allergy, sticky sensation, epitheliopathy (< 1%).

Systemic: Headache (1.5%); heat sensation, dizziness, somnolence, nausea, stomach discomfort, sneezing, dry nose, rash (< 1%).

Overdosage:

Overdose of an oral preparation of 120 to 180 mg resulted in a temporary sensation of warmth, profuse sweating, diarrhea, lightheadedness and a feeling of stomach distension; no permanent adverse effects were observed. Side effects reported following oral administration of 0.1 to 10 mg included a feeling of warmth or flushing, headache, dizziness, fatigue, sweating, nausea, loose stools and urinary frequency/urgency. Consider emesis in the event of accidental ingestion.

Administration and Dosage:

Adults and children > 2 years of age: Instill 1 to 2 drops in each affected eye 4 times daily for up to 3 months.

Rx	**Alomide** (Alcon)	**Solution:** 0.1%	In 10 ml Drop-Tainers.

OLOPATADINE HYDROCHLORIDE

Actions:

Pharmacology: Olopatadine is a relatively selective H_1-receptor antagonist that inhibits, in vivo and in vitro, the Type I immediate hypersensitivity reaction. It has no effect on alpha-adrenergic, dopamine, muscarinic type 1 and 2, and serotonin receptors.

Pharmacokinetics: Olopatadine was shown to have low systemic exposure in man following topical ocular administration. Olopatadine was evaluated in two studies of normal volunteers given 0.15% solution once every 12 hours for 2 weeks. The plasma concentrations were generally below 0.5 ng/ml. Higher concentrations were typically found within 2 hours of dosing and ranged from 0.5 to 1.3 ng/ml. Urinary excretion was the primary route of elimination. The half-life was approximately 3 hours. Approximately 60% to 70% of the parent drug was recovered in the urine, with monodesmethyl and N-oxide detected at low concentrations.

Olopatadine 0.1% was significantly more effective than its vehicle in preventing ocular itching associated with allergic conjunctivitis when challenged with an antigen initially and up to 8 hours after dosing.

Indications:

Allergic conjunctivitis: For the temporary prevention of itching of the eye.

Contraindications:

Hypersensitivity to any component of this product.

Warnings:

For topical ophthalmic use only. Not for injection.

Contact lenses: Instruct patients not to wear contact lenses during treatment with olopatadine.

Pregnancy: Category C. Rats treated at doses 93,750 times and rabbits treated at doses 62,500 times the maximum recommended ocular human use level showed a decrease in the number of live fetuses. There are not adequate and well controlled studies in pregnant women. Use during pregnancy only if the potential benefit justifies the potential risk to the fetus.

Lactation: Olopatadine has been identified in the milk of nursing rats following oral administration. It is not known whether topical ocular administration could result in sufficient systemic absorption to produce detectable quantitites in human breast milk. Exercise caution when administering to a nursing woman.

Children: Safety and effectiveness in pediatric patients less than 3 years of age has not been established.

Adverse Reactions:

Ophthalmic: Burning or stinging; dry eye; foreign body sensation; hyperemia; keratitis; lid edema; pruritis.

Systemic: Headache (7%); asthenia; cold syndrome; pharyngitis; rhinitis; sinusitis; taste perversion.

Patient Information:

To prevent contaminating the dropper tip and solution, take care not to touch the eyelids or surrounding areas with the dropper tip of the bottle.

Keep bottle tightly closed when not in use. Store at controlled room temperature 4° to 30°C (39° to 86°F) .

Administration and Dosage:

The recommended dose is 1 to 2 drops in each affected eye 2 times per day every 6 to 8 hours.

Rx	**Patanol** (Alcon)	**Ophthalmic Solution:** 0.1%[1]	In 5 ml Drop-Tainers.

[1] With 0.01% benzalkonium Cl.

OPHTHALMIC DECONGESTANT/ANTIHISTAMINE COMBINATIONS

In these combinations:

Phenylephrine HCl, naphazoline HCl and *tetrahydrozoline* have decongestant actions. See individual monographs for further information.

Hydroxypropyl methylcellulose and *polyvinyl alcohol* increase the viscosity of the solution, thereby increasing contact time.

Zinc sulfate is an astringent.

Pheniramine maleate and *antazoline* are antihistamines.

Indications:

Itching/Redness: Temporary relief of the minor eye symptoms of itching and redness caused by pollen, animal hair, etc.

Warnings:

Antihistamines: Topical antihistamines are potential sensitizers and may produce a local sensitivity reaction. Because they may produce angle closure, use with caution in persons with a narrow angle or a history of glaucoma.

Administration and Dosage:

Recommendations vary. Refer to manufacturer package insert for instructions.

		Decongestant	Antihistamine	
otc	**Naphazoline HCl & Pheniramine Maleate Solution** (Various, eg, Moore)	naphazoline HCl 0.025%	pheniramine maleate 0.3%	In 15 ml.
otc	**Naphazoline Plus Solution** (Parmed)			In 15 ml.[1]
otc	**Naphcon-A Solution** (Alcon)			In 15 ml Drop-Tainers.[1]
otc	**Opcon-A Solution** (Bausch & Lomb)	naphazoline HCl 0.027%	pheniramine maleate 0.315%	In 15 ml.[2]
otc	**Naphazoline HCl & Antazoline Phosphate Solution** (Various, eg, Moore, Schein, Steris)	naphazoline HCl 0.05%	antazoline phosphate 0.5%	In 5 and 15 ml.
otc	**Vasocon-A Solution** (Ciba Vision)			In 15 ml.[3]

[1] With 0.01% benzalkonium Cl, EDTA.
[2] With 0.5% hydroxypropyl methylcellulose, 0.01% benzalkonium Cl, 0.1% EDTA, boric acid.
[3] With 0.01% benzalkonium Cl, PEG-8000, polyvinyl alcohol, EDTA.

ODF

6

Anti-Inflammatory Agents

CORTICOSTEROIDS

Since their introduction into ocular therapy, corticosteroids have been useful in control of inflammatory and immunologic diseases of the eye. The anti-inflammatory effects of corticosteroids are nonspecific and they inhibit inflammation without regard to cause. In general, corticosteroids appear to be more effective in acute rather than chronic conditions. Degenerative diseases are usually completely refractory to corticosteroid therapy. Corticosteroids are generally not considered appropriate therapy for mild ocular allergies since other modalities can be effective (see the Antiallergy and Decongestant Agents chapter).

The beneficial effects of these agents on inflammation are numerous and include:

- Reduction in capillary permeability and cellular exudation;
- Inhibition of degranulation of mast cells, basophils and neutrophils. Stabilization of intracellular membranes of these cells inhibits release of hydrolytic enzyme and other mediators of inflammation such as histamines, bradykinins and platelet-activating factor;
- Suppression of lymphocyte proliferation;
- Inhibition of phospholipase A synthesis, resulting in decreased synthesis of prostaglandins and leukotrienes; and
- Inhibition of cell-mediated immune responses.

Clinical use and experimental data indicate that corticosteroids differ in their ability to suppress inflammation. This has been attributed, in part, to differences in their ability to penetrate the corneal epithelium. Acetate and alcohol formulations are sparingly soluble in water and are formulated for topical ocular use as suspensions. Phosphate derivatives are highly soluble in aqueous media and are formulated as solutions. The suspension formulations of acetate and alcohol derivatives exhibit biphasic solubility and can therefore better penetrate the lipid-rich layers of the cornea. It has also been suggested that corticosteroid particles in suspension persist in the cul-de-sac for longer periods of time and thus contact of the drug with the ocular surface is prolonged. For topical ocular use, prednisolone (eg, *AK-Pred*), fluorometholone (eg, *FML Liquifilm, Flarex*) and dexamethasone (eg, *Decadron Phosphate*) can be effective in inflammations involving the lids, conjunctiva, cornea, iris and ciliary body. In severe forms of anterior uveitis, topical therapy may require supplementation with periocular injection or systemic corticosteroids.

Chorioretinitis and optic neuritis are usually treated with systemic or periocular administration, or both. Medrysone (*HMS Liquifilm*), which appears to exhibit limited corneal penetration, is recommended for minor reactions involving the lids and conjunctiva. Its efficacy has not been demonstrated in iritis or uveitis.

More recently, a group of compounds with similar anti-inflammatory activity but less propensity to raise intraocular pressure have been synthesized. The first of this group to become available is rimexolone *(Vexol)*. It is presently indicated for treatment of anterior uveitis and for postoperative inflammation following cataract surgery.

The use of corticosteroids in ocular disease remains largely empirical, but some general guidelines include the following:

- Type and location of inflammation determine which route of administration is appropriate;
- Dosage is largely determined by clinical experience and should be reevaluated at frequent intervals during therapy;
- Therapy should be reduced gradually, not discontinued abruptly;
- The minimal effective dose should be used for the shortest time necessary;
- Individualize dosage; and
- Maintain close supervision to assess the effects of therapy on the disease course and possible adverse effects to the patient.

Patient compliance with the drug regimen is important in resolution of the inflammation. Patients should not discontinue use of medication at their own discretion. If suspensions are employed, the patient must shake the bottle sufficiently to maintain the proper concentration of drug.

Adverse effects can occur with all routes of administration and all preparations currently in use. Incidence of adverse effects appears to rise significantly as dosages are increased. Short-term topical ocular therapy usually does not produce significant ocular or systemic side effects.

NONSTEROIDAL ANTI-INFLAMMATORY AGENTS

Nonsteroidal anti-inflammatory drugs (NSAIDs), also referred to as the "aspirin-like" drugs, include the salicylates, as well as indole, pyrazolone and propionic acid derivatives and the fenamates. Following oral administration, these agents relieve discomfort associated with rheumatoid arthritis and lupus erythematosus, as well as reduce fever and alleviate pain that accompanies injury or inflammation.

The mechanism of action of the NSAIDs involves inhibition of cyclo-oxygenase, an enzyme important in synthesis of prostaglandins from their precursor, arachidonic acid. NSAIDs do not inhibit phospholipase A or the lipoxygenase enzyme, which generate the leukotrienes and related compounds that are also involved in the inflammatory response.

Prostaglandins are 20-carbon, unsaturated fatty acid derivatives which are subdivided into groups, designated by letters such as D, E and F. Evidence indicates that they also act as mediators of inflammation in ocular structures. Prostaglandins can cause vasodilation of ocular blood vessels, disrupt the blood-aqueous barrier, and induce neovascularization and miosis. Some of the prostaglandins such as $PGF_{2\alpha}$ and PGD_2 can lower intraocular pressure whereas others (eg, PGF_2) can raise it.

The topical ocular use of NSAIDs includes maintenance of pupillary dilation during surgery, control of inflammation after cataract extraction and following argon laser trabeculoplasty. Also, reactions associated with nonsurgically induced inflammatory disorders of the eye, such as allergic conjunctivitis and pain following RK or excimer laser procedures, respond to topical ocular application. At present, four topical ocular solution formulations are available: flurbiprofen (*Ocufen*), suprofen (*Profenal*), diclofenac (*Voltaren*) and ketorolac (*Acular*).

Siret D. Jaanus, PhD
State University of New York

For More Information

Bartlett JD, Jaanus SD, eds. Clinical Ocular Pharmacology, ed. 3. Boston: Butterworth-Heinemann, 1995.

Bito LZ. Prostaglandins. Old concepts and new perspectives. *Arch Ophthalmol* 1987;105:1036.

Bodor N. The application of soft drug approaches to the design of safer steroids. In: Christophers E, ed. Topical Corticosteroid Therapy. A novel approach to safer drugs. New York: Raven Press, 1988.

Flach AJ. Nonsteroidal anti-inflammatory drugs in ophthalmology. *Int Ophthalmol Clin* 1993;33:1.

Foster CS, et al. Efficacy and safety of rimexolone 1% ophthalmic suspension vs 1% prednisolone acetate in the treatment of uveitis. *Am J Ophthalmol* 1996;122:171–82.

Franzie JP, Leibowitz HM. Steroids. *Int Ophthalmol Clin* 1993;33:9.

Jampol LE. Non-steroidal anti-inflammatory drugs. In: Focal Points 1984: Clinical Modules for Ophthalmology. American Medical Association, 1984.

Leibowitz HM, Kupferman A. Anti-inflammatory medications. *Int Ophthalmol Clin* 1980;20:117.

Taravella MJ, Stulting RD, Mader TH, et al. Calcific band keratopathy associated with the use of topical steroid-phosphate preparations. *Arch Ophthalmol* 1994;112(5):608.

Urban RC, Cotlier E. Corticosteroid-induced cataracts. *Surv Ophthalmol* 1986;31:102.

CORTICOSTEROIDS, TOPICAL

Actions:

Pharmacology: Topical corticosteroids exert an anti-inflammatory action. Aspects of the inflammatory process such as hyperemia, cellular infiltration, vascularization and fibroblastic proliferation are suppressed. Steroids inhibit inflammatory response to inciting agents of mechanical, chemical or immunological nature. Topical corticosteroids are effective in acute inflammatory conditions of conjunctiva, sclera, cornea, lids, iris, ciliary body and anterior segment of the globe; and in ocular allergic conditions. They inhibit edema and capillary dilation. In ocular disease, route depends on site and extent of disorder.

The mechanism of the anti-inflammatory action is thought to be potentiation of epinephrine vasoconstriction, stabilization of lysosomal membranes, retardation of macrophage movement, prevention of kinin release, inhibition of lymphocyte and neutrophil function, inhibition of prostaglandin synthesis and, in prolonged use, decrease of antibody production.

Inhibiting fibroblastic proliferation may prevent symblepharon formation in chemical and thermal burns. Decreased scarring with clearer corneas after topical corticosteroids is a result of inhibiting fibroblast proliferation and vascularization.

Indications:

Inflammatory conditions: Treatment of steroid-responsive inflammatory conditions of the palpebral and bulbar conjunctiva, lid, cornea and anterior segment of the globe, such as: Allergic conjunctivitis; nonspecific superficial keratitis; superficial punctate keratitis; herpes zoster keratitis; iritis; cyclitis; and selected infective conjunctivitis when the inherent hazard of steroid use is accepted to obtain a diminution in edema and inflammation. Rimexolone is also indicated for postoperative inflammation following ocular surgery.

Corneal injury: Also used for corneal injury from chemical, radiation or thermal burns or penetration of foreign bodies.

Graft rejection: May be used to suppress graft rejection after keratoplasty.

Anterior uveitis.

Contraindications:

Acute superficial herpes simplex keratitis; fungal diseases of ocular structures; vaccinia, varicella and most other viral diseases of the cornea and conjunctiva; mycobacterial infection of the eye (eg, ocular tuberculosis); diseases caused by microorganisms; hypersensitivity; after uncomplicated removal of a superficial corneal foreign body.

Medrysone is not for use in iritis and uveitis; its efficacy has not been demonstrated.

Warnings:

Moderate to severe inflammation: Use higher strengths for moderate to severe inflammations. In difficult cases of anterior segment eye disease, systemic therapy may be required. When deeper ocular structures are involved, use systemic therapy.

Ocular damage: Prolonged use may result in glaucoma, elevated IOP, optic nerve damage, defects in visual acuity and fields of vision, posterior subcapsular cataract formation or secondary ocular infections from pathogens liberated from ocular tissues. Check IOP and lens frequently. In diseases causing thinning of cornea or sclera, perforation has occurred with topical steroids.

Mustard gas keratitis or Sjogren's keratoconjunctivitis: Topical steroids not effective.

Infections: Acute, purulent, untreated eye infection may be masked or activity enhanced by steroids. Fungal infections of the cornea have occurred with long-term local steroid applications. Therefore, suspect fungal invasion in any persistent corneal ulceration where a steroid has been, or is being used.

Stromal herpes simplex keratitis treatment with steroid medication requires great caution; frequent slit-lamp microscopy is mandatory.

Pregnancy: Category C. Use only when clearly needed and when potential benefits outweigh potential hazards.

Lactation: It is not known whether topical steroids are excreted in breast milk. Exercise caution when administering to a nursing mother.

Children: Safety and efficacy have not been established in children.

Precautions:

Sulfite sensitivity: Some of these products contain sulfites which may cause allergic-type reactions (eg, hives, itching, wheezing, anaphylaxis) in certain susceptible persons. Although the overall prevalence of sulfite sensitivity in the general population is low, it is seen more frequently in asthmatics or in atopic nonasthmatic persons. Specific products containing sulfites are identified in the product listings.

Adverse Reactions:

Glaucoma (elevated IOP) with optic nerve damage, loss of visual acuity and field defects; posterior subcapsular cataract formation; secondary ocular infection from pathogens, including herpes simplex liberated from ocular tissues; perforation of globe; exacerbation of viral and fungal corneal infections; transient stinging or burning; blurred vision; discharge; discomfort; ocular pain; foreign body sensation; hyperemia; pruritus (rimexolone). Rarely, filtering blebs have occurred with steroid use after cataract surgery.

Other ocular adverse reactions occurring in < 1% of patients included sticky sensation; increased fibrin; dry eye; conjunctival edema; corneal staining; keratitis; tearing; photophobia; edema; irritation; corneal ulcer; browache; lid margin crusting; corneal edema; infiltrate; corneal erosion.

Miscellaneous: Headache; aggravation or worsening of hypertension; rhinitis; pharyngitis; taste perversion.

Systemic: Systemic side effects may occur with extensive use.

Patient Information:

Medical supervision during therapy is recommended.

To avoid contamination, do not touch applicator tip to any surface. Replace cap after use.

If improvement in the condition being treated does not occur within several days, or if pain, itching or swelling of the eye occurs, notify the physician. Do not discontinue use without consulting physician. Take care not to discontinue prematurely.

Refer to the Dosage Forms and Routes of Administration chapter for more complete information on administration and use.

Administration and Dosage:

Treatment duration varies with type of lesion and may extend from a few days to several weeks, depending on therapeutic response. Relapse may occur if therapy is reduced too rapidly; taper over several days. Relapses, more common in chronic active lesions than in self-limited conditions, usually respond to retreatment.

Suspensions and solutions: Refer to specific product labeling, since dosage depends on product and indication.

Generally, instill 1 or 2 drops into the conjunctival sac every hour during the day and every 2 hours during the night. When a favorable response is observed, reduce dosage to 1 drop every 4 hours. Later, 1 drop 3 or 4 times daily may suffice to control symptoms. Shake suspension well before use. For postoperative inflammation, instill 1 to 2 drops 4 times daily beginning 24 hours after surgery; continue throughout the first 2 weeks of the postoperative period.

Ointments: Apply a thin coating (approximately 0.5 to 1 inch) in the lower conjunctival sac 3 or 4 times a day. When a favorable response is observed, reduce the number of daily applications to twice, and later to once a day as a maintenance dose if sufficient to control symptoms.

Ointments are particularly convenient when an eye pad is used and may be the preparation of choice when prolonged contact of drug with ocular tissues is needed.

For product information on Steroid/Antibiotic Combinations, see the Anti-infective Agents chapter.

Individual drug monographs are on the following pages.

DEXAMETHASONE

Complete prescribing information is found in the Corticosteroids group monograph.

Administration and Dosage:

Storage: Store upright at 8° to 27°C (46° to 80°F).

Rx	**Dexamethasone Sodium Phosphate** (Various, eg, Ciba Vision, Rugby, Steris)	**Solution**: 0.1% dexamethasone phosphate (as sodium phosphate)	In 5 ml.
Rx	**AK-Dex** (Akorn)		In 5 ml.[1]
Rx	**Decadron Phosphate** (Merck)		In 5 ml Ocumeters.[2]
Rx	**Dexamethasone** (Steris)	**Suspension**: 0.1% dexamethasone	In 5 ml.
Rx	**Maxidex** (Alcon)		In 5 and 15 ml Drop-Tainers.[3]
Rx	**Dexamethasone Sodium Phosphate** (Various, eg, Major, Zenith-Goldline)	**Ointment**: 0.05% dexamethasone phosphate (as sodium phosphate)	In 3.5 g.
Rx	**AK-Dex** (Akorn)		In 3.5 g.[4]
Rx	**Decadron Phosphate** (Merck)		In 3.5 g.[5]
Rx	**Maxidex** (Alcon)		In 3.5 g.[5]

[1] With 0.01% benzalkonium chloride, EDTA and hydroxyethylcellulose.
[2] With polysorbate 80, EDTA, 0.1% sodium bisulfite, 0.25% phenylethanol, 0.02% benzalkonium chloride.
[3] With 0.01% benzalkonium chloride, EDTA, 0.5% hydroxypropyl methylcellulose, polysorbate 80.
[4] With lanolin anhydrous, parabens, PEG-400, white petrolatum and mineral oil.
[5] With white petrolatum and mineral oil.

FLUOROMETHOLONE

Complete prescribing information is found in the Corticosteroids group monograph.

Administration and Dosage:

Storage: Store at or below 25°C (77°F); protect from freezing.

Rx	**Fluor-Op** (Ciba Vision)	**Suspension**: 0.1% fluorometholone alcohol	In 5, 10 and 15 ml.[1]
Rx	**FML** (Allergan)		In 1, 5, 10 and 15 ml.[1]
Rx	**Flarex** (Alcon)	**Suspension**: 0.1% fluorometholone acetate	In 2.5, 5 and 10 ml Drop-Tainers.[2]
Rx	**eFLone** (Ciba Vision)		In 5 and 10 ml.[2]
Rx	**FML Forte** (Allergan)	**Suspension**: 0.25% fluorometholone alcohol	In 2, 5, 10 and 15 ml.[3]
Rx	**FML S.O.P.** (Allergan)	**Ointment**: 0.1%	In 3.5 g.[4]

[1] With 0.004% benzalkonium chloride, EDTA, polysorbate 80 and 1.4% polyvinyl alcohol.
[2] With 0.01% benzalkonium chloride, EDTA, hydroxyethylcellulose and tyloxapol.
[3] With 0.005% benzalkonium chloride, EDTA, polysorbate 80 and 1.4% polyvinyl alcohol.
[4] With 0.0008% phenylmercuric acetate, white petrolatum, mineral oil, petrolatum and lanolin alcohol.

MEDRYSONE

Complete prescribing information is found in the Corticosteroids group monograph.

Administration and Dosage:

Storage: Protect from freezing.

Rx	**HMS** (Allergan)	**Suspension:** 1%	In 5 and 10 ml.[1]

[1] With 0.004% benzalkonium chloride, EDTA, 1.4% polyvinyl alcohol and hydroxypropyl methylcellulose.

PREDNISOLONE

Complete prescribing information is found in the Corticosteroids group monograph.

Administration and Dosage:

Storage: Protect from freezing.

Rx	**Pred Mild** (Allergan)	**Suspension:** 0.12% prednisolone acetate	In 5 and 10 ml.[1]
Rx	**Econopred** (Alcon)	**Suspension:** 0.125% prednisolone acetate	In 5 and 10 ml Drop-Tainers.[2]
Rx	**Prednisolone Sodium Phosphate** (Various, eg, Steris)	**Solution:** 0.125% prednisolone sodium phosphate	In 5 and 15 ml.
Rx	**AK-Pred** (Akorn)		In 5 ml.[3]
Rx	**Inflamase Mild** (Ciba Vision)		In 3, 5 and 10 ml.[4]
Rx	**Econopred Plus** (Alcon)	**Suspension:** 1% prednisolone acetate	In 5 and 10 ml Drop-Tainers.[2]
Rx	**Pred Forte** (Allergan)		In 1, 5, 10 and 15 ml.[1]
Rx	**Prednisolone Acetate Ophthalmic** (Falcon)		In 5 and 10 ml.[2]
Rx	**Prednisolone Sodium Phosphate** (Various, eg, Bausch & Lomb, Rugby)	**Solution:** 1% prednisolone sodium phosphate	In 5, 10 and 15 ml.
Rx	**AK-Pred** (Akorn)		In 5 and 15 ml.[3]
Rx	**Inflamase Forte** (Ciba Vision)		In 3, 5, 10 and 15 ml.[4]

[1] With benzalkonium chloride, EDTA, polysorbate 80, hydroxypropyl methylcellulose and sodium bisulfite.
[2] With 0.01% benzalkonium chloride, EDTA, polysorbate 80, hydroxypropyl methylcellulose and glycerin.
[3] With 0.01% benzalkonium chloride, EDTA, hydroxypropyl methylcellulose and sodium bisulfite.
[4] With 0.01% benzalkonium chloride and EDTA.

RIMEXOLONE

Complete prescribing information is found in the Corticosteroids group monograph.

Administration and Dosage:

Storage: Store upright between 4° and 30°C (40° and 86°F).

Rx	**Vexol** (Alcon)	**Suspension**: 1%	In 5 and 10 ml Drop-Tainers.[1]

[1] With 0.01% benzalkonium chloride, polysorbate 80 and EDTA in carbapol gel.

NONSTEROIDAL ANTI-INFLAMMATORY AGENTS (NSAIDS)

Actions:

Pharmacology: Flurbiprofen, suprofen, diclofenac and ketorolac are NSAIDs available as ophthalmic solutions. Flurbiprofen and suprofen are phenylalkanoic acids, diclofenac is a phenylacetic acid and ketoralac tromethamine is a member of the pyrrolo-pyrolle group; they have analgesic, antipyretic and anti-inflammatory activity. Their mechanism of action is believed to be through inhibition of the cyclo-oxygenase enzyme that is essential in the biosynthesis of prostaglandins.

In animals, certain prostaglandins are mediators of intraocular inflammation. Prostaglandins produce disruption of the blood-aqueous humor barrier, vasodilation, increased vascular permeability, leukocytosis and increased intraocular pressure (IOP).

Prostaglandins also appear to play a role in the miotic response produced during ocular surgery by constricting the iris sphincter independently of cholinergic mechanisms. NSAIDs inhibit the miosis induced during the course of cataract surgery.

Nonsteroidal Anti-Inflammatory Ophthalmic Agents

Ophthalmic NSAID	Trade name (manufacturer)	Solution concentration	Ophthalmic indication
Flurbiprofen	*Ocufen* (Allergan)	0.03%	Inhibition of intraoperative miosis
Suprofen	*Profenal* (Alcon)	1%	
Diclofenac	*Voltaren* (Ciba Vision)	0.1%	Treatment of postoperative inflammation following cataract extraction; photophobia following incisional surgery
Ketorolac	*Acular* (Allergan)	0.5%	Relief of ocular itching due to seasonal allergic conjunctivitis; treatment of postoperative inflammation following cataract extraction

Indications:

Flurbiprofen, suprofen: Inhibition of intraoperative miosis.

Diclofenac: Treatment of postoperative inflammation following cataract extraction; treatment of photophobia following incisional refractive surgery.

Ketorolac: Temporary relief of ocular itching due to seasonal allergic conjunctivitis; treatment of postoperative inflammation following cataract extraction.

Off-labeled uses:

Diclofenac: Anti-inflammatory treatment following argon laser trabeculoplasty, treatment of seasonal allergic conjunctivitis, pain associated with radial keratotomy and photorefractive keratectomy.

Flurbiprofen: Inflammation after cataract or glaucoma laser surgery and uveitis syndromes.

Ketorolac: Treatment of pain associated with corneal surgery or trauma; topical treatment of cystoid macular edema.

Suprofen: Topical treatment of contact lens-associated GPC.

Contraindications:

Hypersensitivity to the drugs or any component of the products.

Suprofen: Epithelial herpes simplex keratitis (dendritic keratitis).

Diclofenac, ketorolac: Patients wearing soft contact lenses (see Precautions).

Warnings:

Cross-sensitivity: The potential for cross-sensitivity to acetylsalicylic acid, phenylacetic acid derivatives and other NSAIDs exists. Therefore, use caution when treating individuals who have previously exhibited sensitivities to these drugs.

Bleeding tendencies: Systemic absorption occurs with drugs applied ocularly. With some NSAIDs, there exists the potential for increased bleeding time due to interference with thrombocyte aggregation. There have been reports that ocularly applied NSAIDs may cause increased bleeding of ocular tissues (including hyphemas) in conjunction with ocular surgery. Use with caution in surgical patients with known bleeding tendencies or in patients taking drugs known to cause bleeding (eg, anticoagulants).

Pregnancy: Category C (flurbiprofen, ketorolac, suprofen); Category B (diclofenac). Flurbiprofen is embryocidal, delays parturition, prolongs gestation, reduces weight and slightly retards fetal growth in rats at daily oral doses of ≥ 0.4 mg/kg (approximately 185 times the human daily topical dose).

Oral doses of ketorolac at 1.5 mg/kg (8.8 mg/m^2), which was half of the human oral exposure, administered after gestation day 17 caused dystocia and higher pup mortality in rats. Because of the known effects of prostaglandin-inhibiting drugs on the fetal cardiovascular system, avoid the use of ketorolac during late pregnancy.

Oral doses of suprofen of up to 200 mg/kg/day in animals resulted in an increased incidence of fetal resorption associated with maternal toxicity. There was an increase in stillbirths and a decrease in postnatal survival in pregnant rats treated with ≥ 2.5 mg/kg/day.

Oral diclofenac in mice and rats crosses the placental barrier. In rats, maternally toxic doses were associated with dystocia, prolonged gestation and reduced fetal weights, growth and survival. Because of the known effects of prostaglandin-inhibiting drugs on the fetal cardiovascular system, avoid the use of ophthalmic diclofenac during late pregnancy.

There are no adequate and well controlled studies in pregnant women. Use during pregnancy only if the potential benefits outweigh the potential hazards to the fetus.

Lactation: It is not known whether flurbiprofen is excreted in breast milk. Because of the potential for serious adverse reactions in nursing infants, decide whether to discontinue nursing or to discontinue the drug, taking into account the importance of the drug to the mother.

Suprofen is excreted in breast milk after a single oral dose. Based on measurements of plasma and milk levels in women taking oral suprofen, the milk concentration is about 1% of the plasma level. Because systemic absorption may occur from topical ocular administration, consider discontinuing nursing while on suprofen; its safety in human neonates has not been established.

Exercise caution while ketorolac is administered to a nursing woman.

Children: Safety and efficacy for use in children have not been established.

Precautions:

Wound healing may be delayed with the use of flurbiprofen and diclofenac.

Contact lenses: Patients wearing hydrogel soft contact lenses who have used diclofenac concurrently have experienced ocular irritation manifested by redness and burning.

Ketorolac – Do not administer while patient is wearing contact lenses.

Drug Interactions:

Acetylcholine chloride and carbachol: Although clinical and animal studies revealed no interference, and there is no known pharmacological basis for an interaction, both of these drugs have reportedly been ineffective when used in patients treated with flurbiprofen or suprofen.

Adverse Reactions:

Most frequent: Transient burning and stinging upon instillation (diclofenac 15%, ketorolac ≈ 40%); other minor symptoms of ocular irritation.

Suprofen: Discomfort; itching; redness; allergy, iritis, pain, chemosis, photophobia, irritation, punctate epithelial staining (< 0.5%).

Diclofenac: Keratitis (28%, although most cases occurred in cataract studies prior to drug therapy); elevated IOP (15%, although most cases occurred post-surgery and prior to drug therapy); dry eye complaints (12% in patients undergoing incisional refractive surgery); discharge; corneal deposits; corneal lesions; itching; irritation; blurred vision; fever; pain; insomnia. The following reactions occurred in ≤ 1%: Corneal edema; corneal opacity; eyelid disorder; iritis; injection and lacrimation disorder; asthenia; chills; facial edema; vomiting; viral infection; anterior chamber reaction; ocular allergy; nausea.

Ketorolac: Ocular irritation, allergic reactions; superficial keratitis; superficial ocular infections. The following adverse reactions occurred rarely: Eye dryness; corneal infiltrates; corneal ulcer; visual disturbance (blurred vision).

Overdosage:

Overdosage will not ordinarily cause acute problems. If accidentally ingested, drink fluids to dilute.

Individual drug monographs are on the following pages.

DICLOFENAC SODIUM

Complete prescribing information is found in the NSAIDs group monograph.

Administration and Dosage:

Cataract surgery: Instill 1 drop in the affected eye 4 times daily, beginning 24 hours after cataract surgery and continuing throughout the first 2 weeks of the postoperative period.

Incisional refractive surgery: Within 1 hour prior to incisional refractive surgery, instill 1 drop to the operative eye(s). Instill a second drop within 15 minutes after surgery. Instill 1 drop to the operative eye(s) 4 times daily beginning 4 to 6 hours after surgery and continuing for up to 3 days as needed.

Storage: Store between 15° to 30°C (59° to 86°F). Protect from light.

Rx	**Voltaren** (Ciba Vision)	**Solution:** 0.1%	In 2.5 and 5 ml dropper bottles.[1]

[1] With 1 mg/ml EDTA, boric acid, polyoxyl 35 castor oil, 2 mg/ml sorbic acid and tromethamine.

FLURBIPROFEN SODIUM

Complete prescribing information is found in the NSAIDs group monograph.

Administration and Dosage:

Instill 1 drop approximately every 30 minutes, beginning 2 hours before surgery (total of 4 drops).

Storage: Store at room temperature.

Rx	**Ocufen** (Allergan)	**Solution:** 0.03%	In 2.5, 5 and 10 ml dropper bottles.[1]
Rx	**Flurbiprofen Sodium Ophthalmic** (Various, eg, Bausch & Lomb)		In 2.5 ml.[1]

[1] With 1.4% polyvinyl alcohol, 0.005% thimerosal and EDTA.

KETOROLAC TROMETHAMINE

Complete prescribing information is found in the NSAIDs group monograph.

Administration and Dosage:

Relief of ocular itching: Instill 1 drop (0.25 mg) 4 times a day.

Postoperative inflammation: Instill 1 drop (0.25 mg) in the affected eye(s) 4 times daily beginning 24 hours after cataract surgery and continuing through the first 2 weeks of the postoperative period.

Storage: Store at controlled room temperature 15°to 30°C (59° to 86°F). Protect from light.

Rx	**Acular** (Allergan)	**Solution:** 0.5%	In 5 ml dropper bottles.[1]

[1] With 0.01% benzalkonium Cl, 0.1% EDTA and octoxynol 40.

SUPROFEN

Complete prescribing information is found in the NSAIDs group monograph.

Administration and Dosage:

On the day of surgery, instill 2 drops into the conjunctival sac at 3, 2 and 1 hour prior to surgery. Two drops may be instilled into the conjunctival sac every 4 hours, while awake, the day preceding surgery.

Storage: Store at room temperature.

Rx	**Profenal** (Alcon)	**Solution:** 1%	In 2.5 ml Drop-Tainers.[1]

[1] With 0.005% thimerosal, 2% caffeine and EDTA.

ODF

7

Artificial Tear Solutions And Ocular Lubricants

Availability of synthetic polymers suitable for ocular use has resulted in development of artificial tear solutions, ointments and other formulations to help alleviate ocular discomfort and maintain integrity of the surface epithelium. Ideally, formulations for dry eyes should be compatible with and substitute for components of the tear film, including lipid, aqueous and mucin layers.

SOLUTIONS

Lubricant preparations formulated as artificial tear solutions usually contain inorganic electrolytes, preservatives and water-soluble polymeric systems. Sodium chloride (NaCl), potassium chloride (KCl), various other ions and boric acid help maintain tonicity and pH of the formulations. Preservatives, including benzalkonium chloride, chlorobutanol, thimerosal, EDTA, methylparaben and propylparaben, are included in multi-dose preparations to prevent bacterial contamination. Methylcellulose and its derivatives, polyvinyl alcohol (PVA), povidone (PVP), dextran and propylene glycol can enhance viscosity and promote tear film stability. A more recent advance in artificial tear formulations is the introduction of preservative-free preparations. These formulations can prevent adverse ocular surface effects in patients who use artificial tears frequently or for prolonged periods of time.

In addition to polymers, lipids and vitamins have also been incorporated into ocular lubricants. One formulation, *TearGard*, contains a phospholipid derivative in an aqueous solution of hydroxyethyl cellulose and inorganic buffer. Although it has been suggested that this product can replace all layers of the tear film, these claims remain unsubstantiated due to lack of controlled clinical trials. Retinyl, the alcohol form of vitamin A, is available as a solution for topical use on the eye. The formulation *Viva-Drops* contains vitamin A, polysorbate 80 and EDTA. *Dakrina* contains retinyl palmitate form of vitamin A. Definitive data on the benefits of vitamin-containing formulations in dry eye disorders are not available and large-scale, well controlled masked studies are lacking regarding efficacy of vitamin A or its derivatives in patients with ocular surface disease.

Artificial tear solutions should be administered at dosage frequencies of 4 to 6 hours. However, depending on the severity of the clinical signs and symptoms, they may be used as often as hourly or only occasionally. It is highly recommended that the prescriber of the artificial tear product recommend a specific dosage schedule for the patient, particularly at the start of therapy.

OINTMENTS

Petrolatum, lanolin and mineral oil ointments are the second most frequent approach for ocular lubrication. When placed on the eye, they dissolve at the temperature of the ocular tissue and disperse with the tear fluid. A major advantage is that ointments appear to be retained in the cul-de-sac longer than artificial tear solutions.

Ointments are usually applied directly to the inferior conjunctival sac as a 0.25 to 0.5 inch ribbon. An alternative method is to place the ointment on a cotton-tipped applicator and apply it to the lid margins and lashes. Both blurring of vision and possible irritation are minimized with this method of instillation. Recently, manufacturers have begun to formulate preservative-free ointment preparations. These preparations are less toxic and less allergenic than those containing preservatives.

Ophthalmic lubricant ointments are generally preferred for bedtime use. Depending on the clinical signs and patient symptoms, they may also be used as often as necessary during the day. Since ointments may block access of solution to the ocular surface, solutions should be instilled prior to ointment application.

SOLID DEVICES

Another approach to relief of dry eye symptoms is use of a preservative-free, water-soluble, polymeric insert (*Lacrisert*). The cylindrical rod, which contains 5 mg hydroxypropylcellulose, is placed in the lower cul-de-sac. It then imbibes fluid and swells. As it dissolves, the polymer is released to the ocular surface for 12 to 24 hours.

The device can be beneficial in dry eye syndromes such as keratitis sicca. It is comfortable and well accepted, but some disadvantages are associated with its use. Manual dexterity is required for placement in the cul-de-sac, and the cost to the patient is considerably greater than use of solutions and ointments. A common patient complaint is blurred vision as the rod dissolves, causing the tear film to thicken. Adding fluid drops (eg, isotonic saline) can reduce viscosity and minimize visual complaints.

PUNCTAL PLUGS

Mechanical occlusion of the lacrimal puncta has become an accepted method to block tear drainage and thereby prolong action of natural tears as well as artificial tear preparations. Several types of punctal plugs are currently used including a silicone-based plug and a temporary absorbable collagen implant.

The Freeman Punctal Plug is usually inserted directly into the inferior puncta. The procedure may require topical anesthesia and punctal dilation prior to placement.

The Temporary Punctal/Canalicular Collagen Implant consists of collagen inserts packaged at the edge of a foam strip. The implants are placed halfway into the punctal opening and advanced into the horizontal canaliculus with the aid of a jeweler's forceps and magnification. The procedure can be done with or without an anesthetic. Following placement, the implant swells, impeding tear flow up to 14 days before the implants are totally absorbed.

Punctal occlusion can benefit patients whose symptoms are not relieved by topical therapy alone. Although rare, punctal occlusion can lead to epiphora.

Siret D. Jaanus, PhD
State University of New York

For More Information

Bartlett JD, Jaanus SD, eds. Clinical Ocular Pharmacology, ed. 3. Boston: Butterworth-Heinnemann, 1995.

Bernal DL, Ubels JL. Quantitative evaluation of the corneal epithelial barrier: Effect of artificial tears and preservatives. *Curr Eye Res* 1991;10:645.

Holly FJ. Tear film physiology. *Int Ophthalmol Clin* 1987;27:2.

Lemp MA. Recent developments in dry eye management. *Surv Ophthalmol* 1987;94:1299.

Marquardt R. Therapy of the dry eye. In: Lemp MA, Marquardt R, eds. The Dry Eye. Berlin: Springer-Verlag, 1992, chapter 6.

Norn MS, Opauszki A. Effects of ophthalmic vehicles on the stability of the precorneal tear film. *Acta Ophthalmol* 1977;55:23.

Tuberville AW, et al. Punctal occlusion in tear deficiency syndromes. *Ophthalmology* 1982;89:1170.

Werblin TP, et al. The use of slow-release artificial tears in the long-term management of keratitis sicca. *Ophthalmology* 1981;88:78.

ARTIFICIAL TEAR SOLUTIONS

Actions:

Pharmacology: These products contain: Balanced amounts of salts to maintain ocular tonicity (0.9% NaCl equivalent); buffers to adjust pH; viscosity agents to prolong eye contact time; preservatives for sterility. See the Dosage Forms and Routes of Administration chapter for a description and listing of these ingredients.

Indications:

Ophthalmic lubricants: These products offer tear-like lubrication for the relief of dry eyes and eye irritation associated with deficient tear production, and exposure to wind, sun or other irritants. Also used as ocular lubricants for artificial eyes.

Contraindications:

Hypersensitivity to any component of the product.

Patient Information:

Do not touch the tip of the container or dropper to any surface. Close container immediately after use.

If headache, eye pain, vision changes, continued redness or irritation occurs, or if condition worsens or persists for > 3 days, discontinue use and consult a physician.

May cause mild stinging or temporary blurred vision.

Some of these products should not be used with soft contact lenses.

Administration and Dosage:

Instill 1 to 2 drops into eye(s) 3 or 4 times daily, as needed.

otc	**Adsorbotear** (Alcon)	**Solution:** 0.4% hydroxyethylcellulose, 1.67% povidone, water soluble polymers, 0.004% thimerosal, 0.1% EDTA	In 15 ml.
otc	**Akwa Tears** (Akorn)	**Solution:** 0.01% benzalkonium Cl, 1.4% polyvinyl alcohol, sodium phosphate, EDTA, NaCl	In 15 ml.
otc	**AquaSite** (Ciba Vision)	**Solution:** 0.2% PEG-400, 0.1% dextran 70, polycarbophil, NaCl, EDTA, sodium hydroxide	Preservative free. In 0.6 ml (single-use 24s) and 15 ml.
otc	**Artificial Tears** (Various, eg, Parmed, Rugby, Schein)	**Solution:** 0.01% benzalkonium chloride. May also contain EDTA, NaCl, polyvinyl alcohol, hydroxypropyl methylcellulose	In 15 and 30 ml.
otc	**Artificial Tears Plus** (Various, eg, Rugby, Steris)	**Solution:** 1.4% polyvinyl alcohol, 0.6% povidone, 0.5% chlorobutanol, NaCl	In 15 ml.

otc	**Bion Tears** (Alcon)	**Solution:** 0.1% dextran 70, 0.3% hydroxypropyl methylcellulose 2910, NaCl, KCl, sodium bicarbonate	Preservative free. In single-use 0.45 ml containers (28s).
otc	**Celluvisc** (Allergan)	**Solution:** 1% carboxymethylcellulose, NaCl, KCl, sodium lactate	Preservative free. In 0.3 ml (UD 30s).
otc	**Comfort Tears** (PBH Wesley Jessen)	**Solution:** Hydroxyethylcellulose, 0.005% benzalkonium chloride, 0.02% EDTA	In 15 ml.
otc	**Dakrina** (Dakryon)	**Solution:** Povidone, polyvinyl alcohol, antioxidant retinyl palmitate, boric acid, 0.09% EDTA, 0.001% WSCP, NaCl, KCl	In 15 ml.
otc	**Dry Eyes** (Bausch & Lomb)	**Solution:** 1.4% polyvinyl alcohol, 0.01% benzalkonium chloride, sodium phosphate, EDTA, NaCl	In 15 ml.
otc	**Dry Eye Therapy** (Bausch & Lomb)	**Solution:** 0.3% glycerin, NaCl, KCl, sodium citrate, sodium phosphate	Preservative free. In 0.3 ml (UD 32s).
otc	**Dwelle** (Dakryon)	**Solution:** 0.09% EDTA, NaCl, KCl, boric acid, povidone, 0.001% NPX	In 15 ml.
otc	**Eye-Lube-A** (Optopics)	**Solution:** 0.25% glycerin, EDTA, sodium chloride, benzalkonium Cl	In 15 ml.
otc	**Gen Teal** (Ciba Vision)	**Solution:** Hydroxypropyl methylcellulose, boric acid, NaCl, KCl, phosphoric acid. **Preservative:** Sodium perborate	In 15 ml.
otc	**HypoTears** (Ciba Vision)	**Solution:** 1% polyvinyl alcohol, PEG-400, 1% dextrose, 0.01% benzalkonium Cl, EDTA	In 15 and 30 ml.
otc	**HypoTears PF** (Ciba Vision)	**Solution:** 1% polyvinyl alcohol, PEG-400, 1% dextrose, EDTA	Preservative free. In 0.6 ml (30s).
otc	**Isopto Plain** (Alcon)	**Solution:** 0.5% hydroxypropyl methylcellulose 2910, 0.01% benzalkonium chloride, NaCl, sodium phosphate, sodium citrate	In 15 ml Drop-Tainers.
otc	**Isopto Tears** (Alcon)		In 15 and 30 ml.
otc	**Just Tears** (Blairex)	**Solution:** Benzalkonium chloride, EDTA, 1.4% polyvinyl alcohol, NaCl, KCl	In 15 ml.
otc	**Liquifilm Tears** (Allergan)	**Solution:** 1.4% polyvinyl alcohol, 0.5% chlorobutanol, NaCl	In 15 and 30 ml.
otc	**LubriTears** (Bausch & Lomb)	**Solution:** 0.3% hydroxypropyl methylcellulose 2906, 0.1% dextran 70, EDTA, KCl, NaCl, 0.01% benzalkonium chloride	In 15 ml.
otc	**Moisture Drops** (Bausch & Lomb)	**Solution:** 0.5% hydroxypropyl methylcellulose, 0.1% povidone, 0.2% glycerin, 0.01% benzalkonium chloride, EDTA, NaCl, boric acid, KCl, sodium borate	In 15 and 30 ml.
otc	**Murine** (Ross)	**Solution:** 0.5% polyvinyl alcohol, 0.6% povidone, benzalkonium chloride, dextrose, EDTA, NaCl, sodium bicarbonate, sodium phosphate	In 15 and 30 ml.
otc	**Murocel** (Bausch & Lomb)	**Solution:** 1% methylcellulose, propylene glycol, NaCl, 0.046% methylparaben, 0.02% propylparaben, boric acid, sodium borate	In 15 ml.

otc	**Nature's Tears** (Rugby)	**Solution:** 0.4% hydroxypropyl methylcellulose 2910, KCl, NaCl, sodium phosphate, 0.01% benzalkonium Cl, EDTA	In 15 ml.
otc	**Nu-Tears** (Optopics)	**Solution:** 1.4% polyvinyl alcohol, EDTA, sodium chloride, benzalkonium chloride, KCl	In 15 ml.
otc	**Nu-Tears** II (Optopics)	**Solution:** 1% polyvinyl alcohol, 1% PEG-400, EDTA, benzalkonium chloride	In 15 ml.
otc	**OcuCoat** (Storz Ophthalmics)	**Solution:** 0.1% dextran 70, 0.8% hydroxypropyl methylcellulose, sodium phosphate, KCl, NaCl, 0.01% benzalkonium chloride, dextrose	In 15 ml.
otc	**OcuCoat PF** (Storz Ophthalmics)	**Solution:** 0.1% dextran 70, 0.8% hydroxypropyl methylcellulose, sodium phosphate, KCl, NaCl, dextrose	Preservative free. In 0.5 ml single-dose containers (28s).
otc	**Puralube Tears** (Fougera)	**Solution:** 1% polyvinyl alcohol, 1% PEG 400, EDTA, benzalkonium chloride	In 15 ml.
otc	**Refresh** (Allergan)	**Solution:** 1.4% polyvinyl alcohol, 0.6% povidone, NaCl	Preservative free. In 0.3 ml (UD 30s, 50s).
otc	**Refresh Plus** (Allergan)	**Solution:** 0.5% carboxymethylcellulose sodium, KCl, NaCl	Preservative free. In 0.3 ml single-use containers (30s and 50s).
otc	**Tear Drop** (Parmed)	**Solution:** Polyvinyl alcohol, NaCl, EDTA, 0.01% benzalkonium Cl	In 15 ml.
otc	**TearGard** (Lee)	**Solution:** 0.25% sorbic acid, 0.1% EDTA, hydroxyethylcellulose	Thimerosal free. In 15 ml.
otc	**Teargen** (Zenith-Goldline)	**Solution:** 0.01% benzalkonium Cl, EDTA, NaCl, polyvinyl alcohol	In 15 ml.
otc	**Tearisol** (Ciba Vision)	**Solution:** 0.5% hydroxypropyl methylcellulose, 0.01% benzalkonium chloride, EDTA, boric acid, KCl	In 15 ml.
otc	**Tears Naturale** (Alcon)	**Solution:** 0.1% dextran 70, 0.01% benzalkonium chloride, 0.3% hydroxypropyl methylcellulose, NaCl, EDTA, hydrochloric acid, sodium hydroxide, KCl	In 15 and 30 ml.
otc	**Tears Naturale** II (Alcon)	**Solution:** 0.1% dextran 70, 0.3% hydroxypropyl methylcellulose 2910, 0.001% polyquaternium-1, NaCl, KCl, sodium borate	In 15 and 30 ml Drop-Tainers.
otc	**Tears Naturale Free** (Alcon)	**Solution:** 0.3% hydroxypropyl methylcellulose 2910, 0.1% dextran 70, NaCl, KCl, sodium borate	Preservative free. In 0.6 ml single-use containers.
otc	**Tears Plus** (Allergan)	**Solution:** 1.4% polyvinyl alcohol, NaCl, 0.6% povidone, 0.5% chlorobutanol	In 15 and 30 ml.
otc	**Tears Renewed** (Akorn)	**Solution:** 0.01% benzalkonium chloride, EDTA, 0.1% dextran 70, NaCl, 0.3% hydroxypropyl methylcellulose 2906	In 2, 15 and 30 ml.
otc	**Thera Tears** (Advanced Vision)	**Solution:** 0.25% sodium carboxymethylcellulose, NaCl, KCl, sodium phosphate	Preservative free. In 0.6 ml single-use containers.

otc	**Ultra Tears** (Alcon)	**Solution:** 15 hydroxypropyl methylcellulose 2910, 0.01% benzalkonium chloride, NaCl	In 15 ml.
otc	**Viva-Drops** (Vision Pharm)	**Solution:** Polysorbate 80, sodium chloride, EDTA, retinyl palmitate, mannitol, sodium citrate, pyruvate	Preservative free. In 10 and 15 ml.

OCULAR LUBRICANTS

Actions:

Pharmacology: These products serve as lubricants and emollients.

Indications:

Ophthalmic lubrication: Protection and lubrication of the eye.

Contraindications:

Hypersensitivity to any component of the products.

Patient Information:

Do not touch tube tip to any surface since this may contaminate the product.

Do not use with contact lenses.

If eye pain, vision changes or continued redness or irritation occurs, or if the condition worsens or persists for > 72 hours, discontinue use and contact a physician.

Refer to the Dosage Forms and Routes of Administration for more complete information.

Administration and Dosage:

Pull down the lower lid of affected eye(s) and apply a small amount (0.25 inch) of ointment to the inside of the eyelid.

Storage: Store at room temperature 15° to 30°C (59° to 86°F). Store away from heat.

otc	**Akwa Tears** (Akorn)	**Ointment:** White petrolatum, mineral oil, lanolin	Preservative free. In 3.5 g.
otc	**Dry Eyes** (Bausch & Lomb)		Preservative free. In 3.5 g.
otc	**Artificial Tears** (Rugby)	**Ointment:** White petrolatum, anhydrous liquid lanolin, mineral oil	In 3.5 g.
otc	**Duratears Naturale** (Alcon)		Preservative free. In 3.5 g.
otc	**LubriTears** (Bausch & Lomb)	**Ointment:** White petrolatum, mineral oil, lanolin, 0.5% chlorobutanol	In 3.5 g.

otc	**HypoTears** (Ciba Vision)	**Ointment:** White petrolatum, light mineral oil	Preservative and lanolin free. In 3.5 g.
otc	**Puralube** (Fougera)		In 3.5 g.
otc	**Tears Renewed** (Akorn)		Preservative and lanolin free. In 3.5 g.
otc	**Stye** (Del Pharm)	**Ointment:** 55% white petrolatum, 32% mineral oil, boric acid, stearic acid, wheat germ oil	In 3.5 g.
otc	**Lacri-Lube NP** (Allergan)	**Ointment:** 55.5% white petrolatum, 42.5% mineral oil, 2% petrolatum/lanolin alcohol	Preservative free. In 0.7 g (UD 24s).
otc	**Lacri-Lube S.O.P.** (Allergan)	**Ointment:** 56.8% white petrolatum, 42.5% mineral oil, chlorobutanol, lanolin alcohols	In 3.5 and 7 g.
otc	**Refresh PM** (Allergan)	**Ointment:** 56.8% white petrolatum, 41.5% mineral oil, lanolin alcohols, sodium chloride	Preservative free. In 3.5 g.

ARTIFICIAL TEAR INSERT

Actions:

Pharmacology: The hydroxypropyl cellulose insert acts to stabilize and thicken the precorneal tear film and prolong tear film breakup time, which is usually accelerated in patients with dry eye states. The insert also acts to lubricate and protect the eye.

Signs and symptoms resulting from moderate to severe dry eye syndromes, such as conjunctival hyperemia, corneal and conjunctival staining with rose bengal, exudation, itching, burning, foreign body sensation, smarting, photophobia, dryness and blurred or cloudy vision are reduced. Progressive visual deterioration may be retarded, halted or sometimes reversed.

Pharmacokinetics: Hydroxypropyl cellulose is a physiologically inert substance. Dissolution studies in rabbits showed that the inserts became softer within 1 hour after they were placed in the conjunctival sac. Most dissolved completely in 14 to 18 hours; with a single exception, all had disappeared by 24 hours after insertion. Similar dissolution of inserts was observed during prolonged use (up to 54 weeks).

Clinical trials: In a multicenter crossover study, the 5 mg insert administered into the inferior cul-de-sac once a day during the waking hours was compared with artificial tears used ≥ 4 times daily. There was a prolongation of tear film breakup time and a decrease in foreign body sensation associated with dry eye syndrome in patients during treatment with inserts as compared to artificial tears. Improvement was greater in most patients who used the inserts.

Indications:

Dry eye syndromes, moderate to severe: Keratoconjunctivitis sicca (especially in patients who remain symptomatic after an adequate trial of artificial tear solutions); exposure keratitis; decreased corneal sensitivity; recurrent corneal erosions.

Contraindications:

Hypersensitivity to hydroxypropyl cellulose.

Adverse Reactions:

The following have occurred, but in most instances were mild and transient: Transient blurring of vision; ocular discomfort or irritation; matting or stickiness of eyelashes; photophobia; hypersensitivity; edema of the eyelids; hyperemia.

Patient Information:

May produce transient blurring of vision; exercise caution while operating hazardous machinery or driving a motor vehicle.

If improperly placed in the inferior cul-de-sac, corneal abrasion may result. Patient should practice insertion and removal in physician's office until proficiency is achieved.

Illustrated instructions are included in each package.

If symptoms worsen, remove insert and notify physician.

Administration and Dosage:

Once daily, inserted into inferior cul-de-sac beneath the base of the tarsus, not in apposition to the cornea nor beneath the eyelid at the level of the tarsal plate. Individual patients may require twice-daily use for optimal results.

If not properly positioned, the insert will be expelled into the interpalpebral fissure, and may cause symptoms of a foreign body.

Occasionally, the insert is inadvertently expelled from the eye, especially in patients with shallow conjunctival fornices. Caution the patient against rubbing the eye(s), especially upon awakening, so as not to dislodge or expel the insert. If required, another insert may be used. If transient blurred vision develops, the patient may want to remove the insert a few hours after insertion to avoid this.

Rx	**Lacrisert** (Merck)	**Insert:** 5 mg hydroxpropyl cellulose	Preservative free. In 60s with applicator.

PUNCTAL PLUGS

Actions:

Pharmacology: These flexible silicone plugs partially block the puncta and horizontal canaliculus and eliminate tear loss by this route.

Indications:

Keratitis sicca (dry eye): Treatment of symptoms of dry eye (eg, redness, burning, reflex tearing, itching, foreign body sensation); after eye surgery to prevent complications due to dry eye; to enhance the efficacy of ocular medications; for patients experiencing dry eye-related contact lens problems.

Contraindications:

Hypersensitivity to silicone; eye infection.

Precautions:

Injection path: If injecting an anesthetic agent in the region of the canaliculus, maintain approximately a 5 mm distance between the injection path and the angular vessels.

Dilation: Do not dilate punctal opening > 1.2 mm.

Irritation: If irritation caused by plug insertion persists longer than several days, reexamine the patient and consider plug removal.

Patient Information:

Do not press fingers on or near the eyelid. Use a cotton-tipped swab to remove "sleep" from the corner of eyes.

Do not attempt to replace a plug that has fallen out.

Relief may not occur immediately after insertion; some discomfort and tearing may occur for a few days.

Administration and Dosage:

Plugs must be inserted by a physician or doctor of optometry.

Rx	**Herrick Lacrimal Plug** (Lacrimedics)	**Plug**: Silicone plug	In 0.3 and 0.5 mm sizes (packs of 2 plugs).
Rx	**Punctum Plug** (Eagle Vision, Ciba Vision)		In 0.5, 0.6, 0.7 and 0.8 mm sizes (packs of 2 plugs). Contains one inserter tool.
Rx	**Punctum Plug** (FCI Ophthalmics)		In 0.4, 0.7, 0.8 and 1.0 mm sizes (packs of 2 plugs).

COLLAGEN IMPLANTS

Actions:

Pharmacology: These absorbable implants partially block the puncta and horizontal canaliculus, eliminating tear loss by this route.

Indications:

Dry eyes: For the relief of dry eyes and secondary abnormalities such as conjunctivitis, corneal ulcer, pterygium, blepharitis, keratitis, red lid margins, recurrent chalazion, recurrent corneal erosion, filamentary keratitis and other noninfectious external eye diseases; to enhance the effect of ocular medications; treatment of symptoms of dry eye (eg, redness, burning, reflex tearing, itching, foreign body sensation); after eye surgery to prevent complications; for patients experiencing dry eye-related contact lens problems.

Contraindications:

Tearing secondary to chronic dacryocystitis with mucopurulent discharge; allergy to bovine collagen; inflammation of eyelid; epiphoria.

Patient Information:

Relief may not occur immediately after insertion.

No removal is necessary; implants dissolve within 7 to 10 days.

Reexamination is usually required within 14 days.

Successful treatment may indicate a need for permanent treatment (eg, nondissolvable silicone plugs).

Administration and Dosage:

Implants must be inserted by a physician or doctor of optometry. Placement of implants in all four canaliculi is recommended to prevent a false-negative response.

Rx	**Collagen Implant** (Lacrimedics)	**Implant:** Collagen implant	In 0.2, 0.3, 0.4, 0.5 and 0.6 mm sizes (72s).
Rx	**Temporary Punctal/Canalicular Collagen Implant** (Eagle Vision, Ciba Vision)		In 0.2, 0.3, 0.4, 0.5 and 0.6 mm sizes (72s).

TYLOXAPOL (CLEANING/LUBRICANT FOR ARTIFICIAL EYES)

Actions:

Pharmacology: The cleaning/lubricant solution is a sterile, buffered isotonic solution formulated especially for artificial eye wearers. It contains the antibacterial agent benzalkonium chloride to kill most germs that are commonly found in the eye socket of artificial eye wearers. Tyloxapol, a detergent, liquifies the solid matter so that it is less irritating. Benzalkonium chloride, in addition to its germ-killing action, aids tyloxapol in wetting the artificial eye so that it is completely covered.

Indications:

Cleaner/Lubricant: To lubricate, clean and wet artificial eyes to increase wearing comfort.

Contraindications:

Hypersensitivity to any component of the formulation.

Patient Information:

If irritation persists or increases, discontinue use and consult your physician. Keep container tightly closed. Keep out of the reach of children.

To avoid contamination, do not touch dropper tip to any surface. Replace cap after using.

Administration and Dosage:

Use drops just as ordinary eye drops are used. With the artificial eye in place, apply 1 or 2 drops 3 or 4 times daily. The artificial eye may be removed periodically if advised by your physician, and 2 or 3 drops applied to remove oily or mucous materials. The artificial eye is then rubbed between the fingers and rinsed with tap water. Then 1 or 2 drops may be applied to the artificial eye, either prior to or after reinsertion.

Storage: Store at 8° to 27°C (46° to 80°F).

otc	**Enuclene** (Alcon)	**Solution**: 0.25%	In 15 ml Drop-Tainers.[1]

[1] 0.02% benzalkonium Cl.

ODF

8

ANTI-INFECTIVE AGENTS

ANTIBIOTIC AGENTS

Topical and systemic antibiotics may be utilized in the treatment of ocular infections. The most common ocular infections include blepharitis, conjunctivitis, dacryoadenitis, dacryocystitis, keratitis, orbital cellulitis, endophthalmitis, attendant sinusitis and superficial erysipelas of the skin.

The indigenous flora of the eyelids and conjunctiva are primarily *Staphylococcus aureus* and *Staphylococcus epidermidis,* which can overwhelm the ocular defenses and produce infection. Staphylococcal species are most commonly associated with acute papillary conjunctivitis, chronic blepharitis, dacryocystitis, impetigo, blepharoconjunctivitis, superficial keratitis and endophthalmitis. Corneal ulcers are associated with gram-positive bacteria approximately 75% of the time and gram-negative organisms 25% of the time. Fungal organisms may be seen in up to 10% of corneal ulcers in Florida.

A purulent discharge and papillary conjunctivitis are associated with a bacterial infection. A serous discharge with conjunctival chemosis and itching is more frequently associated with conjunctival allergy. Conjunctival hemorrhages are associated with more virulent organisms such as streptococcosis, Haemophilus or adenovirus. Infiltrative keratitis in the visual axis, decreased vision, hazing of the anterior chamber or hypopyon are harbingers of imminent visual loss and require prompt microbiologic studies for organism identification and proper antibiotic selection. Similar fastidious cultures of the lids or conjunctiva are important for any chronic conjunctivitis.

The table on the following page reflects the sensitivity studies of the Department of Ophthalmology, University of South Florida. Individual laboratory sensitivities may vary. See individual product inserts for more information on susceptible microorganisms.

Topical Ophthalmic Antibiotic Preparations

		Miscellaneous								Quinolones			Aminoglycosides				Sulfonamides			Penicillins			Cephalosporins			
	Organism/Infection	Bacitracin	Gramicidin	Polymyxin B	Erythromycin	Chloramphenicol	Trimethoprim	Oxytetracycline	Vancomycin[3]	Norfloxacin	Ciprofloxacin	Ofloxacin	Neomycin	Gentamicin	Tobramycin	Amikacin[3]	Sodium Sulfacetamide	Sulfisoxazole	Sulfamethoxazole[3]	Ampicillin[3]	Oxacillin[3]	Ticarcillin[3]	Cefotaxime[3]	Ceftazidime[3]	Cefuroxime[3]	Cephalothin[3]
Gram-Positive	Staphylococcus sp	✔	✔			✔	✔		✔	✔	✔	✔		✔	✔	✔										
	S aureus	✔	✔		✔	✔	✔	✔	✔	✔	✔	✔	✔	✔[1]	✔	✔	✔	✔	✔		✔		✔		✔	✔
	Streptococcus sp	✔	✔			✔					✔	✔			✔	✔	✔	✔								
	S pneumoniae	✔	✔		✔	✔	✔	✔		✔	✔	✔			✔	✔	✔	✔					✔			✔
	α-hemolytic streptococci (viridans group)	✔			✔	✔		✔			✔					✔	✔	✔		✔			✔		✔	✔
	β-hemolytic streptococci	✔												✔[1]	✔											
	S pyogenes	✔			✔		✔				✔	✔		✔			✔	✔		✔						✔
	Corynebacterium sp	✔	✔			✔					✔		✔	✔	✔	✔										
Gram-Negative	Escherichia coli			✔		✔	✔	✔		✔	✔	✔	✔	✔	✔		✔	✔								
	Haemophilus aegyptius					✔	✔			✔				✔	✔		✔	✔								
	H ducreyi					✔		✔			✔			✔	✔											
	H influenzae or parainfluenzae		✔	✔	✔		✔	✔		✔	✔	✔	✔	✔	✔					✔						
	Klebsiella sp					✔		✔		✔	✔	✔					✔	✔								
	K pneumoniae			✔			✔	✔		✔	✔	✔		✔	✔											✔
	Neisseria sp	✔				✔					✔		✔	✔	✔											
	N gonorrhoeae	✔			✔[2]					✔	✔	✔					✔									
	Proteus sp					✔	✔			✔	✔	✔	✔	✔	✔		✔	✔					✔	✔	✔	✔
	Acinetobacter calcoaceticus									✔	✔	✔		✔	✔							✔		✔		
	Enterobacter aerogenes			✔		✔	✔	✔		✔	✔	✔	✔	✔	✔	✔						✔		✔		
	Enterobacter sp					✔				✔	✔	✔	✔	✔	✔	✔	✔	✔				✔				
	Serratia marcescens						✔			✔	✔	✔		✔	✔	✔						✔		✔		
	Moraxella sp							✔				✔		✔	✔	✔						✔	✔	✔	✔	
	Chlamydia trachomatis				✔[2]						✔	✔					✔	✔								
	Pasteurella tularensis						✔	✔			✔			✔	✔	✔				✔		✔	✔	✔	✔	
	Pseudomonas aeruginosa			✔						✔	✔	✔			✔	✔						✔		✔		
	Bartonella bacilliformis							✔																		
	Bacteroides sp							✔																		
	Vibrio sp					✔		✔		✔	✔			✔	✔											
	Providencia sp									✔	✔															

[1] Increasing resistance has been seen.
[2] For prophylaxis.
[3] Not available as a commercial ophthalmic preparation.

ANTIFUNGAL AGENT

Natamycin (*Natacyn*) is the only topical ophthalmic antifungal agent available commercially. It is a tetraene polyene antibiotic derived from *Streptomyces natalensis*. It possesses in vitro activity against a variety of yeasts and filamentous fungi, including *Candida*, *Aspergillus*, *Cephalosporium*, *Fusarium* and *Penicillium*.

Amiconazole IV may be used topically if natamycin is not available.

ANTIVIRAL AGENTS

The topical ophthalmic antiviral preparations appear to interfere with viral reproduction by altering DNA synthesis. Vidarabine and trifluridine are effective treatment for herpes simplex infections of the conjunctiva and cornea. Ganciclovir is indicated for use in immunocompromised patients with cytomegalovirus (CMV) retinitis and for prevention of CMV retinitis in transplant patients. Foscarnet and cidofovir are indicated for use only in AIDS patients with CMV retinitis.

Antiviral Agents for Ophthalmic Conditions

Generic name	Trade name (manufacturer)	Preparations	Indications
Cidofovir	*Vistide* (Gilead)	Solution for Injection	Cytomegalovirus (CMV) retinitis
Foscarnet sodium	*Foscavir* (Astra)	Solution for Injection	Cytomegalovirus (CMV) retinitis
Ganciclovir sodium	*Cytovene* (Syntex)	Reconstituted powder Capsules 250 mg	Cytomegalovirus (CMV) retinitis
	Vitrasert (Chiron Vision)	Implant	Cytomegalovirus (CMV) retinitis
Vidarabine	*Vira-A* (Parke-Davis)	Ointment 3%	Herpes simplex types 1 and 2; idoxuridine-resistant herpes
Trifluridine	*Viroptic* (Monarch)	Solution 1%	Herpes simplex types 1 and 2; idoxuridine hypersensitivity; vidarabine-resistant keratitis

Viral infection, especially epidemic keratoconjunctivitis (EKC), is more often associated with a follicular conjunctivitis, a serous conjunctival discharge and preauricular lymphadenopathy. The exceptionally contagious organism causing EKC is not susceptible to antiviral therapy at this time. Pustular lesions of the nose and face, and spade-shaped fascicular keratitis in association with chronic blepharitis, suggesting acne rosacea, warrants a trial of systemic tetracycline (eg, *Achromycin V*) or doxycycline (eg, *Vibramycin*) as both an antibiotic and potentially anti-inflammatory regimen.

J. James Rowsey, MD
University of South Florida

For More Information

Bartlett JD, Jaanus SD, eds. Clinical Ocular Pharmacology, ed. 3. Boston: Butterworth-Heinemann, 1995.

Duane TD, ed. Clinical Ophthalmology. Philadelphia: Lippincott-Raven, 1997.

Kucers A, Bennett NM. The Use of Antibiotics, ed. 4. Philadelphia: J.B. Lippincott Company, 1987.

ANTIBIOTICS

Indications:

Ocular infections: Treatment of superficial ocular infections involving the conjunctiva or cornea (eg, conjunctivitis, keratitis, keratoconjunctivitis, corneal ulcers, blepharitis, blepharoconjunctivitis, acute meibomianitis and dacryocystitis) due to strains of microorganisms susceptible to antibiotics.

Erythromycin: Prophylaxis of ophthalmia neonatorum due to *Neisseria gonorrhoeae* or *Chlamydia trachomatis.*

Chloramphenicol: Use only in those serious infections for which less potentially dangerous drugs are ineffective or contraindicated (see Warnings).

For a listing of the microorganisms usually susceptible to the agents, refer to the Topical Ophthalmic Preparations table.

The table below lists common ocular conditions along with the antibiotics used most often to treat them. These antibiotics are preferred choices before cultures are available.

Antibiotic Treatment for Common Ocular Conditions

	Blepharitis	Conjunctivitis	Keratitis
Bacitracin	X		
Polymixin B	X		
Sodium Sulfacetamide	X		
Trimethoprim		X	
Vancomycin			X
Ciprofloxacin		X	X
Gentamicin			X
Tobramycin		X	
Amikacin		X	
Ofloxacin			X
Ceftazidime			X

Contraindications:

Hypersensitivity to any component of these products; history of hypersensitivity to other quinolones; epithelial herpes simplex keratitis (dendritic keratitis); vaccinia; varicella; mycobacterial infections of the eye; fungal diseases of the ocular structure; use of steroid combinations after uncomplicated removal of a corneal foreign body.

Warnings:

Ciprofloxacin and Ofloxacin Hypersensitivity Reactions: Serious and occasionally fatal hypersensitivity (anaphylactic) reactions, some following the first dose, have been reported in patients receiving systemic quinolones, including ofloxacin. Some reactions were accompanied by cardiovascular collapse, loss of consciousness, angioedema (including laryngeal, pharyngeal or facial edema), airway obstruction, dyspnea, urticaria and itching. A rare occurrence of Stevens-Johnson syndrome, which progressed to toxic epidermal necrolysis, has been reported in a patient who was receiving topical ophthalmic ofloxacin. Discontinue drug if an allergic reaction occurs.

Serious acute hypersensitivity reactions may require immediate emergency treatment. Oxygen and airway management, including intubation, should be administered as clinically indicated.

Sensitization from the topical use of an antibiotic may contraindicate the drug's later systemic use in serious infections. For this reason, topical preparations containing antibiotics not ordinarily administered systemically are preferable. Products with neomycin sulfate may cause cutaneous/conjunctival sensitization.

Cross-sensitivity: Allergic cross-reactions may occur that could prevent future use of any or all of these antibiotics: Kanamycin, neomycin, paromomycin, streptomycin, and possibly, gentamicin.

Hematopoietic toxicity has occurred occasionally with the systemic use of chloramphenicol and rarely with topical administration. It is generally a dose-related toxic effect on bone marrow, and is usually reversible on cessation of therapy. Rare cases of aplastic anemia, bone marrow hypoplasia and death have been reported with prolonged (months to years) or frequent intermittent (over months and years) use of ocular chloramphenicol.

Corneal healing: Ophthalmic ointments may retard corneal epithelial healing.

Pregnancy: Category B (erythromycin, tobramycin), Category C (gentamicin, ciprofloxacin, norfloxacin, ofloxacin, polymyxin B). Safety for use during pregnancy has not been established. Use only when clearly needed and when the potential benefits outweigh the potential hazards to the fetus.

Lactation: It is not known whether ciprofloxacin, norfloxacin or ofloxacin appears in breast milk following ophthalmic use. Exercise caution when administering ciprofloxacin to a nursing mother. Because of the potential for adverse reactions in nursing infants from norfloxacin, ofloxacin, chloramphenicol and tobramycin, decide whether to discontinue nursing or discontinue the drug, taking into account the importance of the drug to the mother.

Children: Tobramycin is safe and effective in children. Safety and efficacy of fluoroquinolones in infants < 1 year of age, and polymyxin B/trimethoprim in infants < 2 months of age have not been established.

Precautions:

Monitoring: Perform culture and susceptibility testing during treatment.

Systemic antibiotics: In all except very superficial infections, supplement the topical use of antibiotics with appropriate systemic medication. Systemic aminoglycoside antibiotics require monitoring the total serum concentration (peak and trough). Recent studies suggest that intracameral antibiotics may be efficacious alone, for the treatment of endophthalmitis with minimally virulent organisms, with visual acuity > 20/400.

Crystalline precipitate: A white crystalline precipitate located in the superficial portion of the corneal defect was observed in ≈ 17% of patients on ciprofloxacin. Onset was within 1 to 7 days after starting therapy. The precipitate resolved in most patients within 2 weeks, and did not preclude continued use nor adversely affect the clinical course or outcome. Streptococcal corneal ulcers are often resistant to ciprofloxacin.

Superinfection: Do not use topical antibiotics in deep-seated ocular infections or in those that are likely to become systemic. Use of antibiotics (especially prolonged or repeated therapy) may result in bacterial or fungal overgrowth of nonsusceptible organisms. Such overgrowth may lead to a secondary infection. Take appropriate measures if superinfection occurs.

Sulfite sensitivity: Some of these products contain sulfites which may cause allergic-type reactions (eg, hives, itching, wheezing, anaphylaxis) in certain susceptible persons. Although the overall prevalence of sulfite sensitivity in the general population is probably low, it is seen more frequently in asthmatics or in atopic nonasthmatic persons. Specific products containing sulfites are identified in the product listings.

Adverse Reactions:

Sensitivity reactions such as transient irritation, burning, discomfort, redness, stinging, itching, inflammation, angioneurotic edema, urticaria, vesicular and maculopapular dermatitis have occurred in some patients.

Chloramphenicol:

Hematological events (including aplastic anemia) have occurred (see Warnings).

Fluoroquinolones:

White crystalline precipitates; lid margin crusting; crystals/scales; foreign body sensation; conjunctival hyperemia; bad/bitter taste in mouth; corneal staining; chemical conjunctivitis; keratopathy/keratitis; allergic reactions; lid and facial edema; tearing; photophobia; corneal infiltrates; nausea; decreased or blurred vision; chemosis; dryness; eye pain; dizziness (rarely).

Aminoglycosides:

Localized ocular toxicity and hypersensitivity, lid itching, lid swelling and conjunctival erythema (< 3% with tobramycin); bacterial/fungal corneal ulcers; nonspecific conjunctivitis; conjunctival epithelial defects; conjunctival hyperemia (gentamicin). Similar reactions may occur with the topical use of other aminoglycoside antibiotics.

Overdosage:

Symptoms: Symptoms of tobramycin overdose include punctate keratitis, erythema, increased lacrimation, edema and lid itching. These may be similar to adverse reactions.

Treatment: A topical overdose of ciprofloxacin may be flushed from the eyes with warm tap water.

Patient Information:

Tilt head back, place medication in conjunctival sac holding the dropper 1 inch from the eye and close eyes. Apply light finger pressure on lacrimal sac for 1 minute following instillation.

May cause temporary blurring of vision or stinging following administration. Notify physician if stinging, burning or itching becomes pronounced or if redness, irritation, swelling, decreasing vision or pain persists or worsens.

To avoid contamination, do not touch tip of container to any surface. Replace cap after using.

In general, patients being treated for bacterial conjunctivitis should not wear contact lenses; however, if the physician considers contact lens use appropriate, wait at least 15 minutes after using any solutions containing benzalkonium chloride before inserting the lens, as it may be absorbed by the lens.

Quinolones: Discontinue use and notify physician at the first sign of a skin rash or other allergic reaction.

Administration and Dosage:

Administration and dosage varies for the individual products. Refer to the individual manufacturer inserts for complete information.

Individual drug monographs are on the following pages.

BACITRACIN

Complete prescribing information is found in the Ophthalmic Antibiotics group monograph.

Administration and Dosage:

Apply directly to conjunctival sac(s) 1 to 3 times daily.

Blepharitis: Carefully remove all scales and crusts and then spread ointment uniformly over lid margins.

Storage: Store at room temperature 15° to 30°C (59° to 86°F).

Rx	**Bacitracin** (Various, eg, Major, Schein, URL, Zenith Goldline)	**Ointment:** 500 units/g	In 3.5 and 3.75 g.
Rx	**AK-Tracin** (Akorn)		Preservative free. In 3.5 g.[1]

[1] With white petrolatum and mineral oil.

POLYMYXIN B SULFATE

Complete prescribing information is found in the Ophthalmic Antibiotics group monograph.

Indications:

For treatment of infections of the eye caused by susceptible strains of *Pseudomonas aeruginosa.*

Administration and Dosage:

Dissolve 500,000 units polymyxin B sulfate in 20 to 50 ml sterile distilled water (Sterile Water for Injection, USP) or sterile physiologic saline (Sodium Chloride Injection, USP) for a 10,000 to 25,000 units per ml concentration.

For the treatment of P aeruginosa infections of the eye: Administer a concentration of 0.1% to 0.25% (10,000 to 25,000 units per ml) 1 to 3 drops every hour, increasing the intervals as response indicates.

Subconjunctival injection of up to 100,000 units/day may be used for the treatment of *P aeruginosa* infections of the cornea and conjunctiva.

Avoid total systemic and ophthalmic instillations of over 25,000 units/kg/day.

Rx	**Polymyxin B Sulfate Sterile** (Roerig)	**Powder for solution:** 500,000 units	In 20 ml vials.

CHLORAMPHENICOL

Complete prescribing information is found in the Ophthalmic Antibiotics group monograph.

Use only in those serious infections for which less potentially dangerous drugs are ineffective or contraindicated (see Warnings).

Administration and Dosage:

Ointment: Place a small amount in the conjunctival sac(s) every 3 hours, or more often if required, day and night for the first 48 hours. Intervals between applications may be increased after the first 2 days. Since chloramphenicol is primarily bacteriostatic, continue therapy for 48 hours after an apparent cure has been obtained.

Storage – Store at room temp 15° to 30°C (59° to 86°F). Store away from heat.

Solution (reconstituted): Instill 2 drops into the affected eye(s) every 3 hours, or more frequently if deemed advisable. Continue administration day and night for the first 48 hours, after which the interval between applications may be increased. Continue treatment for at least 48 hours after the eye appears normal.

Solution Preparation	
Strength of solution desired	Add sterile distilled water
0.5%	5 ml
0.25%	10 ml
0.16%	15 ml

Storage – Store below 30°C (86°F). Reconstituted solutions remain stable at room temperature for 10 days.

Solution: Instill 1 or 2 drops 4 to 6 times a day for the first 72 hours, depending upon the severity of the condition. Intervals between applications may be increased after the first 2 days. Since the action of the drug is primarily bacteriostatic, continue therapy for 48 hours after an apparent cure has been attained.

Storage – Refrigerate at 2° to 8°C (36° to 46°F) until dispensed. Protect from light. Remove from refrigerator for dispensing; discard 21 days thereafter.

Rx	**Chloramphenicol** (Various, eg, Schein, Zenith Goldline)	**Solution**[1]: 5 mg/ml	In 7.5 and 15 ml.
Rx	**AK-Chlor** (Akorn)		In 7.5 and 15 ml.[2]
Rx	**Chloroptic** (Allergan)		In 2.5 and 7.5 ml.[3]
Rx	**Chloramphenicol** (Various, eg, Schein)	**Ointment**: 10 mg/g	In 3.5 g.
Rx	**AK-Chlor** (Akorn)		In 3.5 g.[4]
Rx	**Chloromycetin** (Parke-Davis)		Preservative free. In 3.5 g.[5]
Rx	**Chloroptic S.O.P.** (Allergan)		In 3.5 g.[6]
Rx	**Chloromycetin** (Parke-Davis)	**Powder for solution**: 25 mg/vial	Preservative free. In 15 ml with diluent.

[1] Refrigerate until dispensed.
[2] With 0.5% chlorobutanol, boric acid, sodium borate, hydroxypropyl methylcellulose, sodium hydroxide and hydrochloric acid.
[3] With 0.5% chlorobutanol, PEG-300, polyoxyl 40 stearate and sodium hydroxide or hydrochloric acid.
[4] With white petrolatum, mineral oil and polysorbate 60.
[5] With liquid petrolatum and polyethylene base.
[6] With 0.5% chlorobutanol, white petrolatum, mineral oil, polyoxyl 40 stearate, petrolatum (and) lanolin alcohol and PEG-300.

ERYTHROMYCIN

Complete prescribing information is found in the Ophthalmic Antibiotics group monograph.

Indications:

For the treatment of superficial ocular infections involving the conjunctiva or cornea caused by organisms susceptible to erythromycin.

For prophylaxis of ophthalmia neonatorum due to *Neisseria gonorrhoeae* or *Chlamydia trachomatis.* The Centers for Disease Control and the Committee on Drugs, the Committee on Infectious Diseases of the American Academy of Pediatrics and the Committee on Fetus and Newborn recommend 1% silver nitrate solution in single-use ampules or single-use tubes of an ophthalmic ointment containing 0.5% erythromycin or 1% tetracycline as "effective and acceptable regimens for prophylaxis of gonococcal ophthalmia neonatorum." (For infants born to mothers with clinically apparent gonorrhea, give IV or IM injections of aqueous crystalline penicillin G: A single dose of 50,000 units for term infants or 20,000 units for infants of low birth weight. Topical prophylaxis alone is inadequate for these infants.)

For the prevention of neonatal conjunctivitis due to *C trachomatis,* a condition that may develop one to several weeks after delivery in infants of mothers whose birth canals harbor the organism.

Administration and Dosage:

External ocular infections: Apply directly to the infected area 1 or more times daily, depending on the severity of the infection.

Prophylaxis of neonatal gonococcal or chlamydial conjunctivitis: Instill a thin line of ointment approximately 0.5 to 1 cm in length into each conjunctival sac. Do not flush the ointment from the eye following application. Use a new tube for each infant. Administer to infants born by cesarian section and those delivered vaginally.

Storage: Store at room temperature 15° to 30°C (59° to 86°F).

Rx	**Erythromycin** (Various, eg, Akorn, Bausch & Lomb, Fougera, Rugby, Zenith Goldline)	**Ointment**: 5 mg/g	In 3.5 g.
Rx	**Ilotycin** (Dista)		In 3.5 g.[1]

[1] With white petrolatum, mineral oil and parabens.

GENTAMICIN SULFATE

Complete prescribing information is found in the Ophthalmic Antibiotics group monograph.

Administration and Dosage:

Solution: Instill 1 or 2 drops into the affected eye(s) every 4 hours. In severe infections, dosage may be increased to 2 drops once every hour.

This solution is not for injection. Do not inject subconjunctivally. Do not directly introduce into the anterior chamber.

Storage: Store at 2° to 30°C (36° to 86°F). Store away from heat.

Ointment: Apply a small amount to affected eye(s) 2 to 3 times daily.

Storage: Store at 2° to 30°C (36° to 86°F). Store away from heat.

Rx	**Gentamicin Ophthalmic** (Various, eg, Bausch & Lomb, Rugby, Schein, Zenith Goldline)	**Solution**: 3 mg/ml	In 5 and 15 ml.
Rx	**Garamycin** (Schering)		In 5 ml dropper bottles.[1]
Rx	**Genoptic** (Allergan)		In 1 and 5 ml dropper bottles.[2]
Rx	**Gentacidin** (Ciba Vision)		In 5 ml dropper bottles.[1]
Rx	**Gentak** (Akorn)		In 5 and 15 ml dropper bottles.[1]
Rx	**Gentamicin Ophthalmic** (Various, eg, Major)	**Ointment**: 3 mg/g	In 3.5 g.
Rx	**Garamycin** (Schering)		In 3.5 g.[3]
Rx	**Genoptic S.O.P.** (Allergan)		In 3.5 g.[3]
Rx	**Gentacidin** (Ciba Vision)		In 3.5 g.[4]
Rx	**Gentak** (Akorn)		In 3.5 g.[3]

[1] With 0.1 mg/ml benzalkonium chloride, sodium phosphate and NaCl.
[2] With benzalkonium chloride, 1.4% polyvinyl alcohol, EDTA, sodium phosphate dibasic, NaCl and hydrochloric acid or sodium hydroxide.
[3] With white petrolatum and parabens.
[4] With white petrolatum and mineral oil.

TOBRAMYCIN

Complete prescribing information is found in the Ophthalmic Antibiotics group monograph.

Administration and Dosage:

Solution: Mild to moderate disease - Instill 1 or 2 drops into the affected eye(s) every 4 hours. Not for injection into the eye.

Severe infections – Instill 2 drops into the eye(s) hourly until improvement. Reduce treatment prior to discontinuation.

Ointment: Mild to moderate disease - Apply 0.5 inch ribbon into the affected eye(s) 2 or 3 times daily.

Severe infections – Instill 0.5 inch ribbon into the affected eye(s) every 3 to 4 hours until improvement. Reduce treatment prior to discontinuation.

Storage: Store at 8° to 27°C (46° to 80°F).

Rx	**Tobramycin** (Various, eg, Bausch & Lomb, Steris)	**Solution**: 0.3%	In 5 ml bottle.
Rx	**AKTob** (Akorn)		In 5 ml.[1]
Rx	**Defy** (Akorn)		In 5 ml.
Rx	**Tobrex** (Alcon)		In 5 ml Drop-Tainers.[2]
Rx	**Tobrex** (Alcon)	**Ointment**: 3 mg/g	In 3.5 g.[3]

[1] With 0.01% benzalkonium chloride, boric acid and sodium sulfate.
[2] With 0.01% benzalkonium chloride, tyloxapol and boric acid.
[3] With white petrolatum, mineral oil and 0.5% chlorobutanol.

CIPROFLOXACIN

Complete prescribing information is found in the Ophthalmic Antibiotics group monograph.

Administration and Dosage:

Not for injection into the eye.

Remove contact lenses before using.

For the treatment of corneal ulcers: Instill 2 drops into the affected eye(s) every 15 minutes for the first 6 hours and then 2 drops every 30 minutes for the remainder of the first day. On the second day, instill 2 drops every hour. On the third through the fourteenth day, instill 2 drops every 4 hours. Treatment may be continued after 14 days if corneal re-epithelialization has not occurred.

For the treatment of bacterial conjunctivitis: Instill 1 or 2 drops into the conjunctival sac(s) every 2 hours while awake for 2 days, and 1 or 2 drops every 4 hours while awake for the next 5 days.

Storage: Store at 2° to 30°C (36° to 86°F). Protect from light.

Rx	**Ciloxan** (Alcon)	**Solution:** 0.3% (equivalent to 3 mg base)	In 2.5 and 5 ml Drop-Tainers.[1]

[1] With 0.006% benzalkonium chloride, 4.6% mannitol and 0.05% EDTA.

NORFLOXACIN

Complete prescribing information is found in the Ophthalmic Antibiotics group monograph.

Administration and Dosage:

Bacterial conjunctivitis: Instill 1 or 2 drops into the affected eye(s) 4 times daily for up to 7 days. Depending on the severity of the infection, the dosage for the first day of therapy may be 1 or 2 drops every 2 hours during the waking hours.

Storage: Store at room temperature 15° to 30°C (59° to 86°F). Protect from light.

Rx	**Chibroxin** (Merck)	**Solution:** 3 mg/ml	In 5 ml Ocumeters.[1]

[1] With 0.0025% benzalkonium chloride and EDTA.

OFLOXACIN

Complete prescribing information is found in the Ophthalmic Antibiotics group monograph.

Administration and Dosage:

Not for injection into the eye.

Bacterial conjunctivitis: Instill 1 to 2 drops every 2 to 4 hours for the first 2 days and then 4 times daily into the affected eye for up to 5 additional days.

Bacterial corneal ulcer: Instill 1 to 2 drops every 30 minutes while awake; awaken approximately 4 and 6 hours after retiring and instill 1 to 2 drops for 2 days. Instill 1 to 2 drops while awake for the next 5 to 7 days. Instill 1 to 2 drops 4 times daily through treatment completion.

Storage: Store at 15° to 25°C (59° to 77°F).

Rx	**Ocuflox** (Allergan)	**Solution:** 0.3%	In 1, 5 and 10 ml.[1]

[1] With 0.005% benzalkonium chloride.

COMBINATION ANTIBIOTIC PRODUCTS

Complete prescribing information is found in the Ophthalmic Antibiotics group monograph.

	Product and Distributor	**Polymyxin B Sulfate** (units/g or ml)	**Neomycin Sulfate** (mg/g or ml)	**Bacitracin Zinc** (units/g)	Other Antibiotics	How Supplied
Rx	**Triple Antibiotic Ophthalmic Ointment** (Various, eg, Fougera)	10,000	3.5	400		In 3.5 g.
Rx	**Bacitracin Neomycin Polymyxin B Ointment** (Various, eg, Fougera)					In 3.5 g.
Rx	**AK-Spore Ointment** (Akorn)					Preservative free. White petrolatum, mineral oil. In 3.5 g.
Rx	**Neosporin Ophthalmic Ointment** (Glaxo Wellcome)					White petrolatum. In 3.5 g.
Rx	**Ocutricin Ointment** (Bausch & Lomb)					White petrolatum, mineral oil. In 3.5 g.
Rx	**Neomycin Sulfate- Polymyxin B Sulfate -Gramicidin Solution** (Various, eg, Rugby, Steris Zenith Goldline)	10,000	1.75		0.025 mg/ml gramicidin	In 2 and 10 ml.
Rx	**AK-Spore Solution** (Akorn)					In 2 and 10 ml.[1]
Rx	**Neosporin Ophthalmic Solution** (Glaxo Wellcome)					In 10 ml Drop Dose.[1]
Rx	**Bacitracin Zinc and Polymyxin B Ointment** (Bausch & Lomb)	10,000		500		White petrolatum and mineral oil. In 3.5 g.
Rx	**AK-Poly-Bac Ointment** (Akorn)					Preservative free. White petrolatum, mineral oil. In 3.5 g.
Rx	**Polysporin Ophthalmic Ointment** (Glaxo Wellcome)					White petrolatum. In 3.5 g.
Rx	**Terramycin w/Polymyxin B Ointment** (Roerig)	10,000			5 mg/g oxytetracycline HCl	White and liquid petrolatum. In 3.5 g.
Rx	**Terak Ointment** (Akorn)	10,000			5 mg/g oxytetracycline HCl	White and liquid petrolatum. In 3.5 g.
Rx	**Trimethoprim Sulfate and Polymyxin B Sulfate Ophthalmic Solution** (Bausch & Lomb)	10,000			1 mg/ml trimethoprim	In 10 ml.[2]
Rx	**Polytrim Ophthalmic Solution** (Allergan)	10,000			1 mg/ml trimethoprim	In 10 ml.[2]

[1] With 0.001% thimerosal, 0.5% alcohol, propylene glycol, polyoxyethylene polyoxypropylene.
[2] With 0.004% benzalkonium chloride and NaCl.

STEROID AND ANTIBIOTIC SOLUTIONS AND SUSPENSIONS

Indications:

Inflammatory conditions: For steroid-responsive inflammatory ocular conditions in which a corticosteroid is indicated and in which bacterial infection or risk of infection exists.

For inflammatory conditions of the palpebral and bulbar conjunctiva, cornea and anterior segment of the globe in which the inherent risk of steroid use in certain infective conjunctivitides is accepted to obtain a diminution in edema and inflammation. For chronic anterior uveitis and corneal injury from chemical, radiation or thermal burns, or penetration of foreign bodies.

Administration and Dosage:

Store suspensions upright and shake well before using.

Instill 1 or 2 drops into the affected eye(s) every 3 or 4 hours, or more frequently as required. Taper to discontinuation as inflammation subsides.

Do not prescribe > 20 ml initially; do not refill without further evaluation. For complete dosage instructions, see individual manufacturer inserts.

	Product & Distributor	Steroid (per ml)	Antibiotic (per ml)	Other Content	How Supplied
Rx	**Chloromycetin/Hydrocortisone for Suspension** (Parke-Davis)	0.5% hydrocortisone acetate[1] (2.5% as powder)	0.25% chloramphenicol[1] (1.25% as powder)	Cholesterol, methylcellulose, 0.01% benzethonium chloride, boric acid	In 5 ml w/diluent and dropper.
Rx	**Neomycin/Polymyxin B Sulfate/Hydrocortisone** (Various, eg, Rugby, Schein)	1% hydrocortisone	Neomycin sulfate equivalent to 0.35% neomycin base and 10,000 units polymyxin B sulfate		In 7.5 and 10 ml.
Rx	**AK-Spore H.C. Ophthalmic Suspension** (Akorn)			0.001% thimerosal, cetyl alcohol, glyceryl monostearate, polyoxyl 40 stearate, propylene glycol, mineral oil, NaCl	In 7.5 ml.
Rx	**Cortisporin Suspension** (Glaxo Wellcome)				In 7.5 ml Drop Dose.
Rx	**Terra-Cortril Suspension** (Roerig)	1.5% hydrocortisone acetate	0.5% oxytetracycline (as HCl)	Mineral oil and aluminum tristearate	In 5 ml.

	Product & Distributor	Steroid (per ml)	Antibiotic (per ml)	Other Content	How Supplied
Rx	**Poly-Pred Suspension** (Allergan)	0.5% prednisolone acetate	Neomycin sulfate equivalent to 0.35% neomycin base, 10,000 units polymyxin B sulfate	1.4% polyvinyl alcohol, 0.001% thimerosal, polysorbate 80, propylene glycol	In 5 and 10 ml.
Rx	**Pred-G Suspension** (Allergan)	1% prednisolone acetate	Gentamicin sulfate equivalent to 0.3% gentamicin base	1.4% polyvinyl alcohol, 0.005% benzalkonium chloride, EDTA, hydroxypropyl methylcellulose, polysorbate 80, NaCl	In 2, 5 and 10 ml.
Rx	**Neomycin Sulfate/ Dexamethasone Sodium Phosphate Solution** (Various, eg, Rugby, Schein, Zenith Goldline)	0.1% dexamethasone phosphate (as sodium phosphate)	Neomycin sulfate equivalent to 0.35% neomycin base		In 5 ml.
Rx	**NeoDecadron Solution** (Merck)			Polysorbate 80, EDTA, 0.2% benzalkonium Cl, 0.1% sodium bisulfite	In 5 ml Ocumeters.
Rx	**Neo-Dexameth** (Major)			0.01% benzalkonium Cl, EDTA, polysorbate 80, sodium bisulfite	In 5 ml.
Rx	**AK-Neo-Dex Solution** (Akorn)			0.02% benzalkonium Cl, polysorbate 80, EDTA, 0.1% sodium bisulfite	In 5 ml.
Rx	**TobraDex Suspension** (Alcon)	0.1% dexamethasone	0.3% tobramycin	0.01% benzalkonium Cl, tyloxapol, EDTA, hydroxyethylcellulose, sodium sulfate, NaCl	In 2.5 and 5 ml Drop-Tainers.
Rx	**Neomycin/Polymyxin B Sulfate/Dexamethasone Suspension** (Various, eg, Rugby, Schein, Zenith Goldline)	0.1% dexamethasone	Neomycin sulfate equivalent to 0.35% neomycin base and 10,000 units polymyxin B sulfate		In 5 and 10 ml.
Rx	**Dexacidin Suspension** (Ciba Vision)			Hydroxypropyl methylcellulose, polysorbate 20, 0.04% benzalkonium chloride, NaCl	In 5 ml.
Rx	**AK-Trol Suspension** (Akorn)			0.004% benzalkonium chloride, polysorbate 20, 0.5% hydroxypropyl methylcellulose, NaCl	In 5 ml.
Rx	**Maxitrol Suspension** (Alcon)			0.5% hydroxypropyl methylcellulose, polysorbate 20, 0.004% benzalkonium chloride	In 5 ml Drop-Tainers.

[1] As a prepared solution.

STEROID AND ANTIBIOTIC OINTMENTS

Administration and Dosage:

Apply ointment to the affected eye(s) every 3 or 4 hours, depending on the severity of the condition.

Do not prescribe > 8 g initially, and the prescription should not be refilled until further evaluation. For complete dosage instructions, see individual manufacturer inserts.

	Product & Distributor	Steroid (per g)	Antibiotic (per g)	Other Content	How Supplied
Rx	**Bacitracin Zinc/Neomycin Sulfate/Polymyxin B Sulfate/ Hydrocortisone** (Various, eg, Fougera)	1% hydrocortisone	Neomycin sulfate equivalent to 0.35% neomycin base, 400 units bacitracin zinc, 10,000 units polymyxin B sulfate		In 3.5 g.
Rx	**AK-Spore H.C.** (Akorn)			White petrolatum, mineral oil	Preservative free. In 3.5 g.
Rx	**Cortisporin** (Glaxo Wellcome)			White petrolatum	In 3.5 g.
Rx	**Neotricin HC** (Bausch & Lomb)	1% hydrocortisone acetate	Neomycin sulfate equivalent to 0.35% neomycin base, 400 units bacitracin zinc, 10,000 units polymyxin B sulfate	White petrolatum, mineral oil	In 3.5 g.
Rx	**Pred-G S.O.P.** (Allergan)	0.6% prednisolone acetate	Gentamicin sulfate equivalent to 0.3% gentamicin base	0.5% chlorobutanol, white petrolatum, mineral oil, petrolatum, lanolin alcohol	In 3.5 g.
Rx	**NeoDecadron** (Merck)	0.05% dexamethasone phosphate (as sodium phosphate)	Neomycin sulfate equivalent to 0.35% neomycin base	White petrolatum, mineral oil	In 3.5 g.
Rx	**TobraDex** (Alcon)	0.1% dexamethasone	0.3% tobramycin	0.5% chlorobutanol, white petrolatum, mineral oil	In 3.5 g.

	Product & Distributor	Steroid (per g)	Antibiotic (per g)	Other Content	How Supplied
Rx	**Neomycin/Polymyxin B Sulfate/Dexamethasone** (Various, eg, Fougera, Rugby)	0.1% dexamethasone	Neomycin sulfate equivalent to 0.35% neomycin base, 10,000 units polymyxin B sulfate		In 3.5 g.
Rx	**AK-Trol** (Akorn)			White petrolatum, lanolin oil, mineral oil, parabens	In 3.5 g.
Rx	**Dexacidin** (Ciba Vision)			White petrolatum, mineral oil	In 3.5 g.
Rx	**Dexasporin** (Bausch & Lomb)			White petrolatum, mineral oil	In 3.5 g.
Rx	**Maxitrol** (Alcon)			White petrolatum, anhydrous liquid lanolin, parabens	In 3.5 g.

SULFONAMIDES

Actions:

Pharmacology: Sulfonamides are bacteriostatic against a wide range of susceptible gram-positive and gram-negative microorganisms. Through competition with para-aminobenzoic acid (PABA), they restrict synthesis of folic acid which bacteria require for growth.

Pharmacokinetics: Sulfonamides do not appear to be appreciably absorbed from mucous membranes.

Microbiology: Topically applied sulfonamides are considered active against susceptible strains of the following common bacterial eye pathogens: *Escherichia coli, Staphylococcus aureus, Streptococcus pneumoniae, Streptococcus* (viridans group), *Haemophilus influenzae, Klebsiella* sp and *Enterobacter* sp.

Topically applied sulfonamides do not provide adequate coverage against *Neisseria* sp, *Serratia marcescens* and *Pseudomonas aeruginosa.* A significant percentage of staphylococcal isolates are completely resistant to sulfa drugs.

Indications:

Ocular infections: For conjunctivitis, corneal ulcer and other superficial ocular infections due to susceptible microorganisms.

Trachoma: As an adjunct to systemic sulfonamide therapy in the treatment of trachoma.

Contraindications:

Hypersensitivity to sulfonamides or any component of the product; infants < 2 months of age; in epithelial herpes simplex keratitis (dendritic keratitis), vaccinia, varicella and many other viral diseases of the cornea and conjunctiva; mycobacterial infection or fungal diseases of the ocular structures; after uncomplicated removal of a corneal foreign body (steroid combinations).

Warnings:

Staphylococcus species: A significant percentage of isolates are resistant to sulfa drugs.

Hypersensitivity: Severe sensitivity reactions have been identified in individuals with no prior history of sulfonamide hypersensitivity (see Adverse Reactions).

Pregnancy: Category C. Safety for use during pregnancy has not been established. Use only when clearly needed and when potential benefits outweigh potential hazards to the fetus.

Lactation: Systemic sulfonamides are excreted in breast milk.

Children: Safety and efficacy not established. Contraindicated in infants < 2 months of age.

Precautions:

For topical ophthalmic use only. Not for injection.

Epithelial healing: Ophthalmic ointments may retard corneal wound healing.

Sensitization may occur when a sulfonamide is readministered, regardless of route. Cross-sensitivity between different sulfonamides may occur. If signs of sensitivity or other untoward reactions occur, discontinue use of the preparation.

PABA present in purulent exudates inactivates sulfonamides.

Dry eye: Use with caution in patients with severe dry eye.

Superinfection: Use of antibiotics (especially prolonged or repeated therapy) may result in bacterial or fungal overgrowth of nonsusceptible organisms. Such overgrowth may lead to a secondary infection. Take appropriate measures if this occurs.

Sulfite sensitivity: May cause allergic-type reactions (eg, hives, itching, wheezing, anaphylaxis) in certain susceptible persons. Although overall prevalence in the general population is probably low, it is more common in asthmatics or in atopic nonasthmatics. Specific products containing sulfites are identified in product listings.

Drug Interactions:

Silver preparations are incompatible with these solutions.

Adverse Reactions:

Headache; local irritation; itching; periorbital edema, burning and transient stinging; bacterial and fungal corneal ulcers. As with all sulfonamide preparations, severe sensitivity reactions include rare occurrences of Stevens-Johnson syndrome, exfoliative dermatitis, toxic epidermal necrolysis, photosensitivity, fever, skin rash, GI disturbance and bone marrow depression; fatalities have occurred.

Patient Information:

For topical use only.

To avoid contamination, do not touch tip of container to any surface.

Keep bottle tightly closed when not in use. Do not use if solution has darkened.

Notify physician if improvement is not seen after several days, if condition worsens, or if pain, increased redness, itching or swelling of the eye occurs or persists for > 48 hours. Do not discontinue use without consulting physician.

Administration and Dosage:

Usual duration of treatment is 7 to 10 days.

Solutions:

Conjunctivitis or other superficial ocular infections – Instill 1 to 2 drops into the lower conjunctival sac(s) every 1 to 4 hours initially according to severity of infection. Dosages may be tapered by increasing the time interval between doses as the condition responds.

Trachoma – Instill 2 drops every 2 hours. Concomitant systemic sulfonamide therapy is indicated.

Storage – Protect from light. On long standing, solutions will darken in color and should be discarded.

Ointments: Apply a small amount (0.25 inch) into the lower conjunctival sac(s) 3 to 4 times daily and at bedtime. Dosages may be tapered by increasing the time interval between doses as the condition responds. Or apply 0.5 to 1 inch into the conjunctival sac(s) at night in conjunction with the use of drops during the day, or before an eye is patched.

Storage – Store away from heat.

SULFISOXAZOLE DIOLAMINE

Complete prescribing information is found in the Sulfonamides group monograph.

Rx	**Gantrisin** (Roche)	**Solution**: 4%	With 1:100,000 phenylmercuric nitrate. In 15 ml with dropper.

SULFACETAMIDE SODIUM

Complete prescribing information is found in the Sulfonamides group monograph.

Rx	**Sulfacetamide Sodium** (Various, eg, Bausch & Lomb, Fougera, Geneva, Moore, Optopics, Rugby, Schein, Steris, URL, Zenith Goldline)	**Solution**: 10%	In 15 ml.
Rx	**AK-Sulf** (Akorn)		In 2, 5 and 15 ml.[1]
Rx	**Bleph-10** (Allergan)		In 2.5, 5 and 15 ml.[2]
Rx	**Ocusulf-10** (Optopics)		In 2, 5 and 15 ml.[3]
Rx	**Sodium Sulamyd** (Schering)		In 5 and 15 ml.[1]
Rx	**Sulf-10** (Ciba Vision)		In 1 ml Dropperettes[4] and 15 ml dropper bottles.[5]
Rx	**Isopto Cetamide** (Alcon)	**Solution**: 15%	In 5 and 15 ml Drop-Tainers.[6]
Rx	**Sulfacetamide Sodium** (Various, eg, Schein, Steris)	**Solution**: 30%	In 15 ml.
Rx	**Sodium Sulamyd** (Schering)		In 15 ml.[7]

Rx	**Sodium Sulfacetamide** (Various, eg, Fougera, Moore, URL)	**Ointment**: 10%	In 3.5 g
Rx	**AK-Sulf** (Akorn)		In 3.5 g.[8]
Rx	**Bleph-10** (Allergan)		In 3.5 g.[9]
Rx	**Cetamide** (Alcon)		In 3.5 g.[10]
Rx	**Sodium Sulamyd** (Schering)		In 3.5 g.[11]

[1] With 3.1 mg sodium thiosulfate pentahydrate, 5 mg methylcellulose, 0.5 mg methylparaben and 0.1 mg propylparaben per ml.
[2] With 1.4% polyvinyl alcohol, 0.005% benzalkonium chloride, polysorbate 80, sodium thiosulfate and EDTA.
[3] With parabens, 1.4% polyvinyl alcohol and sodium thiosulfate.
[4] With sodium thiosulfate and 0.005% thimerosal.
[5] With 0.1% hydroxypropyl methylcellulose 2208, sodium thiosulfate and 0.01% thimerosal.
[6] With 0.05% methylparaben, 0.01% propylparaben, 0.5% hydroxypropyl methylcellulose 2910 and 0.3% sodium thiosulfate.
[7] With 1.5 mg sodium thiosulfate pentahydrate, 0.5 mg methylparaben and 0.1 mg propylparaben per ml.
[8] With 0.5 mg methylparaben, 0.1 mg propylparaben, 0.25 mg benzalkonium chloride and petrolatum base per g.
[9] With 0.0008% phenylmercuric acetate, white petrolatum, mineral oil, petrolatum and lanolin alcohol.
[10] With 0.05% methylparaben, 0.01% propylparaben, white petrolatum, anhydrous liquid lanolin and mineral oil.
[11] With 0.5 mg methylparaben, 0.1 mg propylparaben, 0.25 mg benzalkonium chloride and petrolatum base per g.

SULFONAMIDE/DECONGESTANT COMBINATION

Complete prescribing information is found in the Sulfonamides group monograph.

In this combination, phenylephrine HCl, an alpha sympathetic receptor agonist, produces vasoconstriction.

Administration and Dosage:

Instill 1 or 2 drops into the lower conjunctival sac(s) every 2 or 3 hours during the day, less often at night.

Storage: Keep tightly closed. Protect from light.

Rx	**Vasosulf** (Ciba Vision)	**Solution**: 15% sodium sulfacetamide and 0.125% phenylephrine HCl	With sodium thiosulfate, poloxamer 188 and parabens. In 5 and 15 ml.

STEROID AND SULFONAMIDE COMBINATIONS, SUSPENSIONS AND SOLUTIONS

The information for steroid preparations and sulfonamide preparations must be considered when using these products. See individual monographs.

Indications:

Inflammation/Infection: For corticosteroid-responsive inflammatory ocular conditions for which a corticosteroid is indicated and where superficial bacterial ocular infection or a risk of infection exists.

Administration and Dosage:

Solutions/Suspensions: Instill 1 to 3 drops into the conjunctival sac(s) every 1 to 4 hours during the day and at bedtime until a favorable response is obtained.

Do not prescribe > 20 ml initially, and the prescription should not be refilled without further evaluation.

For complete dosage instructions, see individual manufacturer inserts.

> *Storage* – Protect from light. Do not freeze. Shake suspensions well before using. Do not use if solution or suspension has darkened. Clumping may occur on long standing at high temperatures.

Ointments: Apply a small amount (≈ ¼ inch ribbon) into the conjunctival sac(s) 3 or 4 times daily and once at bedtime (or once or twice at night) until a favorable response is obtained.

Do not prescribe > 8 g initially, and the prescription should not be refilled without further evaluation.

For complete dosage instructions, see individual manufacturer inserts.

> *Storage* – Keep tightly closed. Store away from heat.

	Product & Distributor	Steroid	Sulfonamide	Other Content	How Supplied
Rx	**FML-S Suspension** (Allergan)	0.1% fluorometholone	10% sodium sulfacetamide	EDTA, 1.4% polyvinyl alcohol, 0.006% benzalkonium chloride, polysorbate 80, povidone, sodium thiosulfate, sodium chloride	In 5 and 10 ml.
Rx	**Blephamide Suspension** (Allergan)	0.2% prednisolone acetate	10% sodium sulfacetamide	EDTA, 1.4% polyvinyl alcohol, polysorbate 80, sodium thiosulfate, benzalkonium chloride	In 2.5, 5 and 10 ml.
Rx	**Isopto Cetapred Suspension** (Alcon)	0.25% prednisolone acetate	10% sodium sulfacetamide	0.5% hydroxypropyl methylcellulose 2910, EDTA, polysorbate 80, sodium thiosulfate, 0.025% benzalkonium chloride, 0.05% methylparaben, 0.01% propylparaben	In 5 and 15 ml Drop-Tainers.
Rx	**AK-Cide Suspension** (Akorn)	0.5% prednisolone acetate	10% sodium sulfacetamide	5 mg phenethyl alcohol, tyloxapol, sodium thiosulfate, 0.25 mg benzalkonium chloride and EDTA per ml	In 5 ml dropper bottle.
Rx	**Metimyd Suspension** (Schering)			0.5% phenylethyl alcohol, 0.025% benzalkonium chloride, sodium thiosulfate, EDTA, tyloxapol	In 5 ml.
Rx	**Sulfacetamide Sodium and Prednisolone Sodium Phosphate** (Schein)	0.25% prednisolone sodium phosphate	10% sodium sulfacetamide	0.01% mg thimerosal, EDTA, boric acid	In 5 and 10 ml.
Rx	**Sulster Solution** (Akorn)			0.01% mg thimerosal, EDTA	In 5 and 10 ml.
Rx	**Vasocidin Solution** (Ciba Vision)			EDTA, 0.01% thimerosal, poloxamer 407	In 5 and 10 ml.

STEROID AND SULFONAMIDE COMBINATIONS, OINTMENTS

	Product & Distributor	Steroid	Sulfonamide	Other Content	How Supplied
Rx	**Blephamide** (Allergan)	0.2% prednisolone acetate	10% sodium sulfacetamide	0.0008% phenylmercuric acetate, mineral oil, white petrolatum, lanolin alcohol	In 3.5 g.
Rx	**Cetapred** (Alcon)	0.25% prednisolone acetate	10% sodium sulfacetamide	Mineral oil, white petrolatum, lanolin oil, 0.05% methylparaben, 0.01% propylparaben	In 3.5 g.
Rx	**AK-Cide** (Akorn)	0.5% prednisolone acetate	10% sodium sulfacetamide	0.5 mg methylparaben, 0.1 mg propylparaben per g, mineral oil, white petrolatum	In 3.5 g applicator tube.
Rx	**Metimyd** (Schering)			Mineral oil, white petrolatum, 0.05% methylparaben, 0.01% propylparaben	In 3.5 g.
Rx	**Vasocidin** (Ciba Vision)			Mineral oil, white petrolatum	In 3.5 g.

SILVER NITRATE

Actions:

Pharmacology: Silver nitrate ophthalmic solution is an anti-infective. In weak solutions, it is used as a germicide and astringent to mucous membranes. The germicidal action is due to precipitation of bacterial proteins by liberated silver ions.

Indications:

Ophthalmic neonatorum: Prevention of gonorrheal ophthalmia neonatorum.

Contraindications:

Hypersensitivity to any component of the formulation.

Warnings:

Neonatal chlamydial conjunctivitis: Silver nitrate has **not** been effective for the prevention of neonatal chlamydial conjunctivitis.

Cauterization of cornea: A 1% solution is considered optimal. Use with caution, since cauterization of the cornea and blindness may result, especially with repeated applications.

Caustic/Irritant: Silver nitrate is caustic and irritating to the skin and mucous membranes.

Precautions:

Staining: Handle solutions carefully since they tend to stain skin and utensils. Stains may be removed from linen by applications of iodine tincture followed by sodium thiosulfate solution.

Drug Interactions:

Sulfonamide preparations are incompatible with silver preparations.

Adverse Reactions:

A mild chemical conjunctivitis should result from a properly performed Credé prophylaxis using silver nitrate. A more severe chemical conjunctivitis occurs in ≤ 20% of cases.

Overdosage:

When ingested, silver nitrate is highly toxic to the GI tract and CNS. Swallowing can cause severe gastroenteritis that may be fatal. Sodium chloride may be used by gastric lavage to remove the chemical.

When a solution of ≥ 2% silver nitrate concentration is used in the eye, conjunctivitis may be produced. Irrigate the eye with an isotonic solution of sodium chloride after solutions of silver nitrate stronger than 1% are instilled.

Administration and Dosage:

Immediately after birth, clean the child's eyelids with sterile absorbent cotton or gauze and sterile water. Use a separate pledget for each eye; wash unopened lids from the nose outward until free of blood, mucus or meconium. Next, separate the lids and instill 2 drops of 1% solution. Elevate lids away from the eyeball so that a lake of silver nitrate may lie for ≥ 30 seconds between them, contacting the entire conjunctival sac.

The American Academy of Pediatrics has endorsed a statement from the Committee on Ophthalmia Neonatorum of the National Society for the Prevention of Blindness, which does not recommend irrigation of the eyes following instillation of the silver nitrate.

Storage: Do not freeze. Do not use when cold. Protect from light.

Rx	**Silver Nitrate** (Lilly)	**Solution:** 1%	With acetic acid and sodium acetate. In 100s (wax ampules).

ZINC SULFATE SOLUTION

Indications:

Astringent: A mild astringent for temporary relief of minor eye irritation.

Warnings:

Irritation/Eye pain: If irritation persists or increases, or if eye pain or a change in vision occurs, discontinue use and consult physician.

Administration and Dosage:

Instill 1 to 2 drops into eye(s) up to 4 times daily. If solution discolors or becomes cloudy, do not use.

otc	**Eye-Sed** (Scherer)	**Solution:** 0.25%	In 15 ml.[1]

[1] With 0.05% tetrahydrozoline HCl, EDTA, benzalkonium Cl and NaCl.

NATAMYCIN

Actions:

Pharmacology: Natamycin, a tetraene polyene antibiotic, is derived from *Streptomyces natalensis.* It possesses in vitro activity against a variety of yeast and filamentous fungi, including *Candida, Aspergillus, Cephalosporium, Fusarium* and *Penicillium.* The mechanism of action appears to be through binding of the molecule to the fungal cell membrane. The polyenesterol complex alters membrane permeability, depleting essential cellular constituents. Although activity against fungi is dose-related, natamycin is predominantly fungicidal. It is not effective in vitro against gram-negative or gram-positive bacteria.

Pharmacokinetics: Topical administration appears to produce effective concentrations within the corneal stroma, but not in intraocular fluid. Absorption from the GI tract is very poor. Systemic absorption should not occur after topical administration.

Indications:

Fungal blepharitis, conjunctivitis and keratitis caused by susceptible organisms. Natamycin is the initial drug of choice in *Fusarium solani* keratitis.

Contraindications:

Hypersensitivity to any component of the formulation.

Warnings:

Pregnancy: Catagory C. Safety for use during pregnancy has not been established. Use only when clearly needed and when potential benefits outweigh potential hazards to the fetus.

Lactation: It is not known if natamycin is excreted in breast milk. Use with caution in nursing women.

Children: Safety and efficacy have not been established

Precautions:

For topical use only. Not for injection.

Fungal endophthalmitis: The effectiveness of topical natamycin as a single agent in fungal endophthalmitis has not been established.

Resistance: Failure of keratitis to improve following 7 to 10 days of administration suggests that the infection may be caused by a microorganism not susceptible to natamycin. Base continuation of therapy on clinical reevaluation and additional laboratory studies.

Toxicity: Adherence of the suspension to areas of epithelial ulceration or retention in the fornices occurs regularly. Should suspicion of drug toxicity occur, discontinue the drug.

Diagnosis/Monitoring: Determine initial and sustained therapy of fungal keratitis by the clinical diagnosis (laboratory diagnosis by smear and culture of corneal scrapings) and by response to the drug. Whenever possible, determine the in vitro activity of natamycin against the responsible fungus. Monitor tolerance to natamycin at least twice weekly.

Adverse Reactions:

One case of conjunctival chemosis and hyperemia, thought to be allergic in nature, was reported.

Patient Information:

Refer to the Dosage Forms and Routes of Administration chapter for more complete information.

Administration and Dosage:

Fungal keratitis: Instill 1 drop into the conjunctival sac at 1 or 2 hour intervals. The frequency of application can usually be reduced to 1 drop 6 to 8 times daily after the first 3 to 4 days. Generally, continue therapy for 14 to 21 days, or until there is resolution of active fungal keratitis. In many cases, it may help to reduce the dosage gradually at 4 to 7 day intervals to ensure that the organism has been eliminated.

Fungal blepharitis and conjunctivitis: 4 to 6 daily applications may be sufficient.

Shake well before each use.

Storage: Store at room temperature 8° to 24°C (46° to 75°F) or refrigerate at 2° to 8°C (36° to 46°F). Do not freeze. Avoid exposure to light and excessive heat.

Rx	**Natacyn** (Alcon)	**Suspension**: 5%	With 0.02% benzalkonium chloride. In 15 ml.

VIDARABINE (Adenine Arabinoside; Ara-A)

Actions:

Pharmacology: The antiviral mechanism of action has not been established. Vidarabine appears to interfere with the early steps of viral DNA synthesis. It is rapidly deaminated to arabinosylhypoxanthine (Ara-Hx), the principal metabolite. Ara-Hx also possesses in vitro antiviral activity less than that of vidarabine. In contrast to topical idoxuridine, vidarabine demonstrated less cellular toxicity in regenerating corneal epithelium of rabbits.

Pharmacokinetics:

Absorption – Systemic absorption is not expected to occur following ocular administration and swallowing lacrimal secretions. In laboratory animals, vidarabine is rapidly deaminated in the GI tract to Ara-Hx.

Distribution – Because of its low solubility, trace amounts of both vidarabine and Ara-Hx can be detected in the aqueous humor only if there is an epithelial defect in the cornea. If the cornea is normal, only trace amounts of Ara-Hx can be recovered from the aqueous humor.

Microbiology: Vidarabine possesses in vitro and in vivo antiviral activity against herpes simplex types 1 and 2, varicella-zoster and vaccinia viruses. Except for rhabdovirus and oncornavirus, it does not display antiviral activity against other RNA or DNA viruses, including adenovirus.

Indications:

Acute keratoconjunctivitis and recurrent epithelial keratitis due to herpes simplex virus types 1 and 2.

Superficial keratitis caused by herpes simplex virus which has not responded to topical idoxuridine, or when toxic or hypersensitivity reactions to idoxuridine have occurred.

Contraindications:

Hypersensitivity to vidarabine; sterile trophic ulcers. Corticosteroids alone are normally contraindicated in herpes simplex virus eye infections.

Warnings:

Efficacy in other conditions: Vidarabine is not effective against RNA virus, adenoviral ocular infections, bacterial, fungal or chlamydial infections of the cornea, or trophic ulcers. Effectiveness against stromal keratitis and uveitis due to herpes simplex virus has not been established.

Corticosteroids alone are normally contraindicated in herpes simplex virus eye infections. If vidarabine is coadministered with topical corticosteroid therapy, consider corticosteroid-induced ocular side effects such as glaucoma or cataract formation and progression of bacterial or viral infection.

Temporary visual haze may be produced with vidarabine.

Carcinogenesis: In female mice treated with IM vidarabine, there was an increase in liver tumor incidence; some male mice developed kidney neoplasia.

In rats, intestinal, testicular and thyroid neoplasia occurred with greater frequency among the vidarabine-treated animals.

Mutagenesis: In vitro, vidarabine can be incorporated into mammalian DNA and can induce mutation. In vivo studies have not been conclusive; however, vidarabine may be capable of producing mutagenic effects in male germ cells.

Vidarabine has caused chromosome breaks and gaps when added to human leukocytes in vitro. While the significance is not fully understood, there is a well known correlation between the ability of various agents to produce such effects and their ability to produce heritable genetic damage.

Pregnancy: Category C. A 10% ointment applied to 10% of the body surface during organogenesis induced fetal abnormalities in rabbits. The possibility of embryonic or fetal damage in pregnant women is remote. The topical ophthalmic dose is small, and the drug is relatively insoluble. Its ocular penetration is very low. However, a safe dose for a human embryo or fetus has not been established, and there are no adequate and well controlled studies in pregnant women. Therefore, use only if the potential benefit outweighs the potential risk to the fetus.

Lactation: It is not known whether vidarabine is excreted in breast milk. Excretion of vidarabine in breast milk is unlikely because the drug is rapidly deaminated in the GI tract. However, it is still recommended that either nursing or the drug be discontinued, taking into account the importance of the drug to the mother.

Precautions:

Viral resistance to vidarabine has not been observed, although this possibility exists.

Adverse Reactions:

Lacrimation; foreign body sensation; conjunctival infection; burning; irritation; superficial punctate keratitis; pain; photophobia; punctal occlusion; sensitivity.

Uveitis, stromal edema, secondary glaucoma, trophic defects, corneal vascularization and hyphema have occurred but may be disease-related.

Overdosage:

The rapid deamination to Ara-Hx should preclude any difficulty. No untoward effects should result from ingestion of the entire contents of a tube. Overdosage by ocular instillation is unlikely because any excess is quickly expelled from the conjunctival sac. Avoid too frequent administration.

Patient Information:

May cause sensitivity to bright light; this may be minimized by wearing sunglasses.

Notify physician if improvement is not seen after 7 days, if condition or pain worsens, or if a decrease in vision, burning or irritation of the eye occurs. Do not discontinue use without consulting physician.

Refer to the Dosage Forms and Routes of Administration chapter for more complete information.

Administration and Dosage:

Administer approximately 0.5 inch of ointment into the lower conjunctival sac(s) 5 times daily at 3 hour intervals.

If there are no signs of improvement after 7 days, or if complete re-epithelialization has not occurred in 21 days, consider other forms of therapy. Some severe cases may require longer treatment.

After re-epithelialization has occurred, treat for an additional 7 days at a reduced dosage (such as twice daily) to prevent recurrence.

Concomitant therapy: Topical corticosteroids (prednisolone or dexamethasone) have been administered concurrently with vidarabine without an increase in adverse reactions, although their advantages and disadvantages must be considered (see Warnings).

Rx	**Vira-A** (Parke-Davis)	**Ointment:** 3% vidarabine monohydrate (equivalent to 2.8% vidarabine)	In a liquid petrolatum base. In 3.5 g.

TRIFLURIDINE (Trifluorothymidine)

Actions:

Pharmacology: A fluorinated pyrimidine nucleoside with in vitro and in vivo activity against herpes simplex virus types 1 and 2, and vaccinia virus. Some strains of adenovirus are also inhibited in vitro. Trifluridine interferes with DNA synthesis in cultured mammalian cells. However, its antiviral mechanism of action is not completely known.

Pharmacokinetics:

> *Absorption* – Intraocular penetration occurs after topical instillation. Decreased corneal integrity or stromal or uveal inflammation may enhance the penetration into the aqueous humor. Systemic absorption following therapeutic dosing appears negligible.

Indications:

Primary keratoconjunctivitis and recurrent epithelial keratitis due to herpes simplex virus types 1 and 2.

Epithelial keratitis that has not responded clinically to topical idoxuridine, or when ocular toxicity or hypersensitivity to idoxuridine has occurred. In a smaller number of patients resistant to topical vidarabine, trifluridine was also effective.

Contraindications:

Hypersensitivity reactions or chemical intolerance to trifluridine.

Warnings:

Efficacy in other conditions: The clinical efficacy in the treatment of stromal keratitis and uveitis due to herpes simplex or ophthalmic infections caused by vaccinia virus and adenovirus, or in the prophylaxis of herpes simplex virus keratoconjunctivitis and epithelial keratitis has not been established by well controlled clinical trials. Not effective against bacterial, fungal or chlamydial infections of the cornea or trophic lesions.

Dosage/Frequency: Do not exceed the recommended dosage or frequency of administration.

Mutagenesis: Trifluridine has exerted mutagenic, DNA-damaging and cell-transforming activities in various standard in vitro test systems. Although the significance of these test results is not clear or fully understood, it is possible that mutagenic agents may cause genetic damage in humans.

Pregnancy: Category C. Fetal toxicity consisting of delayed ossification of portions of the skeleton occurred at dose levels of 2.5 and 5 mg/kg/day in rats and rabbits. In addition, both 2.5 and 5 mg/kg/day produced fetal death and resorption in rabbits. There are no adequate and well controlled studies in pregnant women. Use during pregnancy only if the potential benefit justifies the risk to the fetus.

Lactation: It is unlikely that trifluridine is excreted in breast milk after ophthalmic instillation because of the relatively small dosage (≤ 5 mg/day), its dilution in body fluids and its extremely short half-life (≈ 12 minutes). However, do not prescribe for nursing mothers unless the potential benefits outweigh the potential risks.

Precautions:

Viral resistance, although documented in vitro, has not been reported following multiple exposure to trifluridine; this possibility may exist.

Adverse Reactions:

The most frequent adverse reactions reported are mild, transient burning or stinging upon instillation (4.6%) and palpebral edema (2.8%). Other adverse reactions in decreasing order of reported frequency were: Superficial punctate keratopathy; epithelial keratopathy; hypersensitivity reaction; stromal edema; irritation; keratitis sicca; hyperemia and increased intraocular pressure.

Overdosage:

Local: Overdosage by ocular instillation is unlikely because any excess solution is quickly expelled from the conjunctival sac.

Systemic: No untoward effects are likely to result from ingestion of the entire contents of a bottle. Single IV doses of 15 to 30 mg/kg/day in children and adults with neoplastic disease produce reversible bone marrow depression as the only potentially serious toxic effect and only after three to five courses of therapy.

Patient Information:

Transient stinging may occur upon installation.

Notify physician if improvement is not seen after 7 days, if condition worsens or if irritation occurs. Do not discontinue use without consulting physician.

Refer to the Dosage Forms and Routes of Administration chapter for more complete information.

Administration and Dosage:

Instill 1 drop onto the cornea of the affected eye(s) every 2 hours while awake for a maximum daily dosage of 9 drops until the corneal ulcer has completely re-epithelialized. Following re-epithelialization, treat for an additional 7 days with 1 drop every 4 hours while awake for a minimum daily dosage of 5 drops.

If there are no signs of improvement after 7 days, or if complete re-epithelialization has not occurred after 14 days, consider other forms of therapy. Avoid continuous administration for periods > 21 days because of potential ocular toxicity.

Storage/Stability: Store under refrigeration, 2° to 8°C (36° to 46°F).

Rx	**Trifluridine** (Schein)	**Solution:** 1%	In aqueous solution with NaCl and 0.001% thimerosal. In 7.5 ml Drop-Dose.
Rx	**Viroptic** (Monarch)		

GANCICLOVIR (DHPG) CAPSULES AND POWDER FOR INJECTION

Warning:

The clinical toxicity of ganciclovir includes granulocytopenia, anemia and thrombocytopenia. In animal studies, ganciclovir was carcinogenic, teratogenic and caused aspermatogenesis.

Ganciclovir IV is indicated for use only in the treatment of cytomegalovirus (CMV) retinitis in immunocompromised patients and for the prevention of CMV disease in transplant patients at risk for CMV disease.

Because oral ganciclovir is associated with a risk of more rapid rate of CMV retinitis progression, use only in those patients for whom this risk is balanced by the benefit associated with avoiding daily IV infusions.

Actions:

Pharmacology: Ganciclovir, a synthetic guanine derivative active against cytomegalovirus (CMV), is an acyclic nucleoside analog of 2′-deoxyguanosine that inhibits replication of herpes viruses both in vitro and in vivo. Sensitive human viruses include CMV, herpes simplex virus-1 and -2, herpes virus type 6, Epstein-Barr virus, varicella-zoster virus and hepatitis B virus.

Ganciclovir must be converted to the corresponding triphosphate in order to exert its antiviral activity. In herpes simplex virus-infected cells, the initial conversion to the monophosphate is catalyzed by a viral thymidine kinase. In contrast, in CMV-infected cells, a protein kinase homologue may be responsible for the initial phosphorylation of ganciclovir. Cellular kinases, in CMV-infected cells, subsequently phosphorylate ganciclovir monophosphate to the diphosphate and active triphosphate moieties. Levels of ganciclovir triphosphate are as much as 100-fold greater in CMV-infected cells than in uninfected cells, indicating a preferential phosphorylation of ganciclovir in virus-infected cells. Ganciclovir triphosphate, once formed, appears quite stable and persists for days in the CMV-infected cell. The antiviral activity of ganciclovir triphosphate is believed to be the result of inhibition of viral DNA synthesis by two known modes: (1) Competitive inhibition of viral DNA polymerases; and (2) direct incorporation into viral DNA, resulting in eventual termination of viral DNA elongation. The cellular DNA polymerase alpha is also inhibited, but at a higher concentration than required for inhibition of viral DNA polymerase.

The median concentration of ganciclovir which effectively inhibits the replication of either laboratory strains or clinical isolates of CMV (ED_{50}) has ranged from 0.02 to 3.48 mcg/ml. The relationship of in vitro sensitivity of CMV to ganciclovir and clinical response has not been established. Ganciclovir inhibits mammalian cell proliferation in vitro at higher concentrations: IC_{50} values range from 30 to 725 mcg/ml, with the exception of bone marrow-derived colony-forming cells which are more sensitive with IC_{50} values ranging from 0.028 to 0.7 mcg/ml.

Pharmacokinetics:

Absorption – The absolute bioavailability of oral ganciclovir under fasting conditions was ≈ 5% and following food it was 6% to 9%. When given with a meal containing 602 calories and 46.5% fat, the steady-state area under serum concentration vs time curve (AUC) increased and there was a significant prolongation of time to peak serum concentrations (see Drug Interactions).

At the end of a 1 hour IV infusion of 5 mg/kg, total AUC ranged between 22.1 and 26.8 mcg•hr/ml and C_{max} ranged between 8.27 and 9 mcg/ml.

Distribution – The steady-state volume of distribution after IV administration was 0.74 L/kg. Cerebrospinal fluid concentrations obtained 0.25 and 5.67 hours post-dose in three patients who received 2.5 mg/kg ganciclovir IV every 8 or 12 hours ranged from 0.31 to 0.68 mcg/ml, representing 24% to 70% of the respective plasma concentrations. Binding to plasma proteins was 1% to 2% over ganciclovir concentrations of 0.5 and 51 mcg/ml.

Metabolism – Following oral administration of a single 1000 mg dose, 86% of the administered dose was recovered in the feces and 5% was recovered in the urine. No metabolite accounted for 1% to 2% recovered in urine or feces.

Excretion – When administered IV, ganciclovir exhibits linear pharmacokinetics over the range of 1.6 to 5 mg/kg and when administered orally, it exhibits linear kinetics up to a total daily dose of 4 g/day. Renal excretion of unchanged drug by glomerular filtration and active tubular secretion is the major route of elimination. In patients with normal renal function, 91.3% of IV ganciclovir was recovered unmetabolized in the urine. Systemic clearance of IV ganciclovir was 3.52 ml/min/kg while renal clearance was 3.2 ml/min/kg, accounting for 91% of the systemic clearance. After oral administration, steady state is achieved within 24 hours. Renal clearance following oral administration was 3.1 ml/min/kg. Half-life was 3.5 hours following IV administration and 4.8 following oral use.

Renal function impairment – Because the major elimination pathway for ganciclovir is renal, dosage must be reduced according to creatinine clearance (Ccr; see Administration and Dosage). The pharmacokinetics following IV administration were evaluated in 10 immunocompromised patients with renal impairment who received doses ranging from 1.25 to 5 mg/kg.

IV Ganciclovir Pharmacokinetics in Patients with Renal Impairment

Ccr (ml/min)	Dose (mg/kg)	Clearance (ml/min)	Half-life (hours)
50-79 (n = 4)	3.2-5	128	4.6
25-49 (n = 3)	3-5	57	4.4
< 25 (n = 3)	1.25-5	30	10.7

The pharmacokinetics following oral administration were evaluated in eight solid organ transplant recipients; dose was modified according to estimated Ccr.

Oral Ganciclovir in Patients with Renal Impairment

Ccr (ml/min)	Dose (mg/kg)	AUC_{0-24} (mcg•hr/ml)	Half-life (hours)
50-69 (n = 4)	1000 mg q 8 hr	49.1 ± 12.2	NC[1]
25-49 (n = 1)	1000 mg every day	27.4	18.2
10-24 (n = 1)	500 mg every day	10.7	15.7
< 10 (n = 2)	500 mg 3 times weekly[2]	25.6 ± 5.9	NC[1]

[1] NC = Not calculated; half-life exceeded sampling interval.
[2] After hemodialysis.

Hemodialysis reduces plasma concentrations of ganciclovir by about 50% after both IV and oral administration.

Race – The effects of race were studied in subjects receiving a dose regimen of 1000 mg every 8 hours. Although the numbers of African Americans (16%) and Hispanics (20%) were small, there appeared to be a trend towards a lower steady-state C_{max} and $AUC_{0\text{-}8}$ in these subpopulations as compared to Caucasians.

Children – At an IV dose of 4 or 6 mg/kg in 27 neonates (aged 2 to 49 days), the pharmacokinetic parameters were, respectively, C_{max} of 5.5 and 7 mcg/ml, systemic clearance of 3.14 and 3.56 ml/min/kg and half-life of 2.4 hours for both.

Clinical trials:

IV – Immunocompromised patients – Of 314 immunocompromised patients enrolled in an open label study of the treatment of life- or sight-threatening CMV disease, 121 patients had a positive culture for CMV within 7 days prior to treatment.

Virologic Response to IV Ganciclovir Treatment			
Culture source	No. patients cultured	No. (%) patients responding	Median days to response
Urine	107	93 (87%)	8
Blood	41	34 (83%)	8
Throat	21	19 (90%)	7
Semen	6	6 (100%)	15

Transplant recipients – In 149 CMV seropositive heart allograft recipients and 72 CMV culture positive allogeneic bone marrow transplant recipients, ganciclovir prevented recrudescence of CMV shedding in the heart allograft patients and suppressed CMV shedding in the bone marrow allograft patients.

Patients with Positive CMV Cultures Following IV Ganciclovir				
	Heart allograft		Bone marrow allograft	
Time	Ganciclovir	Placebo	Ganciclovir	Placebo
Pre-Treatment	2%	8%	100%	100%
Week 2	3%	16%	6%	68%
Week 4	5%	43%	0%	80%

Oral – The antiviral activity of ganciclovir capsules was confirmed in two randomized, controlled trials comparing IV vs oral ganciclovir for the maintenance treatment of CMV retinitis in patients with acquired immunodeficiency syndrome (AIDS). Only a small proportion of patients remained culture-positive during maintenance therapy with either IV or oral ganciclovir. There were no statistically significant differences in the rates of positive cultures between the treatment groups. The antiviral effect of oral ganciclovir in the patients in the two studies is summarized in the following table:

Patients with Positive CMV Following Oral Ganciclovir				
	Patients with newly diagnosed CMV retinitis[1]		Patients with stable, previously treated CMV retinitis[2]	
	IV	Oral	IV	Oral[3]
At start of maintenance	13.5%	24.3%	3%	3.6%
Anytime during maintenance	6.3%	9.1%	2.2%	7.1%

[1] 3 weeks of treatment with IV ganciclovir before start of maintenance.
[2] 4 weeks to 4 months treatment with IV ganciclovir before start of maintenance.
[3] Data from 6 times daily and 3 times daily regimens pooled.

Viral resistance – CMV resistance to ganciclovir in individuals with AIDS and CMV retinitis who have not previously been treated with ganciclovir does occur but appears to be infrequent. Viral resistance has been observed in patients receiving prolonged treatment with ganciclovir IV. However, due to the limited number of viral isolates tested, it is difficult to estimate the overall frequency of reduced sensitivity in patients receiving ganciclovir. Nonetheless, consider the possibility of viral resistance in patients who show poor clinical response or experience persistent viral excretion during therapy. The principal mechanism of resistance to ganciclovir in CMV is the decreased ability to form the active triphosphate moiety. Mutations in the viral DNA polymerase have also been reported to confer viral resistance to ganciclovir. In two randomized controlled trials, the incidence of reduced sensitivity appeared to be no more common during treatment with oral ganciclovir than during IV treatment.

Indications:

IV:

CMV retinitis – Treatment of CMV retinitis in immunocompromised patients, including patients with AIDS.

CMV disease – Prevention of CMV disease in transplant recipients at risk for CMV disease.

Oral: Alternative to the IV formulation for maintenance treatment of CMV retinitis in immunocompromised patients, including patients with AIDS, in whom retinitis is stable following appropriate induction therapy and for whom the risk of more rapid progression is balanced by the benefit associated with avoiding daily IV infusions.

Unlabeled uses: Ganciclovir may also be beneficial in some immunocompromised patients in the treatment of other CMV infections (eg, pneumonitis, gastroenteritis, hepatitis [see Warnings]).

Contraindications:

Hypersensitivity to ganciclovir or acyclovir.

Warnings:

CMV disease: Safety and efficacy have not been established for congenital or neonatal CMV disease nor for the treatment of established CMV disease other than retinitis nor for use in non-immunocompromised individuals. The safety and efficacy of oral ganciclovir have not been established for treating any manifestation of CMV disease other than maintenance treatment of CMV retinitis.

Diagnosis of CMV retinitis is ophthalmologic and should be made by indirect ophthalmoscopy. Other conditions in the differential diagnosis of CMV retinitis include candidiasis, toxoplasmosis, histoplasmosis, retinal scars and cotton wool spots, any of which may produce a retinal appearance similar to CMV. The diagnosis may be supported by culture of CMV from urine, blood, throat, etc, but a negative CMV culture does not rule out CMV retinitis.

Retinal detachment has been observed in subjects with CMV retinitis both before and after initiation of therapy with ganciclovir. Its relationship to therapy is unknown. Retinal detachment occurred in 11% of patients treated with IV ganciclovir and in 8% of patients treated with oral ganciclovir. Patients with CMV retinitis should have frequent ophthalmologic evaluations to monitor the status of their retinitis and to detect any other retinal pathology.

Hematologic: Do not administer if the absolute neutrophil count is < $500/mm^3$ or the platelet count is < $25{,}000/mm^3$. Granulocytopenia (neutropenia), anemia and thrombocytopenia have been observed in patients treated with ganciclovir. The frequency and severity of these events vary widely in different patient populations (see Adverse Reactions). Therefore, use with caution in patients with pre-existing cytopenias or with a history of cytopenic reactions to other drugs, chemicals or irradiation. Granulocytopenia usually occurs during the first or second week of treatment, but may occur at any time during treatment. Cell counts usually begin to recover within 3 to 7 days of discontinuing drug. Colony-stimulating factors have increased neutrophil and WBC counts in patients receiving IV ganciclovir for CMV retinitis.

Renal function impairment: Use ganciclovir with caution because the half-life and plasma/serum concentrations of ganciclovir will be increased due to reduced renal clearance (see Administration and Dosage).

Hemodialysis reduces plasma levels of ganciclovir by approximately 50%.

Carcinogenesis/Mutagenesis/Fertility impairment: In mice, daily oral doses of 1000 mg/kg may have caused an increased incidence of tumors in the preputial gland of males, nonglandular mucosa of the stomach of males and females, and reproductive tissues (ovaries, uterus, mammary gland, clitoral gland and vagina) and liver in females. A slightly increased incidence of tumors occurred in the preputial gland (males) and nonglandular mucosa (males and females) of the stomach in mice given 20 mg/kg/day. Consider ganciclovir a potential carcinogen in humans.

Ganciclovir caused point mutations and chromosomal damage in mammalian cells in vitro and in vivo. Because of the mutagenic and teratogenic potential of ganciclovir, advise women of childbearing potential to use effective contraception during treatment. Similarly, advise men to practice barrier contraception during and for at least 90 days following treatment with ganciclovir.

Animal data indicate that ganciclovir causes inhibition of spermatogenesis and subsequent infertility. Ganciclovir caused decreased fertility in male mice and hypospermatogenesis in mice and dogs. These effects were reversible at lower doses and irreversible at higher doses. Although data in humans have not been obtained regarding this effect, it is considered probable that ganciclovir, at the recommended doses, causes temporary or permanent inhibition of spermatogenesis. Animal data also indicate that suppression of fertility in females may occur. Ganciclovir caused decreased mating behavior, decreased fertility and an increased incidence of embryolethality in female mice following IV doses approximately 1.7 times the mean drug exposure in humans.

Elderly: The pharmacokinetic profile in elderly patients has not been established. Since elderly individuals frequently have a reduced glomerular filtration rate, pay particular attention to assessing renal function before and during administration of ganciclovir (see Administration and Dosage).

Pregnancy: Category C. Ganciclovir is embryotoxic in rabbits and mice following IV administration and teratogenic in rabbits. Fetal resorptions were present in at least 85% of rabbits and mice administered 2 times the human exposure. Effects observed in rabbits included: Fetal growth retardation, embryolethality, teratogenicity and maternal toxicity. Teratogenic changes included cleft palate, anophthalmia/microphthalmia, aplastic organs (kidney and pancreas), hydrocephaly and brachygnathia. In mice, effects observed were maternal/fetal toxicity and embryolethality.

Daily IV doses given to female mice prior to mating, during gestation and during lactation caused hypoplasia of the testes and seminal vesicles in the month-old male offspring, as well as pathologic changes in the nonglandular region of the stomach.

Ganciclovir may be teratogenic or embryotoxic at dose levels recommended for human use. There are no adequate and well controlled studies in pregnant women. Use during pregnancy only if the potential benefits justify the potential risk to the fetus.

Lactation: It is not known whether ganciclovir is excreted in breast milk. However, because carcinogenic and teratogenic effects occurred in animals treated with ganciclovir, the possibility of serious adverse reactions from ganciclovir in nursing infants is considered likely. Instruct mothers to discontinue nursing if they are receiving ganciclovir. The minimum interval before nursing can safely be resumed after the last dose of ganciclovir is unknown.

Children: Safety and efficacy in children have not been established. The use of ganciclovir in children warrants extreme caution to the probability of long-term carcinogenicity and reproductive toxicity. Administer to children only after careful evaluation and only if the potential benefits of treatment outweigh the risks. Oral ganciclovir has not been studied in children < 13 years of age.

There has been very limited clinical experience using IV ganciclovir for the treatment of CMV retinitis in patients < 12 years of age. Two children (9 and 5 years of age) showed improvement or stabilization of retinitis for 23 and 9 months, respectively. These children received induction treatment with 2.5 mg/kg 3 times daily followed by maintenance therapy with 6 to 6.5 mg/kg once a day, 5 to 7 days per week. When retinitis progressed during once-daily maintenance therapy, both children were treated with the 5 mg/kg twice-daily regimen. Two other children (2.5 and 4 years of age) who received similar induction regimens showed only partial or no response to treatment. Another child, a 6-year-old with T-cell dysfunction, showed stabilization of retinitis for 3 months while receiving continuous infusions of IV ganciclovir at doses of 2 to 5 mg/kg/24 hours. Continuous infusion treatment was discontinued due to granulocytopenia.

Eleven of the 72 patients in the placebo controlled trial in bone marrow transplant recipients were children, ranging from 3 to 10 years of age (5 treated with IV ganciclovir and 6 with placebo). Five of the pediatric patients treated with ganciclovir received 5 mg/kg IV twice daily for up to 7 days; 4 patients went on to receive 5 mg/kg once daily up to day 100 post-transplant. Results were similar to those observed in adult transplant recipients treated with IV ganciclovir. Two of the 6 placebo-treated pediatric patients developed CMV pneumonia vs none of the 5 treated with ganciclovir. The spectrum of adverse events in the pediatric group was similar to that observed in the adult patients.

The spectrum of adverse reactions reported in 120 immunocompromised pediatric clinical trial participants with serious CMV infections receiving IV ganciclovir were similar to those reported in adults. Granulocytopenia (17%) and thrombocytopenia (10%) were the most common adverse events reported.

Precautions:

Monitoring: Due to the frequency of neutropenia, anemia and thrombocytopenia in patients receiving ganciclovir, it is recommended that complete blood counts and platelet counts be performed frequently, especially in patients in whom ganciclovir or other nucleoside analogs have previously resulted in leukopenia, or in whom neutrophil counts are < 1000/mm^3 at the beginning of treatment. Because dosing with ganciclovir must be modified in patients with renal impairment, and because of the incidence of increased serum creatinine levels that have been observed in transplant recipients treated with IV ganciclovir, patients should have serum creatinine or creatinine clearance values followed carefully.

Large doses/Rapid infusion: The maximum single dose administered was 6 mg/kg by IV infusion over 1 hour. Larger doses have resulted in increased toxicity. It is likely that more rapid infusions would also result in increased toxicity (see Overdosage).

Phlebitis/Pain at injection site: Initially, reconstituted solutions of IV ganciclovir have a high pH (pH 11). Despite further dilution in IV fluids, phlebitis or pain may occur at the site of IV infusion. Take care to infuse solutions containing ganciclovir only into veins with adequate blood flow to permit rapid dilution and distribution.

Hydration: Since ganciclovir is excreted by the kidneys and normal clearance depends on adequate renal function, administration of ganciclovir should be accompanied by adequate hydration.

Photosensitivity: Photosensitization (photoallergy or phototoxicity) may occur; therefore, caution patients to take protective measures against exposure to ultraviolet or sunlight (ie, sunscreens, protective clothing) until tolerance is determined.

Drug Interactions:

Ganciclovir Drug Interactions			
Precipitant drug	Object drug*		Description
Ganciclovir	Cytotoxic drugs	↑	Cytotoxic drugs that inhibit replication of rapidly dividing cell populations such as bone marrow, spermatogonia and germinal layers of skin and GI mucosa may have additive toxicity when administered concomitantly with ganciclovir. Therefore, consider the concomitant use of drugs such as dapsone, pentamidine, flucytosine, vincristine, vinblastine, adriamycin, amphotericin B, trimethoprim/sulfamethoxazole combinations or other nucleoside analogs only if potential benefits outweigh the risks.
Imipenem-cilastatin	Ganciclovir	↑	Generalized seizures occurred in patients who received ganciclovir and imipenem-cilastatin. Do not use these drugs concomitantly unless the potential benefits outweigh the risks.
Nephrotoxic drugs	Ganciclovir	↑	Increases in serum creatinine were observed following concurrent use of ganciclovir and either cyclosporine or amphotericin B (see Warnings).
Probenecid	Ganciclovir	↑	Ganciclovir AUC increased 53% (range, -14% to 299%) in the presence of probenecid. Renal clearance of ganciclovir decreased 22% (range, -54% to -4%), which is consistent with an interaction involving competition for renal tubular secretion.
Ganciclovir	Didanosine	↑	Steady-state didanosine AUC increased 111% (range, 10% to 493%) when didanosine was administered either 2 hours prior to or simultaneously with ganciclovir. A decrease in steady-state ganciclovir AUC of 21% (range, -44% to 5%) was observed when didanosine was administered 2 hours prior to administration of ganciclovir, but ganciclovir AUC was not affected by the presence of didanosine when the two drugs were administered simultaneously.
Didanosine	Ganciclovir	↓	
Ganciclovir	Zidovudine	↑	Mean steady-state ganciclovir AUC decreased 17% (range, -52% to 23%) in the presence of zidovudine. Steady-state zidovudine AUC increased 19% (range, -11% to 74%) in the presence of ganciclovir. Because both drugs can cause granulocytopenia and anemia, many patients will not tolerate combination therapy at full dosage.
Zidovudine	Ganciclovir	↓	

* ↑ = Object drug increased. ↓ = Object drug decreased.

Drug/Food interactions: When ganciclovir was administered orally with food at a total daily dose of 3 g/day (either 500 mg every 3 hours 6 times daily or 1000 mg 3 times daily), the steady-state absorption as measured by AUC and C_{max} were similar following both regimens. When ganciclovir capsules were given with a meal containing 602 calories and 46.5% fat at a dose of 1000 mg every 8 hours to 20 HIV-positive subjects, the steady-state AUC increased by 22% (range, 6% to 68%) and there was a significant prolongation of time to peak serum concentrations (T_{max}) from 1.8 to 3 hours and a higher C_{max} (0.85 vs 0.96 mcg/ml).

Adverse Reactions:

AIDS patients:

Selected Adverse Reactions Reported in ≥ 5% of Subjects: Oral vs IV Ganciclovir Maintenance Treatment		
Adverse reaction	Oral (3000 mg/day) (n = 326)	IV (5 mg/kg/day) (n = 179)
Body as a whole		
Fever	38%	48%
Abdominal pain	17%	19%
Infection	9%	13%
Chills	7%	10%
Sepsis	4%	15%
GI		
Diarrhea	41%	44%
Nausea	26%	25%
Anorexia	15%	14%
Vomiting	13%	13%
Flatulence	6%	3%
Hemic/Lymphatic		
Leukopenia	29%	41%
Anemia	19%	25%
Thrombocytopenia	6%	6%
CNS		
Neuropathy	8%	9%
Paresthesia	6%	10%
Other		
Rash	15%	10%
Sweating	11%	12%
Pruritus	6%	5%
Vitreous disorder	6%	4%
Pneumonia	6%	8%
Catheter-related		
Total catheter events	6%	22%
Catheter infection	4%	9%
Catheter sepsis	1%	8%
Neutropenia (ANC/mm^3)	(n = 320)	(n = 175)
< 500	18	25
500 to < 750	17	14
750 to < 1000	19	26
Total ANC ≤ 1000	54	66
Anemia hemoglobin (g/dl)	(n = 320)	(n = 175)
< 6.5	2	5
6.5 to < 8	10	16
8 to < 9.5	25	26
Total Hb < 9.5	36	46

Overall, subjects treated with IV ganciclovir experienced lower minimum acid-neutralizing capacities (ANCs) and hemoglobin levels, consistent with more neutropenia and anemia, compared with those who received oral ganciclovir.

For the majority of subjects, maximum serum creatinine levels were < 1.5 mg/dl and no difference was noted between IV and oral ganciclovir for the occurrence of renal impairment. Serum creatinine elevations > 2.5 mg/dl occurred in < 2% of all subjects and no significant differences were noted in the time from the start of maintenance to the occurrence of elevations in serum creatinine values.

Transplant recipients:

Granulocytopenia/Thrombocytopenia with IV Ganciclovir				
	Heart allograft[1]		Bone marrow allograft[2]	
Hematologic Effect	Ganciclovir (n = 76)	Placebo (n = 73)	Ganciclovir IV (n = 57)	Control (n = 55)
Neutropenia				
Minimum ANC < 500/mm^3	4%	3%	12%	6%
Minimum ANC 500 - 1000/mm^3	3%	8%	29%	17%
Total ANC ≤ 1000/mm^3	7%	11%	41%	23%
Thrombocytopenia				
Platelet count < 25,000/mm^3	3%	1%	32%	28%
Platelet count 25,000 - 50,000/mm^3	5%	3%	25%	37%
Total Platelet 50,000/mm^3	8%	4%	57%	65%

[1] Mean duration of treatment = 28 days.
[2] Mean duration of treatment = 45 days.

Elevated Serum Creatinine with IV Ganciclovir						
	Heart allograft		Bone marrow allograft			
Maximum serum creatinine levels	Ganciclovir IV (n = 76)	Placebo (n = 73)	Ganciclovir IV (n = 20)	Control (n = 20)	Ganciclovir IV (n = 37)	Placebo (n = 35)
Serum creatinine ≥ 2.5 mg/dl	18%	4%	20%	0%	0%	0%
Serum creatinine ≥ 1.5 - < 2.5 mg/dl	58%	69%	50%	35%	43%	44%

General: Other adverse reactions are listed as follows:

Body as a whole: Asthenia (6%); headache (4%); injection site inflammation, pain (2%); abdomen enlarged, abscess, back pain, cellulitis, chest pain, chills, fever, drug level increased (ganciclovir), edema, face edema, injection site abscess/edema/hemorrhage/pain/phlebitis, lab test abnormality, malaise, photosensitivity reaction, neck pain/rigidity (≤ 1%).

GI: Abnormal liver function test, dyspepsia, nausea, vomiting (2%); constipation, dysphagia, eructation, fecal incontinence, hemorrhage, hepatitis, melena, mouth ulceration, tongue disorder (≤ 1%).

Hematologic: Eosinophilia, hypochromic anemia, marrow depression, pancytopenia (≤ 1%).

Respiratory: Cough increased, dyspnea (≤ 1%).

CNS: Abnormal dreams, abnormal gait, abnormal thinking, agitation, amnesia, anxiety, ataxia, coma, confusion, depression, dizziness, dry mouth, euphoria, hypertonia, hypesthesia, insomnia, libido decreased, manic reaction, nervousness, psychosis, seizures, somnolence, tremor, trismus (≈ 5%).

Dermatologic: Acne, alopecia, dry skin, fixed eruption, herpes simplex, maculopapular rash, skin discoloration, urticaria, vesiculobullous rash (≤ 1%).

Special senses: Abnormal vision, amblyopia, blindness, conjunctivitis, deafness, eye pain, glaucoma, retinitis, photophobia, taste perversion, tinnitus (≤ 1%).

Metabolic/Nutritional: Increased alkaline phosphatase, creatine phosphokinase, lactic dehydrogenase, AST, ALT (≤ 1%); hypokalemia, pancreatitis, decreased blood sugar (≤ 1%).

Cardiovascular: Arrhythmia, deep thrombophlebitis, hypertension, hypotension, vasodilatation (≤ 1%).

GU: Breast pain, creatinine clearance decreased/increased, hematuria, increased BUN, kidney failure, kidney function abnormal, urinary frequency, urinary tract infection.

Musculoskeletal: Myalgia, myasthenia (≤ 1%).

Miscellaneous: Phlebitis (2%); migraine.

The following adverse reactions may be fatal: Pancreatitis, sepsis and multiple organ failure.

Adverse reactions reported in post-market surveillance –

Reported on two or more occasions – Acidosis, anaphylactic reaction, cardiac arrest, cataracts, cholestasis, cholangitis, congenital anomaly, encephalopathy, hyponatremia, impotence, infertility, intracranial hypertension, leukemia, lymphoma, myocardial infarction, pericarditis, Stevens-Johnson syndrome, stroke, transverse myelitis, unexplained death.

Reported once – Allograft rejection, arthritis, asthma, bleeding disorder, cachexia, corneal erosion, cyanosis, diplopia, dry eyes, dysethesia, ear infection, elevated triglyceride levels, endocarditis, exfoliative dermatitis, exacerbation of psoriasis, facial palsy, gangrene, gingival hypertrophy, Guillain-Barre syndrome, hemolytic-uremic syndrome, hypernatremia, hypomagnesemia, icterus, inappropriate serum ADH, increased sweating, irritability, loss of memory, loss of sense of smell, multiple organ failure, myelopathy, myocarditis, nephritis, ophthalmoplegia, parathyroid disorder, Parkinsonism-like reaction, pneumothorax, peripheral ischemia, perforated intestine, pneumonia, proteinuria, pseudotumor cerebri, pulmonary fibrosis, pulmonary embolism, respiratory distress syndrome, rhabdomyolysis, sperm production abnormal, testicular hypotrophy, thyroid disorder, Wolff-Parkinson-White syndrome.

Overdosage:

IV: Overdosage with IV ganciclovir has been reported in 17 patients (13 adults and 4 children < 2 years of age). Five patients experienced no adverse events following overdosage at the following doses: 7 doses of 11 mg/kg over a 3 day period (adult), single dose of 3500 mg (adult), single dose of 500 mg (72.5 mg/kg) followed by 48 hours of peritoneal dialysis (4-month-old), single dose of approximately 60 mg/kg followed by exchange transfusion (18-month-old), 2 doses of 500 mg instead of 31 mg (21 month old).

Irreversible pancytopenia developed in one adult with AIDS and CMV colitis after receiving 3000 mg IV ganciclovir on each of two consecutive days. He experienced worsening GI symptoms and acute renal failure which required short-term dialysis. Pancytopenia developed and persisted until his death from a malignancy several months later. Other adverse events reported following overdosage include: Persistent bone marrow suppression (one adult with neutropenia and thrombocytopenia after a single dose of 6000 mg), reversible neutropenia or granulocytopenia (four adults, overdoses ranging from 8 mg/kg daily for 4 days to a single dose of 25 mg/kg), hepatitis (one adult receiving 10 mg/kg daily, and one 2 kg infant after a single 40 mg dose), renal toxicity (one adult with transient worsening of hematuria after a single 500 mg dose, and one adult with elevated creatinine [5.2 mg/dl] after a single 5000 to 7000 mg dose) and seizure (one adult with known seizure disorder after 3 days of 9 mg/kg). In addition, one adult received 0.4 ml (instead of 0.1 ml) by intravitreal injection, and experienced temporary loss of vision and central retinal artery occlusion secondary to increased intraocular pressure related to the injected fluid volume.

Oral: There have been no reports of overdosage with oral ganciclovir. Doses as high as 6000 mg/day did not result in overt toxicity other than transient neutropenia.

Treatment: Dialysis may be useful in reducing serum concentrations. Adequate hydration should be maintained. Consider the use of hematopoietic growth factors.

Patient Information:

Ganciclovir is not a cure for CMV retinitis, and immunocompromised patients may continue to experience progression of retinitis during or following treatment. Advise patients to have regular ophthalmologic examinations at a minimum of every 6 weeks while being treated.

The major toxicities of ganciclovir are granulocytopenia and thrombocytopenia. Dose modifications may be required, including possible discontinuation. Emphasize the importance of close monitoring of blood counts while on therapy.

Patients with AIDS may be receiving zidovudine. Treatment with zidovudine and ganciclovir will not be tolerated by many patients and may result in severe granulocytopenia.

Advise patients that ganciclovir may cause infertility. Advise women of childbearing potential that ganciclovir should not be used during pregnancy; use effective contraception during ganciclovir treatment. Similarly, advise men to practice barrier contraception during and for at least 90 days following ganciclovir treatment.

Although there is no information, consider ganciclovir a potential carcinogen.

Transplant recipients: Counsel transplant recipients regarding the high frequency of impaired renal function, particularly in patients receiving concomitant administration of nephrotoxic agents such as cyclosporine and amphotericin B.

Administration and Dosage:

IV: Do not administer by rapid or bolus IV injection. The toxicity may be increased as a result of excessive plasma levels. Do not exceed the recommended infusion rate. IM or SC injection of reconstituted ganciclovir may result in severe tissue irritation due to high pH.

CMV retinitis (normal renal function):

Induction – The recommended initial dose is 5 mg/kg (given IV at a constant rate over 1 hour) every 12 hours for 14 to 21 days. Do not use oral ganciclovir for induction treatment.

Maintenance –

IV – Following induction treatment, the recommended maintenance dose is 5 mg/kg given as a constant rate IV infusion over 1 hour once daily 7 days per week, or 6 mg/kg once daily 5 days per week.

Oral – Following induction treatment, the recommended maintenance dose of oral ganciclovir is 1000 mg 3 times daily with food. Alternatively, the dosing regimen of 500 mg 6 times daily every 3 hours with food, during waking hours, may be used.

For patients who experience progression of CMV retinitis while receiving maintenance treatment with either formulation of ganciclovir, reinduction treatment is recommended.

Prevention of CMV disease in transplant recipients: The recommended initial dose of IV ganciclovir for patients with normal renal function is 5 mg/kg (given IV at a constant rate over 1 hour) every 12 hours for 7 to 14 days, followed by 5 mg/kg once daily 7 days per week or 6 mg/kg once daily 5 days per week.

The duration of treatment with IV ganciclovir in transplant recipients is dependent on the duration and degree of immunosuppression. In controlled clinical trials in bone marrow allograft recipients, treatment was continued until day 100 to 120 post-transplantation. CMV disease occurred in several patients who discontinued treatment with ganciclovir prematurely. In heart allograft recipients, the onset of newly diagnosed CMV disease occurred after treatment with ganciclovir was stopped at day 28 post-transplant, suggesting that continued dosing may be necessary to prevent late occurrence of CMV disease in this patient population.

Renal impairment:

IV – Refer to the following table for recommended doses and adjust the dosing interval as indicated.

IV Ganciclovir Dose in Renal Impairment				
Creatinine clearance (ml/min)	Ganciclovir induction dose (mg/kg)	Dosing interval (hours)	Ganciclovir maintenance dose (mg/kg)	Dosing interval (hours)
≥ 70	5	12	5	24
50 to 69	2.5	12	2.5	24
25 to 49	2.5	24	1.25	24
10 to 24	1.25	24	0.625	24
< 10	1.25	3 times per week following hemodialysis	0.625	3 times per week following hemodialysis

Hemodialysis: Dosing for patients undergoing hemodialysis should not exceed 1.25 mg/kg 3 times per week, following each hemodialysis session. Give shortly after completion of the hemodialysis session, since hemodialysis reduces plasma levels by approximately 50%.

Oral – In patients with renal impairment, modify the dose of oral ganciclovir as follows:

Oral Ganciclovir Dose in Renal Impairment	
Creatinine clearance (ml/min)	Ganciclovir doses
≥70	1000 mg TID or 500 mg q3h, 6x/day
50 to 69	1500 mg QD or 500 mg TID
25 to 49	1000 mg QD or 500 mg BID
10 to 24	500 mg QD
< 10	500 mg 3 times per week, following hemodialysis

Ccr can be related to serum creatinine by the following formula:

$$\text{Males:} \quad \frac{\text{Weight (kg)} \times (140 - \text{age})}{72 \times \text{serum creatinine (mg/dl)}} = \text{Ccr}$$

$$\text{Females:} \quad 0.85 \times \text{above value}$$

Patient monitoring: Due to the frequency of granulocytopenia and thrombocytopenia, it is recommended that neutrophil counts and platelet counts be performed frequently, especially in patients in whom ganciclovir or other nucleoside analogs have previously resulted in leukopenia, or in whom neutrophil counts are < 1000/mm^3 at the beginning of treatment. Because dosing with ganciclovir must be modified in patients with renal impairment, and because of the incidence of increased serum creatinine levels that have been observed in transplant recipients treated with IV ganciclovir, patients should have serum creatinine or Ccr values followed carefully.

Reduction of dose: Dose reductions are required for patients with renal impairment and for those with neutropenia or thrombocytopenia. Therefore, perform frequent white blood cell counts. Severe neutropenia (ANC < 500/mm^3) or severe thrombocytopenia (platelets < 25,000/mm^3) require a dose interruption until evidence of marrow recovery is observed (ANC > 750/mm^3).

Preparation of IV solution: Each 10 ml clear glass vial contains ganciclovir sodium equivalent to 500 mg of the free base form of ganciclovir and 46 mg of sodium. Prepare the contents of the vial for administration in the following manner:

Reconstituted solution –

1. Reconstitute lyophilized ganciclovir by injecting 10 ml of Sterile Water for Injection, USP, into the vial. Do not use bacteriostatic water for injection containing parabens; it is incompatible with ganciclovir and may cause precipitation.

2. Shake the vial to dissolve the drug.

3. Visually inspect the reconstituted solution for particulate matter and discoloration prior to proceeding with infusion solution. Discard the vial if particulate matter or discoloration is observed.

4. Reconstituted solution in the vial is stable at room temperature for 12 hours. Do not refrigerate.

Infusion solution – Based on patient weight, remove the appropriate volume of the reconstituted solution (ganciclovir concentration 50 mg/ml) from the vial and add to an acceptable (see below) infusion fluid (typically 100 ml) for delivery over the course of 1 hour. Infusion concentrations > 10 mg/ml are not recommended. The following infusion fluids have been determined to be chemically and physically compatible with ganciclovir IV solution: 0.9% Sodium Chloride, 5% Dextrose, Ringer's Injection and Lactated Ringer's Injection, USP.

Handling and disposal: Exercise caution in the handling and preparation of ganciclovir. Solutions of IV ganciclovir are alkaline (pH 11). Avoid direct contact with the skin or mucous membranes of the powder contained in ganciclovir capsules or of ganciclovir IV solutions. If such contact occurs, wash thoroughly with soap and water; rinse eyes thoroughly with plain water. Do not open or crush ganciclovir capsules.

Because ganciclovir shares some of the properties of antitumor agents (ie, carcinogenicity and mutagenicity), give consideration to handling and disposal according to guidelines issued for antineoplastic drugs.

Storage/Stability: Reconstituted solution in the vial is stable at room temperature for 12 hours. Do not refrigerate. Because nonbacteriostatic infusion fluid must be used with ganciclovir IV solution, the infusion solution must be used within 24 hours of dilution to reduce the risk of bacterial contamination. Refrigerate the infusion solution. Freezing is not recommended.

Rx	**Cytovene** (Syntex)	**Capsules**: 250 mg	In 180s.
		Powder for injection, lyophilized: 500 mg/vial ganciclovir (as sodium)	In 10 ml vials.

GANCICLOVIR INTRAVITREAL IMPLANT

Actions:

Pharmacology: Ganciclovir is a synthetic nucleoside analog of 2'-deoxyguanosine that inhibits replication of herpes viruses both in vitro and in vivo. Sensitive human viruses include cytomegalovirus (CMV), herpes simplex virus-1 and -2 (HSV-1, HSV-2), Epstein-Barr virus (EBV) and varicella-zoster virus (VZV).

The median concentration of ganciclovir which effectively inhibits the replication of human CMV (ED_{50}) has ranged from 0.2 to 3 mcg/ml. The relationship of in vitro sensitivity of CMV to ganciclovir and clinical response has not been established. Ganciclovir inhibits mammalian cell proliferation in vitro at higher concentrations: ID_{50} values range from 10 to 60 mcg/ml, with the exception of bone marrow-derived colony-forming cells, which are more sensitive with ID_{50} values greater than 10 mcg/ml of the cell types tested.

In vitro sensitivity testing of CMV isolates from patients receiving intravenous ganciclovir has shown emergence of viral resistance. Because the prevalence of resistant isolates is unknown, there is a possibility that some patients may be infected with strains of CMV resistant to ganciclovir. Consequently, consider the possibility of viral resistance in patients showing poor clinical response.

Pharmacokinetics: In one clinical trial, 26 patients (30 eyes treated) received a total of 39 primary implants and 12 exchange implants (performed 32 weeks after the implant was inserted or earlier if progression of CMV retinitis occurred). Precise in vivo release rates of the ganciclovir implant could not be calculated because most of the exchanged implants were empty upon removal. It was unknown at what time the implant ran out of the drug. However, approximate in vivo release rates ranged from 1 mcg/h to more than 1.62 mcg/h for the exchanged implants.

In another study, in 14 implants (3 exchanged, 11 autopsy) in which the in vivo release rate could be accurately calculated, the mean release rate was 1.4 mcg/h, with a range of 0.5 to 2.88 mcg/h. The mean vitreous drug levels in 8 eyes (4 collected at time of reginal detachment surgery; 2 collected from autopsy eyes within 6 hours of death and prior to fixation; 2 collected from implant exchange) was 4.1 mcg/ml.

Clinical trials: Ganciclovir implant (*Vitrasert*) and intravenous (*Cytovene*) were compared in a randomized, controlled parallel group trial conducted between May 1993 and December 1994 in 188 patients with AIDS and newly diagnosed CMV retinitis. Patients in the intravenous treatment group received an induction dose of 5 mg/kg twice daily for 14 days followed by a maintenance dose of 5 mg/kg once daily. The median time to progression was approximately 210 days for the implant (*Vitrasert*) treatment group, compared to approximately 120 days for the intravenous (*Cytovene*) ganciclovir treatment group.

Indications:

For the treatment of CMV retinitis in patients with acquired immunodeficiency syndrome (AIDS). The implant is for intravitreal implantation only.

Contraindications:

Hypersensitivity to ganciclovir or acyclovir. Patients contraindicated for intraocular surgery (eg, external infection or severe thrombocytopenia).

Warnings:

Diagnosis of CMV retinitis is ophthalmologic and should be made by indirect ophthalmoscopy. Other conditions in the differential diagnosis of CMV retinitis include candidiasis, toxoplasmosis, histoplasmosis, retinal scars and cotton wool spots, any of which may produce a retinal appearance similar to CMV.

CMV retinitis may be associated with CMV disease elsewhere in the body. The implant provides localized therapy limited to the implanted eye. The implant does not provide treatment for systemic CMV disease. Patients should be monitored for extraocular CMV disease.

Surgical procedures involve risk. The following complications may occur with intraocular surgery to place the implant into the vitreous cavity: Vitreous loss, vitreous hemorrhage, cataract formation, retinal detachment, uveitis, endophthalmitis and decrease in visual acuity.

Loss of visual acuity may occur immediately in the implanted eye of almost all patients postoperatively. This decrease is temporary and lasts for approximately 2 to 4 weeks after implantation. This decrease in visual acuity is probably a result of the surgical implant procedure.

The Vitrasert Implant is sterilized by an ethylene oxide-freon mixture, a substance which harms public health and the environment by destroying ozone in the upper atmosphere.

Carcinogenesis/Mutagenesis/Fertility Impairment: In mice, daily oral doses of 1000 mg/kg may have caused an increased incidence of tumors in the preputial gland of males, nonglandular mucosa of the stomach of males and females, and reproductive tissues (ovaries, uterus, mammary gland, clitoral gland and vagina) and liver in females. A slightly increased incidence of tumors occurred in the preputial and harderian glands (males), forestomach in males and females, and liver in females in mice given 20 mg/kg/day. Except for histiocytic sarcoma of the liver, ganciclovir-induced tumors were generally of epithelial or vascular origin. Consider ganciclovir a potential carcinogen in humans.

Ganciclovir caused mutations in lymphoma cells in mice and DNA damage in human lymphocytes in vitro at concentrations between 50 to 500 and 250 to 2000 mcg/ml, respectively. In the mouse micronucleus assay, ganciclovir was clastogenic at doses of 150 and 500 mg/kg (2.8% to 10% human exposure based on AUC), but not 50 mg/kg (exposure approximately comparable to the human, based on AUC). Ganciclovir was not mutagenic in the Ames Salmonella assay at concentrations of 500 to 5000 mcg/ml.

Ganciclovir caused decreased mating behavior, decreased fertility and an increased incidence of embryolethality in female mice following intravenous doses of 90 mg/kg/

day. Decreased fertility in male mice and hypospermatogenesis in mice and dogs occurred following daily oral or intravenous administration of ganciclovir ranging from 0.2 to 10 mg/kg.

Pregnancy: Category C. Ganciclovir is embryotoxic in rabbits and mice following IV administration and teratogenic in rabbits. Fetal resorptions were present in at least 85% of rabbits and mice administered 60 mg/kg/day and 108 mg/kg/day, respectively. Effects observed in rabbits included: Fetal growth retardation, embryolethality, teratogenicity and maternal toxicity. Teratogenic changes included cleft palate, anophthalmia/microphthalmia, aplastic organs (kidney and pancreas), hydrocephaly and brachygnathia. In mice, effects observed were maternal/fetal toxicity and embryolethality.

Daily IV doses of 90/mg/kg administered to female mice prior to mating, during gestation and during lactation caused hypoplasia of the test and seminal vesicles in the month-old male offspring, as well as pathologic changes in the nonglandular region of the stomach.

There are no adequate and well controlled studies in pregnant women. Use during pregnancy only if the potential benefits justify the potential risk to the fetus.

Lactation: It is not known whether ganciclovir is excreted in breast milk. However, because carcinogenic and teratogenic effects occurred in animals treated with ganciclovir, the possibility of serious adverse reactions from ganciclovir in nursing infants is considered likely. Instruct mothers to discontinue nursing if they have a ganciclovir implant.

Children: Safety and effectiveness in children less than 9 years of age have not been established.

Precautions:

As with all intraocular surgery, sterility of the surgical field and the ganciclovir implant should be rigorously maintained. The implant should be handled only by the suture tab in order to avoid damaging the polymer coatings since this could affect release rate of ganciclovir inside the eye. The implant should not be resterilized by any method.

A high level of surgical skill is required for implantation. A surgeon should have observed or assisted in surgical implantation of the ganciclovir implant prior to attempting the procedure.

Drug Interactions:

No drug interactions have been observed with the ganciclovir implant. There is limited experience with the use of retinal tamponades in conjunction with the ganciclovir implant.

Adverse Reactions:

The most frequent adverse reactions reported involved the eye.

During first 2 months following implantation: Visual acuity loss of 3 lines or more, vitreous hemorrhage and retinal detachments (approximately 10% to 20%).

Local: Cataract formation/lens opacities, macular abnormalities, intraocular pressure spikes, optic disk/nerve changes, hyphemas, uveitis (approximately 1% to 5%). Retinopathy, anterior chamber cell and flare, synechia, hemorrhage (other than vitreous), cotton wool spots, keratophalthy, astigmatism, endophthalmitis, microangiopathy, sclerosis, choroiditis, chemosis, phthisis bulbi, angle-closure glaucoma with anterior chamber shallowing, vitreous detachment, vitreous traction, hypotony, severe postoperative inflammation, retinal tear, retinal hole, corneal dellen, choroidal folds, pellet extrusion from scleral wound, gliosis (< 1%).

Patient Information:

The ganciclovir implant is not a cure for CMV retinitis and immunocompromised patients may continue to experience progression of retinitis with the implant. Advise patients to have regular ophthalmic examinations on both eyes at appropriate intervals following implantation.

As with any surgical procedure, risk is involved. Potential complications accompanying implantation may include intraocular infection or inflammation, retinal detachment, cataract formation in the natural crystalline lens.

Immediate and temporary decrease in visual acuity in the implanted eye are experienced by almost all patients following implantation. This lasts approximately 2 to 4 weeks postoperatively and is probably a result of the surgical implant procedure.

Administration and Dosage:

Each implant contains a minimum of 4.5 mg of ganciclovir, and is designed to release the drug over a 5 to 8 month period. Following depletion of ganciclovir from the implant, as evidenced by progression of retinitis, the implant may be removed and replaced.

Handling and disposal: Exercise caution in handling the implant in order to avoid damage to the polymer coating on the implant, which may result in an increased rate of drug release from the implant. The implant should be handled by the suture tab only. Aseptic technique should be maintained at all times prior to and during the surgical implantation procedure.

Because the implant contains ganciclovir, which shares some of the properties of antitumor agents (ie, carcinogenicity and mutogenicity), consideration should be given to handling and disposal of the implant according to guidelines issued for antineoplastic drugs.

Storage/Stability: Store at room temperature 15° to 30°C (59° to 86°F). Do not freeze. Keep away from excessive heat and light.

Rx	**Vitrasert** (Chiron Vision)	**Implant:** Minimum 4.5 mg	In individual unit boxes in a sterile Tyvek package.

FOSCARNET SODIUM (Phosphonoformic acid)

Warning:

Renal impairment, the major toxicity, occurs to some degree in most patients. Continual assessment of a patient's risk and frequent monitoring of serum creatinine with dose adjustment for changes in renal function are imperative.

Foscarnet causes alterations in plasma minerals and electrolytes that have led to seizures. Monitor patients frequently for such changes and their potential sequelae.

Actions:

Pharmacology: Foscarnet is an organic analog of inorganic pyrophosphate that inhibits replication of all known herpes viruses in vitro including cytomegalovirus (CMV), herpes simplex virus types 1 and 2 (HSV-1, HSV-2), human herpes virus 6 (HHV-6), Epstein-Barr virus (EBV) and varicella-zoster virus (VZV).

Foscarnet exerts its antiviral activity by a selective inhibition at the pyrophosphate binding site on virus-specific DNA polymerases and reverse transcriptases at concentrations that do not affect cellular DNA polymerases. Foscarnet does not require activation (phosphorylation) by thymidine kinase or other kinases, and therefore is active in vitro against HSV mutants deficient in thymidine kinase. CMV strains resistant to ganciclovir may be sensitive to foscarnet.

The quantitative relationship between the in vitro susceptibility of human CMV to foscarnet and clinical response to therapy has not been clearly established in man and virus sensitivity testing has not been standardized. If no clinical response to foscarnet is observed, test viral isolates for sensitivity to foscarnet; naturally resistant mutants may emerge under selective pressure both in vitro and in vivo. The latent state of any of the human herpes viruses is not known to be sensitive to foscarnet and viral reactivation of CMV occurs after foscarnet therapy is terminated.

Pharmacokinetics: Foscarnet is 14% to 17% bound to plasma protein at plasma drug concentrations of 1 to 1000 mcM. Plasma foscarnet concentrations in two studies are summarized in the following table:

Foscarnet Plasma Concentrations

Mean dose (Infusion time)	Day of sampling	Mean plasma concentration (mcM)	
		C_{max} (range)	C_{min} (range)
57 ± 6 mg/kg q 8 hr (1 hour)	1	573 (213 to 1305)[1]	78 (< 33 to 139)[3]
47 ± 12 mg/kg q 8 hr (1 hour)	14 or 15	579 (246 to 922)[2]	110 (< 33 to 148)[4]
55 ± 6 mg/kg q 8 hr (hours)	3	445 (306 to 720)[1]	88 (< 33 to 162)[3]
57 ± 7 mg/kg q 8 hr (2 hours)	14 or 15	517 (348 to 789)[2]	105 (43 to 205)[4]

[1] Observed 0.9 to 2.4 hour after start of infusion.
[2] Observed 0.8 to 2.6 hour after start of infusion.
[3] Observed 4 to 8.1 hour after start of infusion.
[4] Observed 6.3 to 8.7 hour after start of infusion.

Mean plasma clearances were 130 ± 44 and 178 ± 48 ml/min/1.73 m^2 in two studies in which foscarnet was given by intermittent infusion and 152 ± 59 and 214 ± 25 ml/min/1.73 m^2 in two studies using continuous infusion. Approximately 80% to 90% of IV foscarnet is excreted unchanged in the urine of patients with normal renal function. Both tubular secretion and glomerular filtration account for urinary elimination of foscarnet. In one study, plasma clearance was less than creatinine clearance (Ccr), suggesting that foscarnet may also undergo tubular reabsorption. In three studies, decreases in plasma clearance of foscarnet were proportional to decreases in Ccr.

Two studies in patients with initially normal renal function who were treated with intermittent infusions showed average drug plasma half-lives of about 3 hours determined on days 1 or 3 of therapy. This may be an underestimate of the effective half-life due to the limited observation period. Plasma half-life increases with the severity of renal impairment. Half-lives of 2 to 8 hours occurred in patients having estimated or measured 24 hour Ccr of 44 to 90 ml/min. Careful monitoring of renal function and dose adjustment is imperative (see Warnings and Administration and Dosage).

Following continuous foscarnet infusion for 72 hours in six HIV-positive patients, plasma half-lives of 0.45 ± 0.32 and 3.3 ± 1.3 hours were determined. A terminal half-life of 18 ± 2.8 hours was estimated from foscarnet urinary excretion over 48 hours after stopping infusion. When foscarnet was given as a continuous infusion to 13 patients with HIV infection for 8 to 21 days, plasma half-lives of 1.4 ± 0.6 and 6.8 ± 5 hours were determined. A terminal half-life of 87.5 ± 41.8 hours was estimated from foscarnet urinary excretion over 6 days after the last infusion; however, renal function at the time of discontinuing the infusion was not known.

Measurements of urinary excretion are required to detect the longer terminal half-life assumed to represent release of foscarnet from bone. In animal studies (mice), 40% of an IV dose is deposited in bone in young animals and 7% in adults. Evidence indicates that foscarnet accumulates in human bone; however, the extent to which this occurs has not been determined. Mean volumes of distribution at steady state range from 0.3 to 0.6 L/kg.

Variable penetration into cerebrospinal fluid (CSF) has been observed. Intermittent infusion of 50 mg/kg every 8 hours for 28 days in 9 patients produced CSF levels of 150 to 260 mcM 3 hours after the end of infusion or 39% to 103% of the plasma levels. In another 4 patients, CSF concentrations were 35% to 69% of the plasma drug level after a dose of 230 mg/kg/day by continuous infusion for 2 to 13 days. However, the CSF:plasma ratio was only 13% in one patient receiving a continuous infusion at a rate of 274 mg/kg/day. Disease-related defects in the blood-brain barrier may be responsible for the variations seen.

Clinical trials: In most clinical studies, treatment for CMV retinitis was begun with an induction dosage of 60 mg/kg every 8 hours for the first 2 to 3 weeks, followed by a once-daily maintenance at doses ranging from 60 to 120 mg/kg.

A prospective, randomized, masked, controlled clinical trial was conducted in 24 patients with acquired immunodeficiency syndrome (AIDS) and CMV retinitis. Patients received induction treatment of 60 mg/kg every 8 hours for 3 weeks, followed by maintenance treatment with 90 mg/kg/day until retinitis progression (appearance of a new lesion or advancement of the border of a posterior lesion > 750 microns in diameter). The 13 patients randomized to treatment with foscarnet had a significant delay in progression of CMV retinitis compared to untreated controls. Median times to retinitis progression from study entry were 93 days (range, 21 to > 364) and 22 days (range, 7 to 42), respectively.

In another prospective clinical trial of CMV retinitis in AIDS patients, 33 were treated with 2 to 3 weeks of foscarnet induction (60 mg/kg 3 times a day) and then randomized to two maintenance dose groups, 90 and 120 mg/kg/day. Median times from study entry to retinitis progression were 96 days (range, 14 to > 176) and 140 days (range, 16 to > 233), respectively. This was not statistically significant.

Indications:

Treatment of CMV retinitis in patients with AIDS.

Contraindications:

Hypersensitivity to foscarnet.

Warnings:

Mineral and electrolyte imbalances: Foscarnet has been associated with changes in serum electrolytes including hypocalcemia (15%), hypophosphatemia (8%), hyperphosphatemia (6%), hypomagnesemia (15%) and hypokalemia (16%). Foscarnet is associated with a transient, dose-related decrease in ionized serum calcium, which may not be reflected in total serum calcium. This effect most likely is related to foscarnet's chelation of divalent metal ions such as calcium. Therefore, advise patients to report symptoms of low ionized calcium such as perioral tingling, numbness in the extremities and paresthesias. Be prepared to treat these as well as severe manifestations of electrolyte abnormalities, such as tetany and seizures. The rate of infusion may affect the transient decrease in ionized calcium; slowing the rate may decrease or prevent symptoms.

Transient changes in calcium or other electrolytes (including magnesium, potassium or phosphate) may also contribute to a patient's risk for cardiac disturbances and seizures (see Neurotoxicity and Seizures). Therefore, use particular caution in patients with altered calcium or other electrolyte levels before treatment, especially those with neurologic or cardiac abnormalities and those on other drugs known to influence minerals and electrolytes (see Monitoring and Drug Interactions).

Neurotoxicity and seizures: Foscarnet was associated with seizures in 18/189 (10%) of AIDS patients in five controlled studies. Three patients were not taking foscarnet at the time of seizure. In most cases (15/18), the patients had an active CNS condition (eg, toxoplasmosis, HIV encephalopathy) or a history of CNS diseases. The rate of seizures did not increase with duration of treatment. Three cases were associated with overdoses of foscarnet (see Overdosage).

Statistically significant risk factors associated with seizures were low baseline absolute neutrophil count (ANC), impaired baseline renal function and low total serum calcium. Several cases of seizures were associated with death. However, seizures did not always necessitate drug discontinuation. Ten of fifteen patients with seizures while on the drug continued or resumed foscarnet following treatment of their underlying disease, electrolyte disturbances or dose decreases. If factors predisposing to seizures are present, carefully monitor electrolytes, including calcium and magnesium (see Monitoring).

Other CMV infections: Safety and efficacy have not been established for the treatment of other CMV infections (eg, pneumonitis, gastroenteritis); congenital or neonatal CMV disease; or non-immunocompromised individuals.

Renal function impairment: The major toxicity of foscarnet is renal impairment, which occurs to some degree in most patients. Approximately 33% of 189 patients with AIDS and CMV retinitis who received IV foscarnet in clinical studies developed significant impairment of renal function, manifested by a rise in serum creatinine concentration to ≥ 2 mg/dl. Therefore, use foscarnet with caution in all patients, especially those with a history of renal function impairment. Patients vary in their sensitivity to foscarnet-induced nephrotoxicity, and initial renal function may not be predictive of the potential for drug-induced renal impairment.

Renal impairment is most likely to become clinically evident as assessed by increasing serum creatinine during the second week of induction therapy at 60 mg/kg 3 times a day. Renal impairment, however, may occur at any time in any patient during treatment; therefore, monitor renal function carefully (see Monitoring).

Elevations in serum creatinine are usually, but not uniformly, reversible following discontinuation or dose adjustment. Recovery of renal function after foscarnet-induced impairment usually occurs within 1 week of drug discontinuation. However, of 35 patients who experienced grade II renal impairment (serum creatinine 2 to 3 times the upper limit of normal), two died with renal failure within 4 weeks of stopping foscarnet and three others died with renal insufficiency still present < 4 weeks after drug cessation.

Because of foscarnet's potential to cause renal impairment, dose adjustment for decreased baseline renal function and any change in renal function during treatment is necessary. In addition, it may be beneficial for adequate hydration to be established (eg, by inducing diuresis) prior to and during administration.

Mutagenesis: Foscarnet showed genotoxic effects in an in vitro transformation assay at concentrations > 0.5 mcg/ml and an increased frequency of chromosome aberrations in the sister chromatid exchange assay at 1000 mcg/ml. A high dose of foscarnet (350 mg/kg) caused an increase in micronucleated polychromatic erythrocytes in mice at doses that produced exposures comparable to that anticipated clinically.

Elderly: Since these individuals frequently have reduced glomerular filtration, pay particular attention to assessing renal function before and during administration (see Administration and Dosage).

Pregnancy: Category C. Daily SC doses up to 75 mg/kg administered to female rats prior to and during mating, during gestation and 21 days postpartum caused a slight increase (< 5%) in the number of skeletal anomalies compared with the control group. Daily SC doses up to 75 mg/kg (one-third the maximal daily human exposure) administered to rabbits and 150 mg/kg (one-eighth the maximal daily human exposure) administered to rats during gestation caused an increase in the frequency of skeletal anomalies/variations. These studies are inadequate to define the potential teratogenicity at levels to which women will be exposed. There are no adequate and well controlled studies in pregnant women. Use during pregnancy only if clearly needed.

Lactation: It is not known whether foscarnet is excreted in breast milk; however, in lactating rats administered 75 mg/kg, foscarnet was excreted in maternal milk at concentrations three times higher than peak maternal blood concentrations. Exercise caution if foscarnet is administered to a nursing woman.

Children: The safety and efficacy of foscarnet in children have not been studied. Foscarnet is deposited in teeth and bone, and deposition is greater in young and growing animals. Foscarnet adversely affects development of tooth enamel in mice and rats. The effects of this deposition on skeletal development have not been studied. Since deposition in human bone also occurs, it is likely that it does so to a greater degree in developing bone in children. Administer to children only after careful evaluation and only if the potential benefits for treatment outweigh the risks.

Precautions:

Monitoring: The majority of patients will experience some decrease in renal function due to foscarnet administration. Therefore it is recommended that Ccr, either measured or estimated using the modified Cockcroft and Gault equation based on serum creatinine, be determined at baseline, 2 to 3 times per week during induction therapy and at least once every 1 to 2 weeks during maintenance therapy, with foscarnet dose adjusted accordingly (see Dose Adjustment). More frequent monitoring may be required for some patients. It is also recommended that a 24 hour Ccr be determined at baseline and periodically thereafter to ensure correct dosing. Discontinue foscarnet if Ccr drops to < 0.4 ml/min/kg.

Due to foscarnet's propensity to chelate divalent metal ions and alter levels of serum electrolytes, closely monitor patients for such changes. It is recommended that a schedule similar to that recommended for serum creatinine (see above) be used to monitor serum calcium, magnesium, potassium and phosphorus. Particular caution is advised in patients with decreased total serum calcium or other electrolyte levels before treatment, as well as in patients with neurologic or cardiac abnormalities, and in patients receiving other drugs known to influence serum calcium levels. Correct any clinically significant metabolic changes. Also, patients who experience mild (eg, perioral numbness or paresthesias) or severe symptoms (eg, seizures) of electrolyte abnormalities should have serum electrolyte and mineral levels assessed as close in time to the event as possible.

Careful monitoring and appropriate management of electrolytes, calcium, magnesium and creatinine are of particular importance in patients with conditions that may predispose them to seizures (see Warnings).

Diagnosis of CMV retinitis should be made by indirect ophthalmoscopy. Other conditions in the differential diagnosis of CMV retinitis include candidiasis, toxoplasmosis and other diseases producing a similar retinal pattern, any of which may produce a retinal appearance similar to CMV. For this reason it is essential that the diagnosis of CMV retinitis be established by an ophthalmologist familiar with the retinal presentation of these conditions. The diagnosis of CMV retinitis may be supported by culture of CMV from urine, blood, throat or other sites, but a negative CMV culture does not rule out CMV retinitis.

Toxicity/Local irritation: In controlled clinical studies, the maximum single-dose administered was 120 mg/kg by IV infusion over 2 hours. It is likely that larger doses, or more rapid infusions, would result in increased toxicity. Take care to infuse solutions containing foscarnet only into veins with adequate blood flow to permit rapid dilution and distribution, and avoid local irritation (see Administration and Dosage). Local irritation and ulcerations of penile epithelium have occurred in male patients receiving foscarnet, possibly related to the presence of drug in urine. One case of vulvovaginal ulceration in a female has occurred. Adequate hydration with close attention to personal hygiene may minimize the occurrence of such events.

Anemia occurred in 33% of patients. This anemia was usually manageable with transfusions and required discontinuation of foscarnet in < 1% (1/189) of patients in the studies. Granulocytopenia occurred in 17% of patients; however, only 1% (2/189) were terminated from these studies because of neutropenia.

Drug Interactions:

Nephrotoxic drugs: The elimination of foscarnet may be impaired by drugs that inhibit renal tubular secretion. Because of foscarnet's tendency to cause renal impairment, avoid the use of foscarnet in combination with potentially nephrotoxic drugs such as aminoglycosides, amphotericin B and IV pentamidine unless the potential benefits outweigh the risks to the patient.

Pentamidine: Concomitant treatment of four patients with foscarnet and IV pentamidine may have caused hypocalcemia; one patient died with severe hypocalcemia. Toxicity associated with concomitant use of aerosolized pentamidine has not been reported.

Zidovudine: Foscarnet was used concomitantly with zidovudine in approximately one-third of patients in the US studies. Although the combination was generally well tolerated, additive effects on anemia may have occurred. However, no evidence of increased myelosuppression was seen.

Foscarnet decreases serum levels of ionized calcium. Exercise particular caution when other drugs known to influence serum calcium levels are used concurrently.

Adverse Reactions:

The most frequently reported events were: Fever (65%); nausea (47%); anemia (33%); diarrhea (30%); abnormal renal function including acute renal failure, decreased Ccr and increased serum creatinine (27%); vomiting, headache (26%); seizure (10%) (see Warnings and Precautions).

Adverse events categorized as "severe" were: Death (14%); abnormal renal function (14%); marrow suppression (10%); anemia (9%); seizures (7%). Although death was specifically attributed to foscarnet in only one case, other complications of foscarnet (ie, renal impairment, electrolyte abnormalities, seizures) may have contributed to patient deaths (see Warnings and Precautions).

Application site: Injection site pain or inflammation (1% to 5%).

Central and peripheral nervous system: Headache, paresthesia, dizziness, involuntary muscle contractions, hypoesthesia, neuropathy, seizures (including grand mal; see Warnings) (≥ 5%); tremor, ataxia, dementia, stupor, generalized spasms, sensory disturbances, meningitis, aphasia, abnormal coordination, leg cramps, EEG abnormalities (see Warnings) (1% to 5%); vertigo, coma, encephalopathy, abnormal gait, hyperesthesia, hypertonia, visual field defects, dyskinesia, extrapyramidal disorders, hemiparesis, hyperkinesia, vocal cord paralysis, paralysis, paraplegia, speech disorders, tetany, hyporeflexia, hyperreflexia, neuralgia, neuritis, peripheral neuropathy, cerebral edema, nystagmus (< 1%).

Neoplasms: Lymphoma-like disorder, sarcoma (1% to 5%); malignant lymphoma, skin hypertrophy (< 1%).

Reproductive: Perineal pain in women, penile inflammation (< 1%).

Urinary: Alterations in renal function, including serum creatinine, decreased Ccr and abnormal renal function (see Warnings) (≥ 5%); albuminuria, dysuria, polyuria, urethral disorder, urinary retention, urinary tract infections, acute renal failure, nocturia (1% to 5%); hematuria, glomerulonephritis, micturition disorders/frequency, toxic nephropathy, nephrosis, urinary incontinence, renal tubular disorders, pyelonephritis, urethral irritation, uremia (< 1%).

Body as a whole: Fever, fatigue, rigors, asthenia, malaise, pain, infection, sepsis, death (≥ 5%); back/chest pain, edema, influenza-like symptoms, bacterial/fungal infections, moniliasis, abscess (1% to 5%); hypothermia, leg edema, peripheral edema, syncope, ascites, substernal chest pain, abnormal crying, malignant hyperpyrexia, herpes simplex, viral infection, toxoplasmosis (< 1%).

GI: Anorexia, nausea, diarrhea, vomiting, abdominal pain (≥ 5%); constipation, dysphagia, dyspepsia, rectal hemorrhage, dry mouth, melena, flatulence, ulcerative stomatitis, pancreatitis (1% to 5%); enteritis, enterocolitis, glossitis, proctitis, stomatitis, tenesmus, increased amylase, pseudomembranous colitis, gastroenteritis, oral leukoplakia, oral hemorrhage, rectal disorders, colitis, duodenal ulcer, hematemesis, paralytic ileus, esophageal ulceration, ulcerative proctitis, tongue ulceration (< 1%).

Hematologic: Anemia, granulocytopenia, leukopenia (see Precautions) (≥ 5%); thrombocytopenia, platelet abnormalities, thrombosis, WBC abnormalities, lymphadenopathy (1% to 5%); pulmonary embolism, coagulation disorders, decreased coagulation factors, epistaxis, decreased prothrombin, hypochromic anemia, pancytopenia, hemolysis, leukocytosis, cervical lymphadenopathy, lymphopenia (< 1%).

Metabolic/Nutritional: Mineral/electrolyte imbalances (see Warnings), including hypokalemia, hypocalcemia, hypomagnesemia, hypo- or hyperphosphatemia (≥ 5%); hyponatremia, decreased weight, increased alkaline phosphatase, LDH and BUN, acidosis, cachexia, thirst, hypercalcemia (1% to 5%); dehydration, glycosuria, increased creatine phosphokinase, diabetes mellitus, abnormal glucose tolerance, hypervolemia, hypochloremia, periorbital edema, hypoproteinemia (< 1%).

Psychiatric: Depression, confusion, anxiety (≥ 5%); insomnia, somnolence, nervousness, amnesia, agitation, aggressive reaction, hallucination (1% to 5%); impaired concentration, emotional lability, psychosis, suicide attempt, delirium, personality disorders, sleep disorders (< 1%).

Respiratory: Coughing, dyspnea (≥ 5%); pneumonia, sinusitis, pharyngitis, rhinitis, respiratory disorders or insufficiency, pulmonary infiltration, stridor, pneumothorax, hemoptysis, bronchospasm (1% to 5%); bronchitis, laryngitis, respiratory depression, abnormal chest x-ray, pleural effusion, pulmonary hemorrhage, pneumonitis (< 1%).

Dermatologic: Rash, increased sweating (≥ 5%); pruritus, skin ulceration, seborrhea, erythematous rash, maculopapular rash, skin discoloration, facial edema (1% to 5%); acne, alopecia, dermatitis, anal pruritus, genital pruritus, aggravated psoriasis, psoriaform rash, skin disorders, dry skin, urticaria, verruca (< 1%).

Special senses: Vision abnormalities (≥ 5%); taste perversions, eye abnormalities, eye pain, conjunctivitis (1% to 5%); diplopia, blindness, retinal detachment, mydriasis, photophobia, deafness, earache, tinnitus, otitis (< 1%).

Cardiovascular: Hypertension, palpitations, ECG abnormalities including sinus tachycardia, first-degree AV block and non-specific ST-T segment changes, hypotension, flushing, cerebrovascular disorder (see Warnings) (1% to 5%); cardiomyopathy, cardiac failure/arrest, bradycardia, extrasystole, arrhythmias, atrial arrhythmias/fibrillation, phlebitis, superficial thrombophlebitis of arm, mesenteric vein thrombophlebitis (< 1%).

Hepatic: Abnormal A-G ratio, abnormal hepatic function, increased AST and ALT (1% to 5%); cholecystitis, cholelithiasis, hepatitis, cholestatic hepatitis, hepatosplenomegaly, jaundice (< 1%).

Musculoskeletal: Arthralgia, myalgia (1% to 5%); arthrosis, synovitis, torticollis (< 1%).

Endocrine: Antidiuretic hormone disorders, decreased gonadotropins, gynecomastia (< 1%).

Overdosage:

Symptoms: In controlled clinical trials, overdosage was reported in 10 patients. All 10 patients experienced adverse events and all except one made a complete recovery. One patient died after receiving a total daily dose of 12.5 g for 3 days instead of the intended 10.9 g. The patient suffered a grand mal seizure and became comatose. Three days later the patient died with the cause of death listed as respiratory/cardiac arrest. The other nine patients received doses ranging from 1.14 times to 8 times their recommended doses with an average of 4 times their recommended doses. Overall, three patients had seizures, three patients had renal function impairment, four patients had paresthesias either in limbs or periorally, and five patients had documented electrolyte disturbances primarily involving calcium and phosphate.

Treatment: There is no specific antidote. Hemodialysis and hydration may be of benefit in reducing drug plasma levels in patients who receive an overdosage, but these have not been evaluated in a clinical trial setting. Observe the patient for signs and symptoms of renal impairment and electrolyte imbalance. Institute medical treatment if clinically warranted.

Patient Information:

Foscarnet is not a cure for CMV retinitis; patients may continue to experience progression of retinitis during or following treatment.

Regular ophthalmologic examinations are necessary. The major toxicities of foscarnet are renal impairment, electrolyte disturbances and seizures; dose modifications and possibly discontinuation may be required.

Close monitoring while on therapy is essential. Advise patients of the importance of perioral tingling, numbness in the extremities or paresthesias during or after infusion as possible symptoms of electrolyte abnormalities. Should such symptoms occur, stop the infusion, obtain appropriate laboratory samples for assessment of electrolyte concentrations and consult physician before resuming treatment. The rate of infusion must be no more than 1 mg/kg/min.

The potential for renal impairment may be minimized by accompanying administration with hydration adequate to establish and maintain diuresis during dosing.

Administration and Dosage:

Caution: Do not administer by rapid or bolus IV injection. Toxicity may be increased as a result of excessive plasma levels. Take care to avoid unintentional overdose by carefully controlling the rate of infusion. Therefore, an infusion pump must be used. In spite of the use of an infusion pump, overdoses have occurred.

Administer by controlled IV infusion, either by using a central venous line or by using a peripheral vein. The standard 24 mg/ml solution may be used without dilution when using a central venous catheter for infusion. When a peripheral vein catheter is used, dilute the 24 mg/ml solution to 12 mg/ml with 5% Dextrose in Water or with a normal saline solution prior to administration to avoid local irritation of peripheral veins. Since the dose is calculated on the basis of body weight, it may be desirable to remove and discard any unneeded quantity from the bottle before starting with the infusion to avoid overdosage. Use solutions thus prepared within 24 hours of first entry into a sealed bottle.

Do not exceed the recommended dosage, frequency or infusion rates. All doses must be individualized for patient's renal function.

Induction treatment: The recommended initial dose for patients with normal renal function is 60 mg/kg, adjusted for individual patient's renal function, given IV at a constant rate over a minimum of 1 hour every 8 hours for 2 to 3 weeks depending on clinical response. An infusion pump must be used to control the rate of infusion. Adequate hydration is recommended to establish diuresis, both prior to and during treatment to minimize renal toxicity (see Warnings), provided there are no clinical contraindications.

Maintenance treatment: 90 to 120 mg/kg/day (individualized for renal function) given as an IV infusion over 2 hours. Because the superiority of the 120 mg/kg/day has not been established in controlled trials, and given the likely relationship of higher plasma foscarnet levels to toxicity, it is recommended that most patients be started on maintenance treatment with a dose of 90 mg/kg/day. Escalation to 120 mg/kg/day may be considered should early reinduction be required because of retinitis progression.

Some patients who show excellent tolerance to foscarnet may benefit from initiation of maintenance treatment at 120 mg/kg/day earlier in their treatment. An infusion pump must be used to control the rate of infusion with all doses. Again, hydration to establish diuresis both prior to and during treatment is recommended to minimize renal toxicity.

Patients who experience progression of retinitis while receiving maintenance therapy may be retreated with the induction and maintenance regimens given above.

Renal function abnormalities: Use with caution in patients with abnormal renal function because reduced plasma clearance of foscarnet will result in elevated plasma levels. In addition, foscarnet has the potential to further impair renal function (see Warnings). Foscarnet has not been specifically studied in patients with Ccr < 50 ml/min or serum creatinine > 2.8 mg/dl. Carefully monitor renal function at baseline and during induction and maintenance therapy with appropriate dose adjustments. If Ccr falls below the limits of the dosing nomograms (0.4 ml/min/kg) during therapy, discontinue foscarnet and monitor the patient daily until resolution of renal impairment is ensured.

Dose adjustment in renal impairment: Individualize foscarnet dosing according to the patient's renal function status. Refer to the table below for recommended doses and adjust the dose as indicated.

To use this dosing guide, actual 24 hour Ccr (ml/min) must be divided by body weight (kg) or the estimated Ccr in ml/min/kg can be calculated from serum creatinine (mg/dl) using the following formula (modified Cockcroft and Gault equation).

$$\text{Males: } \frac{\text{Weight (kg)} \times (140 - \text{age})}{72 \times \text{serum creatinine (mg/dl)}} = \text{Ccr}$$

$$\text{Females: } 0.85 \times \text{above value}$$

Foscarnet Dosing Guide Based on CCR	
Induction	
Ccr (ml/min/kg)	Equivalent to 60 mg/kg dose every 8 hours
≥ 1.6	60
1.5	57
1.4	53
1.3	49
1.2	46
1.1	42
1	39
0.9	35
0.8	32
0.7	28
0.6	25
0.5	21
0.4	18

Foscarnet Dosing Guide Based on Ccr		
	Maintenance	
Ccr (ml/min/kg)	Equivalent to 90 mg/kg dose every 24 hours	Equivalent to 120 mg/kg dose every 24 hours
≥ 1.4	90	120
1.2-1.4	78	104
1-1.2	75	100
0.8-1	71	94
0.6-0.8	63	84
0.4-0.6	57	76

IV incompatibility: Other drugs and supplements can be administered to a patient receiving foscarnet. However, take care to ensure that foscarnet is only administered with normal saline or 5% Dextrose Solution and that no other drug or supplement is administered concurrently via the same catheter. Foscarnet is chemically incompatible with 30% dextrose, amphotericin B, and solutions containing calcium such as Ringer's Lactate and TPN. Physical incompatibility with other IV drugs includes: Acyclovir sodium, ganciclovir, trimetrexate, pentamidine, vancomycin, trimethoprim/sulfamethoxazole, diazepam, midazolam, digoxin, phenytoin, leucovorin and prochlorperazine. Because of foscarnet's chelating properties, a precipitate can potentially occur when divalent cations are administered concurrently in the same catheter.

Rx	**Foscavir** (Astra)	**Injection:** 24 mg/ml	In 250 and 500 ml bottles.

CIDOFOVIR

Warning:

Renal impairment is the major toxicity of cidofovir. To minimize possible nephrotoxicity, IV prehydration with Normal Saline and administration of probenecid must be used with each cidofovir infusion. Monitor renal function (serum creatinine and urine protein) prior to each dose of cidofovir and modify the dose for changes in renal function as appropriate.

Granulocytopenia has been observed in association with cidofovir treatment. Monitor neutrophil counts during cidofovir therapy.

Actions:

Pharmacology: Cidofovir is a nucleotide analog. Cidofovir suppresses cytomegalovirus (CMV) replication by selective inhibition of viral DNA synthesis. Biochemical data support selective inhibition of CMV DNA polymerase by cidofovir diphosphate, the active intracellular metabolite of cidofovir. Cidofovir diphosphate inhibits herpes virus polymerases at concentrations that are 8– to 600–fold lower than those needed to inhibit human cellular DNA polymerases alpha, beta and gamma. Incorporation of cidofovir into the growing viral DNA results in reductions in the rate of viral DNA synthesis.

Resistance – CMV isolates with reduced susceptibility to cidofovir have been selected in vitro in the presence of high concentration of cidofovir. IC_{50} values for selected resistant isolates ranged from 7 to 15 mcg.

Cross-resistance – Cidofovir-resistant isolates selected in vitro following exposure to increasing concentrations of cidofovir were assessed for susceptibility to ganciclovir and foscarnet. All were cross-resistant to ganciclovir, but remained susceptible to foscarnet. Ganciclovir or ganciclovir/foscarnet-resistant isolates that are cross-resistant to cidofovir have been obtained from drug-naive patients and from patients following ganciclovir or ganciclovir/foscarnet therapy. To date, the majority of ganciclovir-resistant isolates are UL97 gene product (phosphokinase) mutants and remain susceptible to cidofovir. However, reduced susceptibility to cidofovir has been reported for DNA polymerase mutants of CMV that are resistant to ganciclovir. To date, all clinical isolates that exhibit high level resistance to ganciclovir, because of mutations in the DNA polymerase gene, have been shown to be cross-resistant to cidofovir. Cidofovir is active against some, but not all, CMV isolates that are resistant to foscarnet. The incidence of foscarnet-resistant isolates that are resistant to cidofovir is not known.

A few triple-drug resistant isolates have been described. Genotypic analysis of two of these triple-resistant isolates revealed several point mutations in the CMV DNA polymerase gene.

Pharmacokinetics: Cidofovir must be administered with probenecid. Renal tubular secretion contributes to the elimination of cidofovir.

Cidofovir Pharmacokinetic Parameters Following 3 and 5 mg/kg Infusions With and Without Probenecid

Parameters	Cidofovir Administered Without Probenecid		Cidofovir Administered With Probenecid	
	3 mg/kg	5 mg/kg	3 mg/kg	5 mg/kg
AUC (mcg•hr/ml)	20	28.3	25.7	40.8
C_{max} (end of infusion) (mcg/ml)	7.3	11.5	9.8	19.6
Vdss (ml/kg)	537		410	
Clearance (ml/min/1.73 m^2)	179		148	
Renal Clearance (ml/min/1.73 m^2)	150		98.6	

In vitro, cidofovir was < 6% bound to plasma or serum proteins over the cidofovir concentration range 0.25 to 25 mcg/ml. CSF concentrations of cidofovir following IV infusion of cidofovir 5 mg/kg with concomitant probenecid and IV hydration were undetectable (< 0.1 mcg/ml, assay detection threshold) at 15 minutes after the end of a 1 hour infusion in one patient whose corresponding serum concentration was 8.7 mcg/ml.

Clinical trials:

Delayed vs immediate therapy – In an open-label trial, previously untreated patients with peripheral CMV retinitis were randomized to either immediate treatment with cidofovir (5 mg/kg once a week for 2 weeks, then 5 mg/kg every other week), or delayed cidofovir treatment until progression of CMV retinitis occurred. Of 25 and 23 patients in the immediate and delayed groups respectively, 23 and 21 were evaluable for retinitis progression as determined by retinal photography. Based on masked readings of retinal photographs, the median (95% confidence internal [CI]) times to retinitis progression were 120 days (40, 134) and 22 days (10, 27) for the immediate and delayed therapy groups, respectively. This difference was statistically significant. Median (95% CI) times to the alternative endpoint of retinitis progression or study drug discontinuation (including adverse events, withdrawn consent and systemic CMV disease) were 52 days (37, 85) and 22 days (13, 27) for the immediate and delayed therapy groups, respectively. This difference was statistically significant.

Indications:

CMV retinitis: For the treatment of CMV retinitis in patients with acquired immunodeficiency syndrome (AIDS).

The safety and efficacy of cidofovir have not been established for treatment of other CMV infections (such as pneumonitis or gastroenteritis), congenital or neonatal CMV disease, or CMV disease in non-HIV-infected individuals.

Contraindications:

Hypersensitivity to cidofovir; a history of clinically severe hypersensitivity to probenecid or other sulfa-containing medications; direct intraocular injection.

Warnings:

Direct intraocular injection may be associated with significant decreases in intraocular pressure and impairment of vision.

Nephrotoxicity: Dose-dependent nephrotoxicity is the major dose-limiting toxicity related to cidofovir administration. Dose adjustment or discontinuation is required for changes in renal function while on therapy. Proteinuria may be an early indicator of cidofovir-related nephrotoxicity. Continued administration of cidofovir may lead to additional proximal tubular cell injury that may result in glycosuria; decreases in serum phosphate, uric acid and bicarbonate; and elevations in serum creatinine. Patients with these adverse events occurring concurrently and meeting a criteria of Fanconi's syndrome have been reported. Renal function may not return to baseline after drug discontinuation.

Hematological toxicity: Neutropenia may occur during cidofovir therapy. Monitor neutrophil count while receiving cidofovir therapy.

Metabolic acidosis: Fanconi's syndrome and decreases in serum bicarbonate associated with evidence of renal tubular damage have been reported. Serious metabolic acidosis, in association with liver failure, pancreatitis, mucormycosis, aspergillus, disseminated mycobacterial infection and progression to death occurred in one patient.

Ocular hypotony: Among the subset of patients monitored for intraocular pressure changes, ocular hypotony ($\geq$ 50% change from baseline) was reported in five patients. Hypotony was reported in one patient with concomitant diabetes mellitus. Risk of ocular hypotony may be increased in patients with preexisting diabetes.

Renal function impairment: It is recommended that cidofovir not be initiated in patients with baseline serum creatinine > 1.5 mg/dl or creatinine clearances $\leq$ 55 ml/min. In these patients, use cidofovir when the potential benefits exceed the potential risks.

Carcinogenesis/Fertility impairment: Mammary adenocarcinomas have occurred in rats and mice, and Zymbal's gland carcinomas have occurred in rats. Studies showed inhibition of spermatogenesis in rats and monkeys. However, no adverse effects on fertility or reproduction were seen following once weekly IV injections of cidofovir in male rats for 13 consecutive weeks.

Elderly: No studies of the safety and efficacy of cidofovir in patients > 60 years of age have been conducted. Because elderly individuals frequently have reduced glomerular filtration, pay particular attention to assessing renal function before and during cidofovir administration.

Pregnancy: Category C. Cidofovir was embryotoxic (reduced fetal body weights) in rats and in rabbits. An increased incidence of fetal external, soft tissue and skeletal anomalies (meningocele, short snout and short maxillary bones) occurred in rabbits. There are no adequate and well controlled studies in pregnant women. Use cidofovir during pregnancy only if potential benefit justifies the potential risk to the fetus.

Lactation: It is not known whether cidofovir is excreted in breast milk. Since many drugs are excreted in breast milk and because of the potential for adverse reactions as well as the potential for tumorigenicity shown for cidofovir in animal studies, do not administer cidofovir to nursing women. The US Public Health Service Centers for Disease Control and Prevention advises HIV-infected women not to breastfeed and to avoid postnatal transmission of HIV to a child who may not yet be infected.

Children: Safety and effectiveness in children have not been studied. The use of cidofovir in children with AIDS warrants extreme caution due to the risk of long-term carcinogenicity and reproductive toxicity. Administer cidofovir to children only after careful evaluation and only if the potential benefits of treatment outweigh the risks.

Precautions:

Monitoring: Monitor serum creatinine, urine protein and white blood cell counts with differential prior to each dose. In patients with proteinuria, administer IV hydration and repeat the test. Periodically monitor intraocular pressure, visual acuity and ocular symptoms.

Drug Interactions:

Nephrotoxic Agents: Avoid concomitant administration of cidofovir and agents with nephrotoxic potential (eg, amphotericin B, aminoglycosides, foscarnet and IV pentamidine).

Adverse Reactions:

Renal: Renal toxicity (53%); proteinuria (80%); serum creatinine elevations (29%) (see Warnings).

Body as a whole: Allergic reaction; face edema; malaise; back, chest, neck pain; sarcoma; sepsis.

Cardiovascular: Hypotension; postural hypotension; pallor; syncope; tachycardia.

GI: Nausea, vomiting (65%); diarrhea (27%); anorexia (22%); abdominal pain (17%); colitis; constipation; tongue discoloration; dyspepsia; dysphagia; flatulence; gastritis; hepatomegaly; abnormal liver function tests; melena; oral candidiasis; rectal disorder; stomatitis; aphthous stomatitis; mouth ulceration; dry mouth.

Hematologic/Lymphatic: Thrombocytopenia; neutropenia (< 750/mm^3; 31%); anemia (20%).

Metabolic/Nutritional: Edema; dehydration; hyperglycemia; hyperlipemia; hypocalcemia; hypokalemia; increased alkaline phosphatase; increased SGOT; increased SGPT; weight loss.

Musculoskeletal: Arthralgia; myasthenia; myalgia.

CNS: Headache (27%); asthenia (46%); amnesia; anxiety; confusion; convulsion; depression; dizziness; abnormal gait; hallucinations; insomnia; neuropathy; paresthesia; somnolence; vasodilation.

Respiratory: Asthma; bronchitis; coughing; dyspnea (22%); hiccough; increased sputum; lung disorder; pharyngitis; pneumonia (9%); rhinitis; sinusitis.

Dermatologic: Alopecia (25%); rash (30%); acne; skin discoloration; dry skin; herpes simplex; pruritus; rash; sweating; urticaria.

Special senses: Amblyopia; conjunctivitis; eye disorder; hypotony (12%) (see Warnings); iritis; retinal detachment; taste perversion; uveitis; abnormal vision.

GU: Decreased creatinine clearance; glycosuria; hematuria; urinary incontinence; urinary tract infection.

Miscellaneous: Fever (57%); infections (24%); chills (24%).

Overdosage:

Overdosage with cidofovir has not been reported; however, hemodialysis and hydration may reduce drug plasma concentrations in patients who receive an overdosage of cidofovir. Probenecid may reduce the potential for nephrotoxicity in patients who receive an overdose of cidofovir through reduction of active tubular secretion.

Patient Information:

Advise patients that cidofovir is not a cure for CMV retinitis, and that they may continue to experience progression of retinitis during and following treatment. Advise patients receiving cidofovir to have regular follow-up ophthalmologic examinations. Patients may also experience other manifestations of CMV disease despite cidofovir therapy.

HIV-infected patients may continue taking antiretroviral therapy. However, because probenecid reduces metabolic clearance of zidovudine, advise those taking zidovudine to temporarily discontinue zidovudine administration or decrease their zidovudine dose by 50% on days of cidofovir administration only.

Inform patients of the major toxicity of cidofovir, namely renal impairment, and that dose modification, including reduction, interruption and possibly discontinuation, may be required. Emphasize close monitoring of renal function (routine urinalysis and serum creatinine) while on therapy.

Emphasize the importance of completing a full course of probenecid with each cidofovir dose. Warn patients of potential adverse events caused by probenecid (eg, headache, nausea, vomiting and hypersensitivity reactions). Hypersensitivity/allergic reactions may include rash, fever, chills and anaphylaxis. Administration of probenecid after a meal or use of antiemetics may decrease the nausea. Prophylactic or therapeutic antihistamines or acetaminophen may be used to ameliorate hypersensitivity reactions.

Cidofovir caused reduced testes weight and hypospermia in animals. Such changes may occur in humans and cause infertility. Advise women of childbearing potential that cidofovir is embryotoxic in animals and not to use the drug during pregnancy. Women of childbearing potential should use effective contraception during and for 1 month following treatment. Men should practice barrier contraceptive methods during and for 3 months following treatment.

Administration and Dosage:

Do not administer by intraocular injection.

Dosage: The recommended dosage, frequency or infusion rate must not be exceeded. Cidofovir must be diluted in 100 ml 0.9% Saline Solution prior to administration. To minimize potential nephrotoxicity, probenecid and IV saline prehydration must be administered with each cidofovir infusion.

Induction treatment: The recommended dose of cidofovir is 5 mg/kg body weight (given as an IV infusion at a constant rate over 1 hour) administered once weekly for 2 consecutive weeks.

Maintenance treatment: The recommended maintenance dose of cidofovir is 5 mg/kg body weight (given as an IV infusion at a constant rate over 1 hour) administered once every 2 weeks.

Probenecid: Probenecid must be administered orally with each cidofovir dose. Two grams must be administered 3 hours prior to the cidofovir dose, and 1 g administered at 2 hours and again at 8 hours after completion of the 1 hour cidofovir infusion (for a total of 4 g).

Ingestion of food prior to each dose of probenecid may reduce drug-related nausea and vomiting. Administration of an antiemetic may reduce the potential for nausea associated with probenecid ingestion. In patients who develop allergic or hypersensitivity symptoms to probenecid, consider the use of an appropriate prophylactic or therapeutic antihistamine or acetaminophen.

Hydration: Patients should receive a total of 1 L of 0.9% Saline Solution IV with each infusion of cidofovir. Infuse the saline solution over a 1 to 2 hour period immediately before the cidofovir infusion. Patients who can tolerate the additional fluid load should receive a second liter. If administered, the second liter of saline should be initiated either at the start of the cidofovir infusion or immediately afterwards, and should be infused over a 1 to 3 hour period.

Nephrotoxicity: For increases in serum creatinine (0.3 to 0.4 mg/dl), reduce the cidofovir dose from 5 mg/kg to 3 mg/kg. Discontinue cidofovir therapy for an increase in serum creatinine of $\geq$ 0.5 mg/dl or development of $\geq$ 3+ proteinuria.

Renal function impairment:

Dosing of Cidofovir with Renal Function Impairment		
Creatinine Clearance (ml/min)	Induction (once weekly for 2 weeks)	Maintenance (once every 2 weeks)
41 - 55	2 mg/kd	2 mg/kg
30 - 40	1.5 mg/kg	1.5 mg/kg
20-29	1 mg/kg	1 mg/kg
≤ 19	0.5 mg/kg	0.5 mg/kg

Storage/Stability: Store at controlled room temperature 20° to 25°C (68° to 77°F).

Admixtures may be stored under refrigeration (2° to 8°C; 36° to 46°F) for no more than 24 hours. Allow refrigerated admixtures to equilibrate to room temperature prior to use.

Rx	**Vistide** (Gilead Sciences)	**Injection**: 75 mg/ml	5 ml amp

ODF

9

AGENTS FOR GLAUCOMA

Glaucoma is a condition of the eye in which there is usually an elevation of the intraocular pressure (IOP) that leads to progressive cupping and atrophy of the optic nerve head, deterioration of the visual fields and ultimately to blindness. *Primary open-angle glaucoma* is the most common type of glaucoma. *Angle-closure glaucoma* and *congenital glaucoma* are treated primarily by surgical methods, although short-term drug therapy is used to decrease IOP prior to surgery.

Drugs used in the therapy of primary open-angle glaucoma include a variety of agents with different mechanisms of action. The therapeutic goal in treating glaucoma is reducing the IOP, a major risk factor in the pathogenesis of glaucomatous visual field loss. The higher the level of IOP, the greater the likelihood of optic nerve damage and glaucomatous visual field loss. Reduction of IOP may be accomplished by: 1) decreasing the rate of production of aqueous humor or 2) increasing the rate of outflow (drainage) of aqueous humor from the eye.

The seven groups of agents used in the therapy of primary open-angle glaucoma are listed in Table 1: Agents for Glaucoma, which summarizes their mechanism of decreasing IOP, effects on pupil size and ciliary muscle and duration of action.

EPINEPHRINES

Epinephrine (eg, *Epifrin*), dipivefrin (*Propine*) have both α and β activity. They lower IOP mainly by increasing aqueous outflow. Epinephrine, usually used as an adjunct to miotic or beta blocker therapy, is also used as primary therapy, especially in young patients who develop intolerable fluctuating myopia or in older patients with lens opacities or cataracts. The combination of a miotic and a sympathomimetic (eg, epinephrine) will have additive effects in lowering IOP.

Dipivefrin HCl is a prodrug which is metabolized to epinephrine in vivo. The IOP-lowering and intraocular effects are qualitatively and quantitatively similar to epinephrine; however, dipivefrin may be better tolerated and have a lower incidence of adverse effects because of its lower concentration.

Table 1: Agents for Glaucoma						
Drug	**Strength**	**Duration (hrs)**	**Decrease aqueous production**	**Increase aqueous outflow**	**Effect on pupil**	**Effect on ciliary muscle**
Epinephrines						
Epinephrine	0.1%-2%	12	+	++	mydriasis	NR
Dipivefrin	0.1%	12	+	++	mydriasis	NR
Alpha-2 Adrenergic Agonists						
Apraclonidine	0.5%–1%	7–12	+++	NR	NR	NR
Brimonidine	0.2%	6-8	++	++	NR	NR
Beta Blockers						
Betaxolol	0.25%–0.5%	12	+++	NR	NR	NR
Carteolol	1%	12	+++	nd	NR	NR
Levobunolol	0.25%–0.5%	12-24	+++	NR	NR	NR
Metipranolol	0.3%	12-24	+++	NR	NR	NR
Timolol	0.25%-0.5%	12-24	+++	NR	NR	NR
Miotics, Direct-Acting						
Carbachol[1]	0.75%-3%	6–8	NR	+++	miosis	accommodation
Pilocarpine[2]	0.25%-10%	4-8	NR	+++	miosis	accommodation
Miotics, Cholinesterase Inhibitors						
Physostigmine	0.25%-0.5%	12-36	NR	+++	miosis	accommodation
Demecarium	0.125%-0.25%	days/wks	NR	+++	miosis	accommodation
Echothiophate	0.03%-0.25%	days/wks	NR	+++	miosis	accommodation
Carbonic Anhydrase Inhibitors						
Acetazolamide[3]	125-500 mg	8-12	+++	NR	NR	NR
Dichlorphenamide[3]	50 mg	6-12	+++	NR	NR	NR
Dorzolamide[4]	2%	≈ 8	+++	NR	NR	NR
Methazolamide[3]	25-50 mg	10-18	+++	NR	NR	NR
Prostaglandins						
Latanoprost	0.005%	12-24	NR	+++	NR	NR

+++ = significant activity
++ = moderate activity
+ = some activity
NR = no activity reported
nd = No data available
[1] Available as intraocular administration during surgery; carbachol also available as a topical agent.
[2] Also available as a gel and an insert; the duration of these doseforms is longer (18 to 24 hours and 1 week, respectively) than the solution.
[3] Systemic agents.
[4] Topical ophthalmic agent.

ALPHA-2 ADRENERGIC AGONISTS

Alpha-2 adrenergic agonists (apraclonidine [*Iopidine*] and brimonidine [*Alphagan*]) are new to the treatment of glaucoma. Apraclonidine is used primarily before or after laser surgery to control or prevent post-surgical elevations of IOP and as short-term adjunctive therapy for patients requiring additional IOP reduction. Approximately 30% of patients on apraclonidine developed an allergic response. Also, the drug lost its effectiveness in approximately 40% of patients after 2 to 3 months of chronic use. Brimonidine, the newer alpha-2 agonist, seems to have a much lower allergic response associated with it and is much more successful as chronic therapy for most patients.

BETA-ADRENERGIC BLOCKING AGENTS

Beta-adrenergic blocking agents (eg, betaxolol [*Betoptic*], carteolol [*Ocupress*], levobunolol [eg, *Betagan Liquifilm*], metipranolol [*OptiPranolol*] and timolol [eg, *Betimol, Timoptic*]) may be used alone or in conjunction with other agents. They may be more effective than either pilocarpine or epinephrine alone and have the advantage of not affecting either pupil size or accommodation. They lower IOP by decreasing the rate of aqueous production.

DIRECT-ACTING MIOTICS

Direct-acting miotics, carbachol [eg, *Isopto Carbachol*], pilocarpine [eg, *Isopto Carpine*]) were considered the first step in glaucoma therapy. They have now yielded to the β-blockers. They are useful adjunctive agents that are additive to either the β-blockers, carbonic anhydrase inhibitors or the sympathomimetics. Dosage and frequency of administration must be individualized. Recent information indicates pilocarpine 2% and carbachol 1.5% every 12 hours with nasolacrimal occlusion (NLO) provide maximum effect. Increasing the concentration and dosage intervals may correct an inadequate response. Concentrations greater than pilocarpine 4% or carbachol 3% are occasionally required in patients with darkly pigmented irides.

CHOLINESTERASE INHIBITOR MIOTICS

Cholinesterase inhibitor miotics include both reversible/short-acting (physostigmine [*Eserine Sulfate*], demecarium [*Humorsol*]), and irreversible/long-acting (echothiophate [*Phospholine Iodide*]) agents which enhance the effects of endogenous acetylcholine by inactivation of the enzyme acetylcholinesterase. These agents are more potent and longer acting than the direct-acting cholinergic agents. Side effects and systemic toxicity are more common and of greater significance. Using a direct-acting cholinergic and a cholinesterase inhibitor provides no improvement in response.

CARBONIC ANHYDRASE INHIBITORS

Carbonic anhydrase inhibitors (eg, acetazolamide [*Diamox*], dichlorphenamide [*Daranide*], methazolamide [eg, *Neptazane*]) are administered systemically. Dorzolamide (*Trusopt*) is administered topically. IOP is lowered by a direct action on the ciliary epithelium to suppress the secretion of aqueous humor (inflow). Usually carbonic anhydrase inhibitors are used as adjunctive therapy.

HYPEROSMOTIC AGENTS

Hyperosmotic agents (eg, mannitol [eg, *Osmitrol*]), urea [*Ureaphil*], glycerin [*Osmoglyn*] and isosorbide [*Ismotic*]) are useful in lowering IOP in acute situations (see the Hyperosmotic Agents chapter). These agents lower IOP by creating an osmotic gradient between the ocular fluids and plasma. These agents are not for chronic use.

PROSTAGLANDINS

Although it has been long recognized that prostaglandins have IOP-lowering effects, side effects such as ocular redness, stinging and burning discouraged use of this class of drug as chronic treatment for glaucoma. The prostaglandin analog latanoprost (*Xalatan*) appears to be fairly well tolerated with a similar side effect profile of timolol in regards to ocular redness, stinging and burning. However, latanoprost does change the iris color in some patients after chronic use. Yellow/blue, yellow/green and blue/gray irises appear to be most susceptible to color change.

Consequently, this drug is approved only as adjunctive therapy. It is as effective or more effective than the beta blockers for lowering IOP and appears to be an acceptable additive with most ocular hypotensive agents.

Thom J. Zimmerman, MD, PhD
University of Louisville

For More Information

Bartlett JD, Jaanus SD, eds. Clinical Ocular Pharmacology, ed. 3. Boston: Butterworth-Heinemann, 1995.

Becker B, Shaffer RN. Diagnosis and Therapy of the Glaucomas, ed. 4. St. Louis: C.V. Mosby Co., 1987.

Chandler PA, Grant WM. Lectures on Glaucoma. Philadelphia: Lea & Febiger, 1965.

Duane TD, ed. Clinical Ophthalmology. Philadelphia: Lippincott-Raven, 1997.

Zimmerman TJ, ed. Textbook of Ocular Pharmacology. Philadelphia: Lippincott-Raven, 1997.

EPINEPHRINES

EPINEPHRINE

Actions:

Pharmacology: Epinephrine, a direct-acting sympathomimetic agent, acts on α and β receptors. Topical application, therefore, causes conjunctival decongestion (vasoconstriction), transient mydriasis (pupillary dilation) and reduction in intraocular pressure (IOP). It is believed IOP reduction is primarily due to increased aqueous outflow. The duration of decrease in IOP is 12 to 24 hours.

Epinephrine is available as the bitartrate hydrochloride and borate salts. These preparations are therapeutically equal when given in equivalent doses of epinephrine base.

Indications:

Glaucoma: Management of open-angle (chronic simple) glaucoma; may be used in combination with miotics, beta blockers (not usually additive), hyperosmotic agents or carbonic anhydrase inhibitors.

Contraindications:

Hypersensitivity to epinephrine or any component of the formulation; narrow- or angle-closure glaucoma; aphakia; patients with a narrow angle but no glaucoma; if the nature of the glaucoma is not clearly established. Do not use while wearing soft contact lenses; discoloration of lenses may occur.

Warnings:

For ophthalmic use only. Not for injection or intraocular use.

Gonioscopy: Since pupil dilation may precipitate an acute attack of angle-closure glaucoma, evaluate anterior chamber angle by gonioscopy prior to beginning therapy.

Anesthesia: Discontinue use prior to general anesthesia with anesthetics that sensitize the myocardium to sympathomimetics (eg, cyclopropane, halothane).

Aphakic patients: Maculopathy with associated decrease in visual acuity may occur in the aphakic eye; if this occurs, promptly discontinue use.

Elderly: Use with caution.

Pregnancy: Category C. Safety for use during pregnancy has not been established. Use only when clearly needed.

Lactation: It is not known whether this drug is excreted in breast milk. Exercise caution when administering to a nursing woman.

Children: Safety and efficacy for use in children have not been established.

Precautions:

Instillation discomfort: Epinephrine is relatively uncomfortable upon instillation. Discomfort lessens as concentration of epinephrine decreases.

Special risk patients: Use with caution in the presence of or history of: Hypertension; diabetes; hyperthyroidism; heart disease; cerebral arteriosclerosis; bronchial asthma.

Hazardous tasks: Epinephrine may cause temporarily blurred or unstable vision after instillation; observe caution while driving, operating machinery or performing other tasks requiring coordination or physical dexterity.

Sulfite sensitivity: Some of these products contain sulfites which may cause allergic-type reactions (eg, hives, itching, wheezing, anaphylaxis) in certain susceptible persons. Although the overall prevalence of sulfite sensitivity in the general population is probably low, it is seen more frequently in asthmatics or atopic nonasthmatics.

Drug Interactions:

Beta-adrenergic blockers, nonselective, administered concomitantly with epinephrine may block the ocular hypotensive effects of epinephrine.

Bretylium may potentiate the action of vasopressors on adrenergic receptors, possibly resulting in arrhythmias.

Guanethidine may increase the pressor response of the direct-acting vasopressors, possibly resulting in severe hypertension.

Halogenated hydrocarbon anesthetics may sensitize the myocardium to the effects of catecholamines. Use of vasopressors may lead to serious arrhythmias; use with extreme caution.

Oxytocic drugs: In obstetrics, if vasopressor drugs are used either to correct hypotension or added to the local anesthetic solution, some oxytocic drugs may cause severe persistent hypertension.

Tricyclic antidepressants: The pressor response of the direct-acting vasopressors may be potentiated by these agents; use with caution.

Drug/Lab test interactions: After prolonged use or epinephrine overdosage, elevated serum lactic acid levels with severe metabolic acidosis may occur. Transient elevations of blood glucose may be associated with epinephrine administration.

Adverse Reactions:

Local: Transient stinging and burning; eye pain/ache; browache; headache; allergic lid reaction; conjunctival hyperemia; conjunctival or corneal pigmentation; ocular irritation (hypersensitivity); localized adrenochrome deposits in conjunctiva and cornea (prolonged use); cystoid macular edema may result from use in aphakic patients.

Systemic: Headache; palpitations; tachycardia; extrasystoles; cardiac arrhythmia; hypertension; faintness.

Overdosage:

If ocular overdosage occurs, flush eye(s) with water or normal saline.

Patient Information:

To avoid contamination, do not touch tip of container to any surface. Replace cap after using.

Do not use if solution is brown or contains a precipitate.

Do not use while wearing soft contact lenses.

Transitory stinging may occur upon initial instillation. Headache or browache may occur.

Patients should immediately report any decrease in visual acuity.

Refer to the Dosage Forms and Routes of Administration chapter for more complete information.

Administration and Dosage:

Instill 1 drop into affected eye(s) twice daily.

More frequent instillation than 1 drop twice daily does not usually elicit any further improvement in therapeutic response.

When used in conjunction with miotics, instill the miotic last.

Storage: Store at 2° to 24°C (36° to 75°F). Keep container tightly sealed. Protect solution from light; store in cool place. Do not freeze. Discard if solution becomes discolored or contains a precipitate.

EPINEPHRINE HYDROCHLORIDE

Rx	**Epinephrine HCl** (Ciba Vision)	**Solution:** 0.1%	In 1 ml Dropperettes (12s).[1]
Rx	**Epifrin** (Allergan)	**Solution:** 0.5% (as base)	In 15 ml dropper bottles.[2]
Rx	**Epifrin** (Allergan)	**Solution:** 1% (as base)	In 15 ml dropper bottles.[2]
Rx	**Glaucon** (Alcon)	**Solution:** 1%	In 10 ml Drop-Tainers.[3]
Rx	**Epifrin** (Allergan)	**Solution:** 2% (as base)	In 15 ml dropper bottles.[2]
Rx	**Glaucon** (Alcon)	**Solution:** 2%	In 10 ml Drop-Tainers.[3]

[1] With 0.5% chlorobutanol and sodium bisulfite.
[2] With benzalkonium chloride, sodium metabisulfite, EDTA and hydrochloric acid.
[3] With 0.01% benzalkonium chloride, sodium metabisulfite, EDTA, sodium chloride, hydrochloric acid and sodium hydroxide.

EPINEPHRYL BORATE

Rx	**Epinal** (Alcon)	**Solution:** 0.5%	In 7.5 ml.[1]
		1%	In 7.5 ml.[1]

[1] With 0.01% benzalkonium chloride, ascorbic acid, acetylcysteine, boric acid and sodium carbonate.

DIPIVEFRIN HYDROCHLORIDE (Dipivalyl epinephrine)

Refer to Agents for Glaucoma Introduction for a general discussion of these products.

Actions:

Pharmacology: Dipivefrin is a prodrug of epinephrine formed by diesterification of epinephrine and pivalic acid, enhancing its lipophilic character and, consequently, penetration into the anterior chamber. Corneal penetration is ≈ 17 times that of epinephrine. Dipivefrin, converted to epinephrine in the eye by enzymatic hydrolysis, appears to act by enhancing outflow facility. It has the same therapeutic effects as epinephrine with fewer local and systemic side effects.

Dipivefrin does not produce the miosis or accommodative spasm that cholinergic agents produce. The blurred vision and night blindness often associated with miotic agents do not occur with dipivefrin. In patients with cataracts the inability to see around lenticular opacities caused by constricted pupil is avoided.

Pharmacokinetics: The onset of action with 1 drop occurs about 30 minutes after treatment, with maximum effect seen at about 1 hour.

Clinical trials: In patients with a history of epinephrine intolerance, only 3% of dipivefrin-treated patients exhibited intolerance, while 55% treated with epinephrine again developed an intolerance. Response to dipivefrin twice daily is less than that to 2% epinephrine twice daily and comparable to 2% pilocarpine 4 times daily. Patients using dipivefrin twice daily had mean IOP reductions ranging from 20% to 24%.

Indications:

Glaucoma: Initial therapy or as an adjunct with other antiglaucoma agents for the control of IOP in chronic open-angle glaucoma.

Contraindications:

Hypersensitivity to dipivefrin or any formulation component; narrow-angles (any dilation of pupil may predispose patient to an attack of angle-closure glaucoma).

Warnings:

Pregnancy: Category B. There are no adequate and well controlled studies in pregnant women. Use only when clearly needed.

Lactation: It is not known whether this drug is excreted in breast milk. Use caution in nursing mothers.

Children: Safety and efficacy for use in children have not been established.

Precautions:

Aphakic patients: Macular edema occurs in up to 30% of aphakic patients treated with epinephrine. Discontinuation generally results in reversal of the maculopathy.

Adverse Reactions:

Cardiovascular: Tachycardia; arrhythmias; hypertension (reported with epinephrine).

Local: Burning and stinging (6%); conjunctival injection (6.5%); follicular conjunctivitis; mydriasis; allergic reactions (infrequent). Epinephrine therapy can lead to adrenochrome deposits in the conjunctiva and cornea.

Dipivefrin 0.1% is less irritating than 1% epinephrine HCl. Only 1.8% of dipivefrin patients reported discomfort due to photophobia, glare or light sensitivity.

Patient Information:

Slight stinging or burning on initial instillation may occur.

Do not try to "catch up" on missed doses by applying more than one dose at a time.

Administration and Dosage:

Initial glaucoma therapy: Instill 1 drop into the eye(s) every 12 hours.

Concomitant therapy: When patients receiving other antiglaucoma agents require additional therapy, add 1 drop of dipivefrin every 12 hours.

Rx	**Dipivefrin HCl** (Various, eg, Falcon, Schein)	**Solution:** 0.1%	In 5, 10 and 15 ml.
Rx	**Propine** (Allergan)		In 5, 10 & 15 ml C Cap Compliance Cap B.I.D.[1]
Rx	**AKPro** (Akorn)		In 2, 5, 10 and 15 ml dropper bottles.[1]

[1] With 0.005% benzalkonium chloride, sodium chloride, EDTA and hydrochloric acid.

ALPHA$_2$-ADRENERGIC AGONISTS

APRACLONIDINE HYDROCHLORIDE

Actions:

Pharmacology: Apraclonidine has the action of reducing elevated, as well as normal, intraocular pressure (IOP) whether accompanied by glaucoma or not. Apraclonidine is a relatively selective α_2-adrenergic agonist that does not have significant membrane stabilizing (local anesthetic) activity. Topical application of apraclonidine reduces IOP and has minimal effect on cardiovascular parameters.

Optic nerve head damage and visual field loss may result from an acute elevation in IOP that can occur after argon laser surgical procedures. The higher the peak or spike of IOP, the greater the likelihood of visual field loss and optic nerve damage, especially in patients with previously compromised optic nerves. The onset of action is usually within 1 hour and the maximum IOP reduction occurs 3 to 5 hours after application of a single dose. Apraclonidine's mechanism of action is not completely established, although its predominant action may be related to a reduction of aqueous formation via stimulation of the alpha-adrenergic system.

Pharmacokinetics: Topical use of apraclonidine 0.5% leads to systemic absorption. Studies of apraclonidine ophthalmic solution 1 drop 3 times daily in both eyes for 10 days in healthy volunteers yielded mean peak and trough concentrations of 0.9 and 0.5 ng/ml, respectively. The half-life of apraclonidine 0.5% was calculated to be 8 hours.

Clinical trials: The clinical utility of apraclonidine 0.5% is most apparent for those glaucoma patients on maximally tolerated medical therapy (ie, patients were using combinations of a topical beta blocker, sympathomimetics, parasympathomimetics and oral carbonic anhydrase inhibitors). Patients with advanced glaucoma and uncontrolled IOP scheduled to undergo laser trabeculoplasty or trabeculectomy surgery were enrolled in a study to determine whether apraclonidine dosed 3 times daily could delay the need for surgery for ≤ 3 months. Apraclonidine treatment resulted in a significantly greater percentage of treatment successes compared with patients treated with placebo.

Indications:

1%: To control or prevent post-surgical elevations in IOP that occur in patients after argon laser trabeculoplasty or iridotomy.

0.5%: Short-term adjunctive therapy in patients on tolerated maximal medical therapy who require additional IOP reduction.

Contraindications:

Hypersensitivity to any component of this medication or to clonidine; concurrent monoamine oxidase inhibitor therapy (see Drug Interactions).

Warnings:

Concomitant therapy: The addition of apraclonidine 0.5% to patients already using two aqueous-suppressing drugs (eg, beta blocker plus carbonic anhydrase inhibitor) as part of their medical therapy may not provide additional benefit. This is because apraclonidine is an aqueous-suppressing drug and the addition of a third aqueous suppressant may not significantly reduce IOP.

Tachyphylaxis: The IOP-lowering efficacy of apraclonidine 0.5% diminishes over time in some patients. This loss of effect, or tachyphylaxis, appears to be an individual occurrence with a variable time of onset and should be closely monitored. The benefit for most patients is < 3 months.

Hypersensitivity: Apraclonidine can lead to an allergic-like reaction characterized wholly or in part by the symptoms of hyperemia, pruritus, discomfort, tearing, foreign body sensation and edema of the lids and conjunctiva. If ocular allergic-like symptoms occur, discontinue therapy.

Renal/Hepatic function impairment: Although the topical use of apraclonidine has not been studied in renal failure patients, structurally related clonidine undergoes a significant increase in half-life in patients with severe renal impairment. Close monitoring of cardiovascular parameters in patients with impaired renal function is advised if they are candidates for topical apraclonidine therapy. Close monitoring of cardiovascular parameters in patients with impaired liver function is also advised as the systemic dosage form of clonidine is partly metabolized in the liver.

Pregnancy: Category C. Apraclonidine has an embryocidal affect in rabbits when given in an oral dose of 3 mg/kg (60 times the maximum recommended human dose). There are no adequate and well controlled studies in pregnant women. Use during pregnancy only if the potential benefit justifies the potential risk to the fetus.

Lactation: It is not known if topically applied apraclonidine is excreted in breast milk. Exercise caution when apraclonidine is administered to a nursing woman. Consider discontinuing nursing for the day(s) on which apraclonidine is used.

Children: Safety and efficacy for use in children have not been established.

Precautions:

Monitoring: Glaucoma patients on tolerated maximal medical therapy who are treated with apraclonidine 0.5% to delay surgery should have their visual fields monitored periodically. Discontinue treatment if IOP rises significantly or is not lowered.

IOP reduction: Apraclonidine is a potent depressor of IOP. An unpredictable decrease of IOP effect in some patients and incidence of ocular allergic responses and systemic side effects may limit the utility of apraclonidine 0.5%. However, patients on tolerated maximal medical therapy may still benefit from the additional IOP reduction provided by the short-term use of apraclonidine 0.5%.

Cardiovascular disease: Acute administration of apraclonidine has had minimal effect on heart rate or blood pressure; however, observe caution in treating patients with severe cardiovascular disease.

Use apraclonidine 0.5% with caution in patients with coronary insufficiency, recent myocardial infarction, cerebrovascular disease, chronic renal failure, Raynaud's disease or thromboangiitis obliterans.

Depression: Caution and monitor depressed patients since apraclonidine has been infrequently associated with causing depression or worsening existing depression.

Vasovagal attack: Consider the possibility of a vasovagal attack occurring during laser surgery; use caution in patients with a history of such episodes.

Corneal changes: Topical ocular administration of apraclonidine 1.5% to rabbits 3 times daily for 1 month resulted in sporadic and transient instances of minimal corneal cloudiness. No corneal changes were observed in humans given at least one dose of apraclonidine 1%.

Drug Interactions:

Apraclonidine Drug Interactions

Precipitant drug	Object drug*		Description
Apraclonidine	Cardiovascular agents	⬇	Since apraclonidine may reduce pulse and blood pressure, caution in using cardiovascular drugs is advised. Patients using cardiovascular drugs concurrently with apraclonidine 0.5% should have pulse and blood pressures frequently monitored.
Apraclonidine	MAO inhibitors	⬆	Apraclonidine should not be used in patients receiving MAO inhibitors (see Contraindications).

* ⬆ = Object drug increased. ⬇ = Object drug decreased.

Adverse Reactions:

In clinical studies the overall discontinuation rate related to apraclonidine was 15%. The most commonly reported events leading to discontinuation included (in decreasing order of frequency): Hyperemia; pruritus; tearing; discomfort; lid edema; dry mouth; foreign body sensation.

The following adverse effects were reported with the use of apraclonidine in laser surgery: Upper lid elevation (1.3%); conjunctival blanching (0.4%); mydriasis (0.4%).

The following additional adverse effects were reported (listed by solution strength):

Ophthalmic:

1% – Conjunctival blanching; upper lid elevation; mydriasis; burning; discomfort; foreign body sensation; dryness; itching; hypotony; blurred or dimmed vision; allergic response; conjunctival microhemorrhage.

0.5% – Hyperemia (13%); pruritus (10%); discomfort (6%); tearing (4%); lid edema, blurred vision, foreign body sensation, dry eye, conjunctivitis, discharge, blanching (< 3%); lid margin crusting, conjunctival follicles, conjunctival edema, edema, abnormal vision, pain, lid disorder, keratitis, blepharitis, photophobia, corneal staining, lid erythema, blepharoconjunctivitis, irritation, corneal erosion, corneal infiltrate, keratopathy, lid scales, lid retraction (< 1%).

GI:

1% – Abdominal pain; diarrhea; stomach discomfort; emesis; dry mouth.

0.5% – Dry mouth (2%); constipation, nausea (< 1%).

Cardiovascular:

1% – Bradycardia; vasovagal attack; palpitations; orthostatic episode.

0.5% – Asthenia (< 3%); peripheral edema, arrhythmia (< 1%). Although there are no reports of bradycardia, consider the possibility.

CNS:

1% – Insomnia; dream disturbances; irritability; decreased libido; headache; paresthesia.

0.5% – Headache (< 3%); somnolence, dizziness, nervousness, depression, insomnia, paresthesia (< 1%).

Hypersensitivity – Use can lead to an allergic-like reaction (see Warnings).

Respiratory:

0.5% – Dry nose (2%); rhinitis, dyspnea, pharyngitis, asthma (< 1%).

Miscellaneous:

1% – Taste abnormalities; nasal burning or dryness; head cold sensation; chest heaviness or burning; clammy or sweaty palms; body heat sensation; shortness of breath; increased pharyngeal secretion; extremity pain or numbness; fatigue; pruritus not associated with rash.

0.5% – Taste perversion (3%); contact dermatitis, dermatitis, chest pain, abnormal coordination, malaise, facial edema (< 1%); myalgia, parosmia (0.2%).

Patient Information:

Do not touch dropper tip to any surface as this may contaminate the contents.

Apraclonidine can cause dizziness and somnolence. Patients who engage in hazardous activities requiring mental alertness should be warned of the potential for a decrease in mental alertness, physical dexterity or coordination while using apraclonidine.

Administration and Dosage:

0.5%: Instill 1 to 2 drops in the affected eye(s) 3 times daily. Since apraclonidine 0.5% will be used with other ocular glaucoma therapies, use an approximate 5 minute interval between instillation of each medication to prevent washout of the previous dose. Not for injection into the eye.

1%: Instill 1 drop in scheduled operative eye 1 hour before initiating anterior segment laser surgery. Instill second drop into same eye immediately upon completion of surgery.

Storage: Store at room temperature. Protect from light and freezing (0.5%).

Rx	**Iopidine** (Alcon)	**Solution**: 0.5%	In 5 ml and 10 ml Drop-Tainers.[1]
		Solution: 1%	In 0.1 ml (2s).[1]

[1] With 0.01% benzalkonium chloride.

BRIMONIDINE TARTRATE

Actions:

Pharmacology: Brimonidine tartrate is a relatively selective alpha-2 adrenergic agonist for ophthalmic use. It has a peak ocular hypotensive effect occurring at 2 hours post-dosing. Fluorophotometric studies in animals and humans suggest that brimonidine tartrate has a dual mechanism of action by reducing aqueous humor production and increasing uveoscleral outflow.

Pharmacokinetics: After ocular administration of a 0.2% solution, plasma concentration peaked within 1 to 4 hours and declined with a systemic half-life of approximately 3 hours. In humans it is systemically metabolized by the liver primarily, with urinary excretion as the major route of elimination of the drug and its metabolites.

Clinical trials: Elevated IOP presents a major risk factor in glaucomatous field loss. The higher the level of IOP, the greater the likelihood of optic nerve damage and visual field loss. Brimonidine tartrate has the action of lowering intraocular pressure with minimal effect on cardiovascular and pulmonary parameters.

Indications:

To lower intraocular pressure in patients with open-angle glaucoma or ocular hypertension. The ability to lower IOP diminishes over time in some patients. This loss of effect appears with a variable time of onset in each patient, and should be closely monitored.

Contraindications:

Hypersensitivity to brimonidine tartrate or any component of this medication. It also is contraindicated in patients receiving monoamine oxidase (MAO) inhibitor therapy.

Warnings:

Pregnancy: Category B. Reproduction studies performed in rats revealed no evidence of impaired fertility or harm to the fetus due to brimonidine tartrate. There are no studies of brimonidine tartrate in pregnant women; however, in animal studies, brimonidine crossed the placenta and entered into the fetal circulation to a limited extent. Brimonidine tartrate should be used during pregnancy only if the potential benefit to the mother justifies the potential risk to the fetus.

Nursing mothers: It is not known whether brimonidine tartrate is excreted in human milk, although in animal studies brimonidine tartrate has been shown to be excreted in breast milk. A decision should be made whether to discontinue nursing or to discontinue the drug, taking into account the importance of the drug to the mother.

Children: Safety and efficacy in children have not been established.

Precautions:

Cardiovascular disease: Although in clinical studies, brimonidine tartrate had minimal effect on blood pressure, caution should be exercised in treating patients with severe cardiovascular disease.

Renal/Hepatic function impairment: Brimonidine tartrate has not been studied in patients with hepatic or renal impairment; caution should be used in treating such patients.

Depression: Caution should be used in patients with depression, cerebral or coronary insufficiency, Raynaud's phenomenon, orthostatic hypotension or thromboangiitis obliterans.

Hazardous tasks: Brimonidine tartrate may cause fatigue and drowsiness in some patients. Observe caution while driving, operating machinery or performing other tasks requiring coordination or physical dexterity.

Drug Interactions:

CNS depressants: The possibility of an additive or potentiating effect with CNS depressants (alcohol, barbiturates, opiates, sedatives or anesthetics) should be considered.

Concomitant therapy: Brimonidine tartrate did not have significant effects on pulse and blood pressure in clinical studies. However, caution is advised in using concomitant drugs such as beta blockers (ophthalmic and systemic), antihypertensives and cardiac glycosides.

Tricyclic antidepressants have been reported to blunt the hypotensive effect of systemic clonidine. It is not known whether the concurrent use of these agents with brimonidine tartrate can lead to an interference in IOP-lowering effect. No data on the level of circulating catecholamines after brimonidine tartrate is instilled are available. Caution is advised in patients taking tricyclic antidepressants, which can affect the metabolism and uptake of circulating amines.

Adverse Reactions:

The most commonly reported adverse events included: Oral dryness, ocular hyperemia, burning and stinging, headache, blurring, foreign body sensation, fatigue/drowsiness, conjunctival follicles, ocular allergic reactions, ocular pruritus, corneal staining/erosion, photophobia, eyelid erythema, ocular ache/pain, ocular dryness, tearing, upper respiratory symptoms, eyelid edema, conjunctival edema, dizziness, blepharitis, ocular irritation, gastrointestinal symptoms, asthenia, conjunctival blanching, abnormal vision, muscular pain, lid crusting, conjunctival hemorrhage, abnormal taste, insomnia, conjunctival discharge, depression, hypertension, anxiety, palpitations, nasal dryness and syncope.

Patient Information:

Do not touch dropper tip to any surface as this may contaminate the contents.

The preservative in brimonidine tartrate, benzalkonium chloride, may be absorbed by soft contact lenses. Patients wearing soft contact lenses should be instructed to wait at least 15 minutes after instilling brimonidine tartrate to insert soft contact lenses.

Brimonidine tartrate may cause fatigue and drowsiness in some patients. Patients who engage in hazardous activities should be cautioned of the potential for a decrease in mental alertness.

Administration and Dosage:

Instill 1 drop of brimonidine tartrate in the affected eye(s) 3 times daily, approximately 8 hours apart.

Storage: Store at or below 25°C (77° F).

Rx	**Alphagan** (Allergan)	**Solution:** 0.2% brimonidine tartrate, 0.05 mg benzalkonium chloride	In 5 and 10 ml dropper bottles.

BETA-ADRENERGIC BLOCKING AGENTS

Actions:

Pharmacology: Timolol, levobunolol, carteolol and metipranolol are noncardioselective (β_1 and β_2) β-blockers; betaxolol is a cardioselective (β_1) β-blocker. Topical β-blockers generally do not have significant membrane-stabilizing (local anesthetic) actions or intrinsic sympathomimetic activity (ISA) except for carteolol which does have ISA.

The exact mechanism of ocular hypotensive action is not established, but it appears to be a reduction of aqueous production. Some studies show a slight increase in outflow facility with timolol and metipranolol.

These agents reduce IOP with little or no effect on pupil size or accommodation. Blurred vision and night blindness often associated with miotics are not associated with these agents. In addition, in patients with cataracts, the inability to see around lenticular opacities when the pupil is constricted, is avoided. These agents, as well as all topically applied ocular agents, may be absorbed systemically (see Warnings).

Pharmacokinetics:

Pharmacokinetics of Ophthalmic β-Adrenergic Blocking Agents				
Drug	β-receptor selectivity	Onset (min)	Maximum effect (hr)	Duration (hr)
Carteolol	β_1 and β_2	nd	nd	12
Betaxolol	β_1	30	2	12
Levobunolol	β_1 and β_2	< 60	2 to 6	12 to 24
Metipranolol	β_1 and β_2	≤ 30	≈ 2	12 to 24
Timolol	β_1 and β_2	30	1 to 2	12 to 24

nd = No data

Clinical trials:

Timolol – In controlled studies of untreated IOP of ≥ 22 mm Hg, timolol 0.25% or 0.5% twice daily caused greater IOP reduction than 4% pilocarpine solution 4 times daily or 2% epinephrine HCl solution twice daily. In comparative studies, mean IOP reduction was 31% to 33% with timolol, 22% with pilocarpine and 28% with epinephrine.

In ocular hypertension, effects of timolol and acetazolamide are additive. Timolol, generally well tolerated, produces fewer and less severe side effects than pilocarpine or epinephrine. Timolol has been well tolerated in patients wearing conventional (PMMA) hard contact lenses.

Betaxolol ophthalmic was compared to ophthalmic timolol and placebo in patients with reactive airway disease. Betaxolol had no significant effect on pulmonary function as measured by Forced Expiratory Volume (FEV_1), Forced Vital Capacity (FVC) and FEV_1/VC. Also, action of isoproterenol was not inhibited. Timolol significantly decreased these pulmonary functions. No evidence of cardiovascular β-blockade during exercise was observed with betaxolol. Mean arterial blood pressure was not affected by any treatment; however, timolol significantly decreased mean heart rate. Betaxolol reduces mean IOP 25% from baseline. In controlled studies, the magnitude and duration of the ocular hypotensive effects of betaxolol and timolol were clinically similar. Clinical observation of glaucoma patients treated with betaxolol solution for up to 3 years shows that the IOP-lowering effect is well maintained.

Betaxolol has been successfully used in glaucoma patients who have undergone laser trabeculoplasty and have needed long-term hypotensive therapy. The drug is well tolerated in glaucoma patients with hard or soft contact lenses and in aphakic patients.

Levobunolol effectively reduced IOP in controlled clinical studies from 3 months to over 1 year when given topically twice daily; IOP was well maintained. The mean IOP decrease is clinically similar to timolol.

Metipranolol reduced the average intraocular pressure approximately 20% to 26% in controlled studies of patients with IOP > 24 mm Hg at baseline. Clinical studies in patients with glaucoma treated ≤ 2 years indicate that an intraocular pressure lowering effect is maintained.

Carteolol produced a median percent IOP reduction of 22% to 25% when given twice daily in clinical trials ranging from 1.5 to 3 months.

Indications:

Glaucoma: Lowering IOP in patients with chronic open-angle glaucoma.

For specific approved indications, refer to individual drug monographs.

Contraindications:

Bronchial asthma, a history of bronchial asthma or severe chronic obstructive pulmonary disease; sinus bradycardia; second-degree and third-degree AV block; overt cardiac failure; cardiogenic shock; hypersensitivity to any component of the products.

Warnings:

Systemic absorption: These agents may be absorbed systemically. The same adverse reactions found with systemic β-blockers may occur with topical use. For example, severe respiratory reactions and cardiac reactions, including death due to bronchospasm in asthmatics, and rarely, death associated with cardiac failure, have been reported with topical β-blockers. These agents may decrease heart rate and blood pressure, and betaxolol has had adverse effects on pulmonary and cardiovascular parameters. Exercise caution with all of these agents.

Cardiovascular: Timolol can decrease resting and maximal exercise heart rate even in healthy subjects.

> *Cardiac failure* – Sympathetic stimulation may be essential for circulation support in diminished myocardial contractility; its inhibition by β-receptor blockade may precipitate more severe failure.
>
> *In patients without history of cardiac failure,* continued depression of myocardium with β-blockers may lead to cardiac failure. Discontinue at the first sign or symptom of cardiac failure.

Non-allergic bronchospasm patients or patients with a history of chronic bronchitis, emphysema, etc, should receive β-blockers with caution; they may block bronchodilation produced by catecholamine stimulation of β_2-receptors.

Major surgery: Withdrawing β-blockers before major surgery is controversial. Beta-receptor blockade impairs the heart's ability to respond to β-adrenergically mediated reflex stimuli. This may augment the risk of general anesthesia. Some patients on β-blockers have had protracted severe hypotension during anesthesia. Difficulty restarting and maintaining heartbeat has been reported. In elective surgery, gradual withdrawal of β-blockers may be appropriate.

The effects of β-blocking agents may be reversed by β-agonists such as isoproterenol, dopamine, dobutamine or norepinephrine.

Diabetes mellitus: Administer with caution to patients subject to spontaneous hypoglycemia or to diabetic patients (especially labile diabetics). Beta-blocking agents may mask signs and symptoms of acute hypoglycemia.

Thyroid: Beta-adrenergic blocking agents may mask clinical signs of hyperthyroidism (eg, tachycardia). Manage patients suspected of developing thyrotoxicosis carefully to avoid abrupt withdrawal of β-blockers which might precipitate thyroid storm.

Cerebrovascular insufficiency: Because of potential effects of β-blockers on blood pressure and pulse, use with caution in patients with cerebrovascular insufficiency. If signs or symptoms suggesting reduced cerebral blood flow develop, consider alternative therapy.

Carcinogenesis: In female mice receiving oral metipranolol doses of 5, 50 and 100 mg/kg/day, the low dose had an increased number of pulmonary adenomas.

Pregnancy: Category C. There have been no adequate and well controlled studies in pregnant women. Use during pregnancy only if the potential benefits outweigh potential hazards to the fetus.

> *Carteolol* – Increased resorptions and decreased fetal weights occurred in rabbits and rats at maternal doses ≈ 1052 and 5264 times the maximum human dose, respectively. A dose-related increase in wavy ribs was noted in the developing rat fetus when pregnant rats received doses ≈ 212 times the maximum human dose.
>
> *Betaxolol* – In oral studies with rats and rabbits, evidence of post-implantation loss was seen at dose levels above 12 mg/kg and 128 mg/kg, respectively. Betaxolol was not teratogenic, however, and there were no other adverse effects on reproduction at subtoxic dose levels.
>
> *Levobunolol* – Fetotoxicity was observed in rabbits at doses 200 and 700 times the glaucoma dose.
>
> *Metipranolol* – Increased fetal resorption, fetal death and delayed development occurred in rabbits receiving 50 mg/kg orally during organogenesis.
>
> *Timolol* – Doses 1000 times the maximum recommended human oral dose were maternotoxic in mice and resulted in increased fetal resorptions. Increased fetal resorptions were also seen in rabbits at 100 times the maximum recommended human oral dose.

Lactation: It is not known whether *betaxolol, levobunolol* or *metipranolol* are excreted in breast milk. Systemic β-blockers and topical *timolol maleate* are excreted in milk. *Carteolol* is excreted in breast milk of animals. Exercise caution when administering to a nursing mother.

Because of the potential for serious adverse reactions from *timolol* in nursing infants, decide whether to discontinue nursing or discontinue the drug taking into account the importance of the drug to the mother.

Children: Safety and efficacy for use in children have not been established.

Precautions:

Angle-closure glaucoma: The immediate objective is to reopen the angle, requiring constriction of the pupil with a miotic. These agents have little or no effect on the pupil. When they are used to reduce elevated IOP in angle-closure glaucoma, use with a miotic.

Muscle weakness: Beta-blockade may potentiate muscle weakness consistent with certain myasthenic symptoms (eg, diplopia, ptosis, generalized weakness). *Timolol* has increased muscle weakness in some patients with myasthenic symptoms.

Long-term therapy: Diminished responsiveness to *betaxolol* and *timolol* after prolonged therapy has occurred. However, in long-term studies (2 and 3 years), no significant differences in mean IOP were observed after initial stabilization.

Sulfite sensitivity: Some of these products contain sulfites which may cause allergic-type reactions (eg, hives, itching, wheezing, anaphylaxis) in certain susceptible persons. Although the overall prevalence of sulfite sensitivity in the general population is probably low, it is seen more frequently in asthmatics or atopic nonasthmatics.

Drug Interactions:

Ophthalmic Beta Blocker Drug Interactions

Precipitant drug	Object drug*		Description
Beta blockers, ophthalmic	Beta blockers, oral	↑	Use topical β-blockers with caution because of the potential for additive effects on systemic β-blockade.
Beta blockers, ophthalmic	Epinephrine, ophthalmic	↔	Use of epinephrine with topical β-blockers is controversial. Some reports indicate initial effectiveness decreases over time. In one case verified by rechallenge, combined use of topical epinephrine and topical timolol appeared to result in hypertension from unopposed α-adrenergic stimulation. However, this combination has been used to reduce IOP.
Beta blockers, ophthalmic	Quinidine	↑	One case of sinus bradycardia has been reported with the coadministration of ophthalmic timolol. The incidence was reaffirmed by a negative rechallenge with the β-blockers alone and positive rechallenge with the combination.
Beta blockers, ophthalmic	Verapamil	↑	Coadministration of ophthalmic timolol has caused bradycardia and asystole.

* ↑ = Object drug increased. ↔ = Undetermined effect.

Other drugs that may interact with systemic β-adrenergic blocking agents may also interact with ophthalmic agents. These agents are listed below.

Antithyroid agents
Calcium channel blockers
Cimetidine
Clonidine
Contraceptives, oral
Digoxin
Disopyramide
Haloperidol
Hydralazine
Insulin
Lidocaine
Morphine
Neuromuscular blockers, nondepolarizing
Nicotine
NSAIDs
Phenobarbital
Phenothiazines
Prazosin
Rifampin
Salicylates
Smoking
Sympathomimetics
Theophylline
Thyroid hormones

Adverse Reactions:

The following have occurred with ophthalmic β_1 *and* β_2 *(nonselective) blockers:*

CNS – Headache; depression.

Cardiovascular – Arrhythmia; syncope; heart block; cerebral vascular accident; cerebral ischemia; congestive heart failure; palpitation.

GI – Nausea.

Dermatologic – Hypersensitivity, including localized and generalized rash.

Respiratory – Bronchospasm (predominantly in patients with preexisting bronchospastic disease); respiratory failure.

Endocrine – Masked symptoms of hypoglycemia in insulin-dependent diabetics (see Warnings).

Ophthalmic – Keratitis; blepharoptosis; visual disturbances including refractive changes (due to withdrawal of miotic therapy in some cases); diplopia; ptosis.

The following adverse reactions have occurred with the individual agent:

Carteolol:

Ophthalmic – Transient irritation, burning, tearing, conjunctival hyperemia, edema (≈ 25%), blurred/cloudy vision; photophobia; decreased night vision; ptosis; blepharoconjunctivitis; abnormal corneal staining; corneal sensitivity.

Systemic – Bradycardia; decreased blood pressure; arrhythmia; heart palpitation; dyspnea; asthenia; headache; dizziness; insomnia; sinusitis; taste perversion.

Betaxolol:

Ophthalmic – Brief discomfort (> 25%); occasional tearing (5%), decreased corneal sensitivity, erythema, itching, corneal punctate staining, keratitis, anisocoria; photophobia (rare).

Systemic – Insomnia; depressive neurosis (rare).

Metipranolol:

Ophthalmic – Transient local discomfort; conjunctivitis; eyelid dermatitis; blepharitis; blurred vision; tearing; browache; abnormal vision; photophobia; edema.

Systemic – Allergic reaction; headache; asthenia; hypertension; myocardial infarction; atrial fibrillation; angina; palpitation; bradycardia; nausea; rhinitis; dyspnea; epistaxis; bronchitis; coughing; dizziness; anxiety; depression; somnolence; nervousness; arthritis; myalgia; rash.

Levobunolol:

Ophthalmic – Transient burning/stinging (25%); blepharoconjunctivitis (5%); iridocyclitis (rare); decreased corneal sensitivity.

Cardiovascular – Effects may resemble timolol.

CNS – Ataxia, dizziness, lethargy (rare).

Dermatologic – Urticaria, pruritus (rare).

Timolol:

Ophthalmic – Ocular irritation including conjunctivitis; blepharitis; keratitis; blepharoptosis; decreased corneal sensitivity; visual disturbances including refractive changes (due, in some cases, to withdrawal of miotics); diplopia; ptosis.

CNS – Dizziness; depression; fatigue; lethargy; hallucinations; confusion.

Cardiovascular – Bradycardia; arrhythmia; hypotension; syncope; heart block; cerebral vascular accident; cerebral ischemia; heart failure; palpitation; cardiac arrest. These generally occur in the elderly or in patients with preexisting cardiovascular problems.

Respiratory – Bronchospasm (mainly in patients with preexisting bronchospastic disease); respiratory failure; dyspnea.

Miscellaneous – Aggravation of myasthenia gravis; alopecia; nail pigmentary changes; nausea; hypersensitivity, including localized and generalized rash; urticaria; asthenia; sexual dysfunction, including impotence, decreased libido; decreased ejaculation; hyperkalemia; masked symptoms of hypoglycemia in insulin-dependent diabetics; diarrhea; paresthesia.

Causal relationship unknown – Hypertension; chest pain; dyspepsia; anorexia; dry mouth; behavioral changes (eg, anxiety, disorientation, nervousness, somnolence, psychic disturbance); aphakic cystoid macular edema; retroperitoneal fibrosis.

Systemic β-adrenergic blocker-associated reactions – Consider potential effects with ophthalmic use (see Warnings).

Overdosage:

If ocular overdosage occurs, flush eye(s) with water or normal saline. If accidentally ingested, efforts to decrease further absorption may be appropriate (gastric lavage).

The most common signs and symptoms of overdosage from systemic β-blockers are bradycardia, hypotension, bronchospasm and acute cardiac failure. If these occur, discontinue therapy and initiate appropriate supportive therapy.

Patient Information:

Refer to the Dosage Forms and Routes of Administration chapter for more complete information.

Transient stinging/discomfort is relatively common; notify physician if severe.

Administration and Dosage:

Concomitant therapy: If IOP is not controlled with these agents, institute concomitant pilocarpine, other miotics, dipivefrin or carbonic anhydrase inhibitors.

Use of epinephrine with topical β-blockers is controversial. Some reports indicate that initial effectiveness of the combination decreases over time (see Drug Interactions).

Monitoring: The IOP-lowering response to betaxolol and timolol may require a few weeks to stabilize. Determine the IOP during the first month of treatment. Thereafter, determine IOP on an individual basis.

Because of diurnal IOP variations in individual patients, satisfactory response to twice-a-day therapy is best determined by measuring IOP at different times during the day. Intraocular pressures $\leq$ 22 mm Hg may not be optimal to control glaucoma in each patient; therefore, individualize therapy.

Individual drug monographs are on the following pages.

BETAXOLOL HYDROCHLORIDE

For complete prescribing information, refer to the Beta-adrenergic Blocking Agents group monograph.

Indications:

Treatment of ocular hypertension and chronic open-angle glaucoma. Betaxolol may be used alone or in combination with other antiglaucoma drugs.

Administration and Dosage:

Usual dose: Instill 1 drop twice daily.

Replacement therapy (single agent): Continue the agent already used and add 1 drop of betaxolol twice daily. The following day, discontinue the previous agent and continue betaxolol. Monitor with tonometry.

Replacement therapy (multiple agents): When transferring from several concomitant antiglaucoma agents, individualize dosage. Adjust 1 agent at a time at intervals of not less than 1 week. One may continue the agents being used and add 1 drop betaxolol twice daily. The next day, discontinue another agent. Decrease or discontinue remaining antiglaucoma agents according to patient response.

Storage: Store at room temperature 15° to 30°C (59° to 86°F). Shake suspension well.

Rx	**Betoptic** (Alcon)	**Solution:** 5.6 mg (equiv. to 5 mg base) per ml (0.5%)	In 2.5, 5, 10 and 15 ml Drop-Tainer bottles.[1]
Rx	**Betoptic S** (Alcon)	**Suspension:** 2.8 mg (equiv. to 2.5 mg base) per ml (0.25%)	In 2.5, 5, 10 and 15 ml Drop-Tainer bottles.[2]

[1] With 0.01% benzalkonium chloride and EDTA.
[2] With 0.01% benzalkonium chloride, mannitol, poly sulfonic acid, carbomer 934P and EDTA.

CARTEOLOL HYDROCHLORIDE

For complete prescribing information, refer to the Beta-adrenergic Blocking Agents group monograph.

Indications:

Treatment of chronic open-angle glaucoma and ocular hypertension. It may be used alone or in combination with other IOP lowering drugs.

Administration and Dosage:

Usual dose: Instill 1 drop in affected eye(s) twice daily. If the patient's IOP is not at a satisfactory level on this regimen, concomitant therapy can be instituted.

Rx	**Ocupress** (Otsuka America)	**Solution:** 1%	In 5 and 10 ml dropper bottles.[1]

[1] With 0.005% benzalkonium chloride.

LEVOBUNOLOL HYDROCHLORIDE

For complete prescribing information, refer to the Beta-adrenergic Blocking Agents group monograph.

Indications:

Lower IOP in chronic open-angle glaucoma or ocular hypertension.

Administration and Dosage:

Usual dose: Instill 1 drop in the affected eye(s) once or twice daily.

Rx	**Levobunolol** (Various, eg, Bausch & Lomb, Pacific Pharma)	**Solution:** 0.25%	In 5 and 10 ml.
Rx	**AKBeta** (Akorn)		In 5 and 10 ml.
Rx	**Betagan Liquifilm** (Allergan)		In 5 and 10 ml dropper bottles with B.I.D. *C Cap.*[1]
Rx	**Levobunolol** (Various, eg, Bausch & Lomb)	**Solution:** 0.5%	In 5, 10 and 15 ml.
Rx	**AKBeta** (Akorn)		In 5, 10 and 15 ml.
Rx	**Betagan Liquifilm** (Allergan)		In 2 ml bottles with B.I.D. and Q.D. *C Cap.*[1]

[1] With 1.4% polyvinyl alcohol, 0.004% benzalkonium chloride, sodium metabisulfite and EDTA.

METIPRANOLOL HYDROCHLORIDE

For complete prescribing information, refer to the Beta-adrenergic Blocking Agents group monograph.

Indications:

Treatment of ocular conditions in which lowering IOP is likely to be of therapeutic benefit, including ocular hypertension and chronic open-angle glaucoma.

Administration and Dosage:

Usual dose: Instill 1 drop in the affected eye(s) twice a day. If the patient's IOP is not at a satisfactory level on this regimen, more frequent administration or a larger dose is of benefit. Concomitant therapy to lower IOP can be instituted.

Rx	**OptiPranolol** (Bausch & Lomb)	**Solution:** 0.3%	In 5 or 10 ml dropper bottles.[1]

[1] With 0.004% benzalkonium chloride and EDTA.

TIMOLOL MALEATE

For complete prescribing information, refer to the Beta-adrenergic Blocking Agents group monograph.

Indications:

Lower IOP in chronic open-angle glaucoma, aphakic glaucoma patients, some patients with secondary glaucoma and in patients with elevated IOP who need ocular pressure lowering. In patients who respond inadequately to multiple antiglaucoma drug therapy, the addition of timolol may produce further IOP reduction.

Administration and Dosage:

Solution:

Initial therapy – Instill 1 drop of 0.25% or 0.5% twice daily. Since the pressure-lowering response may require a few weeks to stabilize, evaluation should include a determination of IOP after approximately 4 weeks of treatment.

Gel: Invert the closed container and shake once before each use; it is not necessary to shake it more than once. Administer other ophthalmics at least 10 minutes before the gel. Dose is 1 drop (0.25% or 0.5%) once daily. Consider concomitant therapy if IOP is not at a satisfactory level. When patients are switched from timolol solution twice daily to the gel once daily, the ocular hypotensive effect should remain constant.

Rx	**Timolol Maleate** (Various, eg, Alcon)	**Solution:** 0.25%	In 5, 10 and 15 ml.
Rx	**Timoptic Maleate** (Merck)		In 2.5, 5, 10 & 15 ml Ocu-meters[1] & UD 60s Ocudose.[2]
Rx	**Betimol** (Ciba Vision)	**Solution:** 0.25% (timolol hemihydrate)	In 2.5, 5, 10 and 15 ml.[1]
Rx	**Timolol Maleate** (Various, eg, Alcon)	**Solution:** 0.5%	In 5, 10 and 15 ml.
Rx	**Timoptic** (Merck)		In 2.5, 5, 10 & 15 ml Ocu- meters[1]& UD 60s Ocudose.[2]
Rx	**Betimol** (Ciba Vision)	**Solution:** 0.5% (timolol hemihydrate)	In 2.5, 5, 10 and 15 ml.[1]
Rx	**Timoptic-XE** (Merck)	**Solution, gel-forming:** 0.25%	In 2.5 and 5 ml.[3]
		0.5%	In 2.5 and 5 ml.[3]

[1] With 0.01% benzalkonium chloride.
[2] Preservative free; use immediately after opening; discard remaining contents.
[3] With 0.012% benzododecinium bromide.

MIOTICS, DIRECT-ACTING

Refer to the Agents for Glaucoma introduction for a general discussion of these products.

Actions:

Pharmacology: The direct-acting miotics are parasympathomimetic (cholinergic) drugs which duplicate the muscarinic effects of acetylcholine. When applied topically, these drugs produce pupillary constriction, stimulate the ciliary muscles and increase aqueous humor outflow facility. Miosis, produced through contraction of the iris sphincter, causes increased tension on the scleral spur (reducing outflow resistance) and opening of the trabecular meshwork spaces facilitating outflow. With the increase in outflow facility, there is a decrease in intraocular pressure (IOP). Topical ophthalmic instillation of acetylcholine causes no discernible response as cholinesterase destroys the molecule more rapidly than it can penetrate the cornea; therefore, acetylcholine is used only intraocularly.

Miosis Induction of Direct-Acting Miotics			
Topical Miotic	Onset	Peak	Duration
Carbachol	10 to 20 min	—	4 to 8 hours
Pilocarpine	10 to 30 min	—	4 to 8 hours

Indications:

Carbachol, topical; pilocarpine:

Glaucoma – To decrease elevated IOP in glaucoma.

Acetylcholine; carbachol, intraocular:

Miosis – To induce miosis during surgery.

See individual monographs for specific indications.

Contraindications:

Hypersensitivity to any component of the formulation; where constriction is undesirable (eg, acute iritis, acute or anterior uveitis, some forms of secondary glaucoma, pupillary block glaucoma, acute inflammatory disease of the anterior chamber).

Warnings:

Corneal abrasion: Use carbachol with caution in the presence of corneal abrasion to avoid excessive penetration.

Pregnancy: Category C (carbachol, pilocarpine). Safety for use during pregnancy has not been established. Use only when clearly needed.

Lactation: It is not known whether these drugs are excreted in breast milk; exercise caution when administering to a nursing woman.

Children: Safety and efficacy for use in children have not been established.

Precautions:

Systemic reactions: Caution is advised in patients with acute cardiac failure, bronchial asthma, peptic ulcer, hyperthyroidism, GI spasm, urinary tract obstruction, Parkinson's disease, recent MI, hypertension or hypotension.

Retinal detachment has been caused by miotics in susceptible individuals, in individuals with preexisting retinal disease, or in those who are predisposed to retinal tears. Fundus examination is advised for all patients prior to initiation of therapy.

Miosis usually causes difficulty in dark adaptation. Advise patients to use caution while night driving or performing hazardous tasks in poor light.

Angle-closure: Although withdrawal of the peripheral iris from the anterior chamber angle by miosis may reduce the tendency for angle-closure, miotics can occasionally precipitate angle closure by increasing resistance to aqueous flow from posterior to anterior chamber.

Pilocarpine ocular system (Ocusert): Carefully consider and evaluate patients with acute infectious conjunctivitis or keratitis prior to use.

Drug Interactions:

Nonsteroidal anti-inflammatory agents, topical: Although studies with acetylcholine chloride or carbachol revealed no interference, and there is no known pharmacological basis for an interaction, there have been reports that both of these drugs have been ineffective when used in patients treated with topical nonsteroidal anti-inflammatory agents.

Adverse Reactions:

Acetylcholine:

Ophthalmic – Corneal edema; clouding; decompensation.

Systemic – Bradycardia; hypotension; flushing; breathing difficulties; sweating.

Carbachol:

Ophthalmic – Transient stinging and burning; corneal clouding; persistent bullous keratopathy; postoperative iritis following cataract extraction with intraocular use; retinal detachment; transient ciliary and conjunctival injection; ciliary spasm with resultant temporary decrease of visual acuity.

Systemic – Headache; salivation; GI cramps; vomiting; diarrhea; asthma; syncope; cardiac arrhythmia; flushing; sweating; epigastric distress; tightness in bladder; hypotension; frequent urge to urinate.

Pilocarpine:

Ophthalmic – Transient stinging and burning; tearing; ciliary spasm; conjunctival vascular congestion; temporal, peri- or supra-orbital headache; superficial keratitis; induced myopia (especially in younger individuals who have recently started administration); blurred vision; poor dark adaptation; reduced visual acuity in poor illumination in older individuals and in individuals with lens opacity. A subtle corneal granularity has occurred with pilocarpine gel. Lens opacity (prolonged use), retinal detachment (rare; see Precautions).

Systemic – Hypertension; tachycardia; bronchiolar spasm; pulmonary edema; salivation; sweating; nausea; vomiting; diarrhea (rare).

Pilocarpine ocular system (Ocusert) Conjunctival irritation, including mild erythema with or without a slight increase in mucus secretion with first use. These symptoms tend to lessen or disappear after the first week of therapy. Ciliary spasm may occur with pilocarpine usage but is not a contraindication to continued therapy unless the induced myopia is debilitating to the patient. Rarely, a sudden increase in pilocarpine effects has been reported during use.

Irritation from pilocarpine has been infrequently encountered and may require cessation of therapy. True allergic reactions are uncommon, but require discontinuation of therapy. Corneal abrasion and visual impairment have occurred.

Overdosage:

Should accidental overdosage in the eye(s) occur, flush with water.

Treatment: Treatment includes usual supportive measures. Observe patients for signs of toxicity (eg, salivation, lacrimation, sweating, nausea, vomiting, diarrhea). If these occur, therapy with anticholinergics (atropine) may be necessary. Bronchial constriction may be a problem in asthmatic patients.

Patient Information:

May sting upon instillation, especially first few doses.

May cause headache, browache and decreased night vision. Use caution while night driving or performing hazardous tasks in poor light.

To avoid contamination, do not touch tip of container to any surface. Replace cap after using. Keep bottle tightly closed when not in use. Discard solution after expiration date. Wash hands immediately after use.

Individual drug monographs are on the following pages.

ACETYLCHOLINE CHLORIDE, INTRAOCULAR

For complete prescribing information, refer to the Miotics, Direct-Acting group monograph. The following section is included here for completeness to show all of the clinical uses of this class of drug.

Indications:

Miosis: To produce complete miosis rapidly in cataract surgery, penetrating keratoplasty, iridectomy and other anterior segment surgery where rapid, complete miosis is desirable.

Administration and Dosage:

Solution: 0.5 to 2 ml produces satisfactory miosis. Solution need not be flushed from the chamber after miosis occurs. Since acetylcholine has a short duration of action, pilocarpine may be applied topically after the operation to maintain miosis.

Preparation of solution: The aqueous solution of acetylcholine chloride is unstable. Prepare solution immediately before use. Do not use solution which is not clear and colorless. Discard any solution that has not been used. Do not gas sterilize.

Storage: Store at room temperature 15° to 30°C (59° to 86°F). Do not freeze.

Rx	**Miochol-E** (Ciba Vision)	**Solution**: 1:100 acetylcholine chloride when reconstituted	In 2 ml dual chamber univial (lower chamber 20 mg lyophilized acetylcholine chloride and 56 mg mannitol; upper chamber 2 ml electrolyte diluent[1] and sterile water for injection).

[1] Sodium chloride, potassium chloride, magnesium chloride hexahydrate, calcium chloride dihydrate.

CARBACHOL, INTRAOCULAR

For complete prescribing information, refer to the Miotics, Direct-Acting group monograph. The following section is included here for completeness to show all of the clinical uses of this class of drug.

Indications:

Miosis: Intraocular use for miosis during surgery.

Administration and Dosage:

For single-dose intraocular use only. Discard unused portion.

Open under aseptic conditions only.

Gently instill no more than 0.5 ml into the anterior chamber before or after securing sutures. Miosis is usually maximal 2 to 5 minutes after application.

Storage: Store at room temperature 15° to 30°C (59° to 86°F).

Rx	**Carbastat** (Ciba Vision)	**Solution**: 0.01%	In 1.5 ml vials.[1]
Rx	**Miostat** (Alcon)		In 1.5 ml vials.[1]

[1] With 0.64% sodium chloride, 0.075% potassium chloride dihydrate, 0.03% magnesium chloride hexahydrate, 0.39% sodium acetate trihydrate, 0.17% sodium citrate dihydrate, sodium hydroxide, hydrochloric acid.

CARBACHOL, TOPICAL

For complete prescribing information, refer to the Miotics, Direct-Acting group monograph.

Indications:

Glaucoma: For lowering intraocular pressure in the treatment of glaucoma.

Administration and Dosage:

Instill 1 drop into eye(s) up to 3 times daily.

Storage: Store at 8° to 27°C (46° to 80°F).

Rx	**Isopto Carbachol** (Alcon)	**Solution**: 0.75%	In 15 and 30 ml Drop-Tainers.[1]
		1.5%	In 15 and 30 ml Drop-Tainers.[1]
		2.25%	In 15 ml Drop-Tainers.[1]
Rx	**Isopto Carbachol** (Alcon)	3%	In 15 and 30 ml Drop-Tainers.[1]
Rx	**Carboptic** (Optopics)		In 15 ml.[2]

[1] With 0.005% benzalkonium chloride, 1% hydroxypropyl methylcellulose, sodium chloride, boric acid and sodium borate.
[2] With benzalkonium chloride, polyvinyl alcohol and sodium phosphate dibasic and monobasic.

PILOCARPINE HYDROCHLORIDE

For complete prescribing information, refer to the Miotics, Direct-Acting group monograph.

Indications:

To lower intraocular pressure (IOP) in glaucoma.

Chronic angle-closure glaucoma.

Acute (angle-closure) glaucoma: Alone, or in combination with β–adrenergic blocking agents, carbonic anhydrase inhibitors, apraclonidine or hyperosmotic agents to decrease IOP and break the attack.

Pre- and postoperative elevated intraocular pressure.

Administration and Dosage:

Solution:

Initial – Instill 1 drop 3 to 4 times daily. The frequency of instillation and the concentration are determined by patient response. Individuals with heavily pigmented irides may require higher strengths.

Gel: Apply a 0.5 inch ribbon in the lower conjunctival sac of affected eye(s) once daily at bedtime. If other glaucoma medication is also used at bedtime, use drops at least 5 minutes before the gel.

Storage: Do not freeze. Store at room temperature; 2° to 26°C (36° to 80°F).

Rx	**Isopto Carpine** (Alcon)	**Solution:** 0.25%	In 15 ml.[1]
Rx	**Pilocarpine HCl** (Various, eg, Rugby)	**Solution:** 0.5%	In 15 and 30 ml.
Rx	**Isopto Carpine** (Alcon)		In 15 and 30 ml.[1]
Rx	**Pilocar** (Ciba Vision)		In 15 ml and twin-pack (2 × 15 ml).[2]
Rx	**Piloptic – 1/2** (Optopics)		In 15 ml.[3]
Rx	**Pilostat** (Bausch & Lomb)		In 15 ml.[4]
Rx	**Pilocarpine HCl** (Various, eg, Alcon, Rugby, Zenith-Goldline)	**Solution:** 1%	In 2, 15 and 30 ml and UD 1 ml.
Rx	**Adsorbocarpine** (Alcon)		In 15 ml.[5]
Rx	**Akarpine** (Akorn)		In 15 ml.
Rx	**Isopto Carpine** (Alcon)		In 15 and 30 ml.[1]
Rx	**Pilocar** (Ciba Vision)		In 15 ml, twin-pack (2 × 15 ml) and 1 ml dropperettes.[2]
Rx	**Piloptic-1** (Optopics)		In 15 ml.[3]
Rx	**Pilostat** (Bausch & Lomb)		In 15 ml and twin pack (2 × 15 ml).[4]
Rx	**Pilocarpine HCl** (Various, eg, Alcon, Rugby, Zenith-Goldline)	**Solution:** 2%	In 2, 15 and 30 ml.
Rx	**Adsorbocarpine** (Alcon)		In 15 ml dropper bottles.[5]
Rx	**Akarpine** (Akorn)		In 15 ml dropper bottles.
Rx	**Isopto Carpine** (Alcon)		In 15 and 30 ml.[1]
Rx	**Pilocar** (Ciba Vision)		In 15 ml, twin-pack (2 × 15 ml) and 1 ml dropperettes.[2]
Rx	**Piloptic-2** (Optopics)		In 15 ml.[3]
Rx	**Pilostat** (Bausch & Lomb)		In 15 ml and twin-pack (2 × 15 ml).[4]

Rx	**Isopto Carpine** (Alcon)	**Solution**: 3%	In 15 and 30 ml.[1]
Rx	**Pilocar** (Ciba Vision)		In 15 ml and twin-pack (2 × 15 ml).[2]
Rx	**Piloptic-3** (Optopics)		In 15 ml.[3]
Rx	**Pilostat** (Bausch & Lomb)		In 15 ml and twin-pack (2 × 15 ml).[4]
Rx	**Pilocarpine HCl** (Various, eg, Alcon, Rugby, Zenith-Goldline)	**Solution**: 4%	In 2, 15 and 30 ml.
Rx	**Adsorbocarpine** (Alcon)		In 15 ml dropper bottles.[5]
Rx	**Akarpine** (Akorn)		In 15 ml dropper bottles.
Rx	**Isopto Carpine** (Alcon)		In 15 and 30 ml.[1]
Rx	**Pilocar** (Ciba Vision)		In 15 ml, twin-pack (2 x 15 ml) and 1 ml dropperettes.[2]
Rx	**Piloptic-4** (Optopics)		In 15 ml.[5]
Rx	**Pilopto-Carpine** (Lebeh Pharmacal)		In 15 ml.
Rx	**Pilostat** (Bausch & Lomb)		In 15 ml and twin-pack (2 × 15) ml.[4]
Rx	**Isopto Carpine** (Alcon)	**Solution**: 5%	In 15 ml.[1]
Rx	**Pilocarpine HCl** (Various, eg, Rugby)	**Solution**: 6%	In 15 ml.
Rx	**Isopto Carpine** (Alcon)		In 15 and 30 ml.[1]
Rx	**Pilocar** (Ciba Vision)		In 15 ml and twin-pack (2 x 15 ml).[3]
Rx	**Piloptic-6** (Optopics)		In 15 ml.[3]
Rx	**Pilostat** (Bausch & Lomb)		In 15 ml.[4]
Rx	**Isopto Carpine** (Alcon)	**Solution**: 8%	In 15 ml.
Rx	**Pilocarpine HCl** (Alcon)		In 2 ml.
Rx	**Isopto Carpine** (Alcon)	**Solution**: 10%	In 15 ml.[1]
Rx	**Pilopine HS** (Alcon)	**Gel**: 4%	In 3.5 g.[6]

[1] With 0.5% hydroxypropyl methylcellulose and 0.01% benzalkonium chloride.
[2] With hydroxypropyl methylcellulose, benzalkonium chloride and EDTA.
[3] With polyvinyl alcohol, benzalkonium chloride and EDTA.
[4] With hydroxypropyl methylcellulose, 0.01% benzalkonium chloride and EDTA.
[5] With 0.004% benzalkonium chloride, EDTA, povidone, PEG and hydroxyethyl cellulose.
[6] With 0.008% benzalkonium chloride, carbopol 940 and EDTA.

PILOCARPINE NITRATE

For complete prescribing information, refer to the Miotics, Direct-Acting group monograph.

Indications:

To control IOP in glaucoma.

For emergency relief of angle-closure glaucoma.

Administration and Dosage:

Glaucoma: Instill 1 drop 2 to 4 times daily. Patient response may vary.

Storage: Do not freeze. Keep out of reach of children.

Rx	**Pilagan** (Allergan)	**Solution**: 1%	In 15 ml.[1]
		2%	In 15 ml.[1]
		4%	In 15 ml.[1]

[1] With 1.4% polyvinyl alcohol, 0.5% chlorobutanol, menthol, camphor, phenol and eucalyptol.

PILOCARPINE OCULAR THERAPEUTIC SYSTEM

Refer to the general discussion in the Miotics, Direct-Acting group monograph.

Actions:

Pharmacology: An elliptical unit designed for continuous release of pilocarpine following placement in the cul-de-sac of the eye.

Pharmacokinetics: Ocusert initially releases the drug at 3 times the rated value in the first hours and declines to the rated value in approximately 6 hours. A total of 0.3 to 0.7 mg pilocarpine is released during this initial 6 hour period (one drop of 2% pilocarpine ophthalmic solution contains 1 mg pilocarpine). During the remainder of the 7 day period, the release rate is within ± 20% of the rated value.

Ocular hypotensive effect is fully developed within 1.5 to 2 hours after placement in cul-de-sac. A satisfactory ocular hypotensive response is maintained around the clock. IOP reduction for the entire week is achieved with the system from either 3.4 or 6.7 mg pilocarpine (20 or 40 mcg/hr times 24 hrs/day times 7 days, respectively), vs 28 mg given as a 2% ophthalmic solution 4 times daily.

During the first several hours after insertion, induced myopia may occur. In contrast to fluctuating and high levels of induced myopia typical of pilocarpine eye drop use, the amount of induced myopia with *Ocusert* decreases after the first several hours to a low baseline level (≤ 0.5 diopters), which persists for the therapeutic life of the system. Pilocarpine-induced miosis approximately parallels induced myopia.

Indications:

IOP reduction: Control of elevated IOP in pilocarpine-responsive patients.

Patient Information:

Patient package insert is available with the product.

Wash hands with soap and water before touching or manipulating the system. If a displaced system contacts unclean surfaces, rinse with cool tap water before replacing. Discard contaminated systems and replace with a fresh unit.

Check for the presence of the system before retiring at night and upon awakening.

Administration and Dosage:

Damaged or deformed systems: Do not place or retain in the eye. Remove and replace systems believed to be associated with an unexpected increase in drug action.

Initiation of therapy: There is no direct correlation between the strength of *Ocusert* used and the strength of pilocarpine eyedrop solutions required to achieve a given level of pressure lowering. It has been estimated that *Ocusert* 20 mcg is roughly equal to 0.5% or 1% drops and 40 mcg is roughly equal to 2% or 3% drops. *Ocusert* reduces the amount of drug necessary to achieve adequate medical control; therefore, therapy may be started with the 20 mcg system, regardless of the strength of pilocarpine solution the patient previously required. Because of the patient's age, family history and disease status or progression, however, therapy may be started with the 40 mcg system. The patient should return during the first week of therapy for evaluation of IOP, and as often thereafter as deemed necessary.

If pressure is satisfactorily reduced with the 20 mcg system, the patient should continue its use, replacing each unit every 7 days. If IOP reduction greater than that achieved by 20 mcg is needed, transfer the patient to the 40 mcg system. If necessary, concurrently use epinephrine, a β-blocker or carbonic anhydrase inhibitor; *Ocusert's* release rate is not influenced by other ophthalmic preparations.

Placement and removal of the system: The system is placed in and removed from the eye by the patient. Since pilocarpine-induced myopia may occur during the first several hours of therapy, place the system into the conjunctival cul-de-sac at bedtime. By morning, the myopia is at a stable level (≤ 0.5 diopters).

In those patients in whom retention is a problem, superior cul-de-sac placement is often more desirable. The unit can be manipulated from lower to upper conjunctival cul-de-sac by gentle digital massage through the eyelid. If possible, move the unit before sleep to the upper conjunctival cul-de-sac for best retention. Should the unit slip out during sleep, its ocular hypotensive effect after loss continues for a period comparable to that following instillation of eyedrops.

Ocusert has been used concomitantly with various ophthalmic medications.

Storage: Refrigerate at 2° to 8°C (36°to 46°F).

Rx	**Ocusert Pilo-20** (Alza)	**Ocular Therapeutic System**: Releases 20 mcg pilocarpine per hour for 1 week	In packs of 8 individ. sterile systems.
Rx	**Ocusert Pilo-40** (Alza)	**Ocular Therapeutic System**: Releases 40 mcg pilocarpine per hour for 1 week	In packs of 8 individ. sterile systems.

CHOLINESTERASE INHIBITORS

Actions:

Pharmacology: These indirect-acting agents inhibit the enzyme cholinesterase, potentiating the action of acetylcholine on the parasympathomimetic end organs. Topical application to the eye produces intense miosis and ciliary muscle contraction. Intraocular pressure (IOP) is reduced by a decreased resistance to aqueous outflow.

Cholinesterase inhibitors are subdivided into reversible and irreversible agents. Reversible agents (eg, physostigmine, demecarium) quickly combine with cholinesterase; the resulting complex is slowly hydrolyzed and the inhibited enzyme is regenerated. The demecarium-enzyme complex is hydrolyzed more slowly than the physostigmine complex; therefore, its duration of action is longer.

Irreversible agents (eg, echothiophate) also bind to cholinesterase; however, the resulting covalent bond is not hydrolyzed. Therefore, cholinesterase is not regenerated. More cholinesterase must be synthesized or supplied from depots elsewhere in the body before ophthalmic action dependent on cholinesterase returns. Echothiophate will depress both plasma and erythrocyte cholinesterase levels in most patients after a few weeks of eyedrop therapy.

These effects are accompanied by increased permeability of the blood-aqueous barrier and vasodilation. Myopia may be induced or, if present, may be augmented by the increased refractive power of the lens that results from the accommodative effect of the drug. Demecarium indirectly produces some of the muscarinic and nicotinic effects of acetylcholine as quantities of the latter accumulate.

Cholinesterase-Inhibiting Miotics

	Miosis		IOP reduction		
Miotics	Onset (minutes)	Duration	Onset (hours)	Peak (hours)	Duration
Reversible					
Physostigmine	20 to 30	12 to 36 hrs	—	2 to 6	12 to 36 hrs
Demecarium	15 to 60	3 to 10 days	—	24	7 to 28 days
Irreversible					
Echothiophate	10 to 30	1 to 4 weeks	4 to 8	24	7 to 28 days

Indications:

Glaucoma: Therapy of open-angle glaucoma.

For other specific indications, refer to the individual monographs.

Contraindications:

Hypersensitivity to cholinesterase inhibitors or any component of the formulation; active uveal inflammation or any inflammatory disease of the iris or ciliary body; glaucoma associated with iridocyclitis.

Demecarium: Pregnancy.

Echothiophate: Most cases of angle-closure glaucoma (due to the possibility of increasing angle-block).

Warnings:

Myasthenia gravis: Because of possible additive adverse effects, administer demecarium and echothiophate only with extreme caution to patients with myasthenia gravis who are receiving systemic anticholinesterase therapy. Conversely, exercise extreme caution in the use of anticholinesterase drugs for the treatment of myasthenia gravis patients who are already undergoing topical therapy with cholinesterase inhibitors.

Surgery: In patients receiving cholinesterase inhibitors, administer succinylcholine with extreme caution before and during general anesthesia (see Drug Interactions). Stop these drugs 4 to 6 weeks prior to ophthalmic surgery to avoid a severe inflammatory response.

Pregnancy: Category X (demecarium). Contraindicated in women who are or who may become pregnant. If this drug is used during pregnancy, or if the patient becomes pregnant while taking this drug, apprise the patient of the potential hazard to the fetus.

Category C (physostigmine, echothiophate). Safety for use during pregnancy has not been established. Use only when clearly needed and when the potential benefits outweigh the potential hazards to the fetus.

Lactation: It is not known whether these drugs are excreted in breast milk. Exercise caution when administering to a nursing woman. Because of the potential for serious adverse reactions in nursing infants, decide whether to discontinue nursing or the drug, taking into account the importance of the drug to the mother.

Children: The occurrence of iris cysts is more frequent in children (see Precautions). Exercise extreme caution in children receiving demecarium who may require general anesthesia. Safety and efficacy for use of physostigmine have not been established.

Precautions:

Concomitant therapy: Cholinesterase inhibitors may be used in combination with adrenergic agents, β-blockers, carbonic anhydrase inhibitors or hyperosmotic agents.

Narrow angle glaucoma: Use with caution in patients with chronic angle-closure (narrow-angle) glaucoma or in patients with narrow angles, because of the possibility of producing pupillary block and increasing angle blockage.

Special risk patients: Use caution in patients with marked vagotonia, bronchial asthma, spastic GI disturbances, peptic ulcer, pronounced bradycardia/hypotension, recent MI, epilepsy, parkinsonism and other disorders that may respond adversely to vagotonic effects.Temporarily discontinue if cardiac irregularities occur.

Ophthalmic ointments may retard corneal healing.

Miosis usually causes difficulty in dark adaptation. Use caution while driving at night or performing hazardous tasks in poor light.

Gonioscopy: Use only when shorter-acting miotics have proved inadequate. Gonioscopy is recommended prior to use of these medications. Routine examination (eg, slit-lamp) to detect lens opacities should accompany therapy.

Concomitant ocular conditions: When an intraocular inflammatory process is present, breakdown of the blood-aqueous barrier from anticholinesterase therapy requires abstention from, or cautious use of, these drugs. Use with great caution where there is a history of quiescent uveitis. After long-term use, blood vessel dilation and resultant greater permeability increase the possibility of hyphema or a severe inflammatory response during or after ophthalmic surgery. Discontinue 4 to 6 weeks before surgery.

Systemic effects: Repeated administration may cause depression of the concentration of cholinesterase in the serum and erythrocytes, with resultant systemic effects. Discontinue if salivation, urinary incontinence, diarrhea, profuse sweating, muscle weakness, respiratory difficulties, shock or cardiac irregularities occur.

Although systemic effects are infrequent, use digital compression of the nasolacrimal ducts immediately before and for 2 minutes after instillation to minimize systemic absorption.

Iris cysts may form, enlarge and obscure vision (more frequent in children). The iris cyst usually shrinks upon discontinuation of the miotic, or following reduction in strength of the drops or frequency of instillation. Rarely, the cyst may rupture or break free into the aqueous humor. Frequent examination for this occurrence is advised.

Sulfite sensitivity: Some of these products contain sulfites which may cause allergic-type reactions (eg, hives, itching, wheezing, anaphylaxis) in certain susceptible persons. Although the overall prevalence of sulfite sensitivity in the general population is probably low, it is seen more frequently in asthmatics or atopic nonasthmatics.

Drug Interactions:

Ophthalmic Cholinesterase Inhibitor Drug Interactions

Precipitant drug	Object drug*		Description
Carbamate/ Organophosphate insecticides, pesticides	Cholinesterase inhibitors	↑	Warn persons on cholinesterase inhibitors who are exposed to these substances (eg, gardeners, organophosphate plant or warehouse workers, farmers) of systemic effects possible from absorption through respiratory tract or skin. Advise use of respiratory masks, frequent washing and clothing changes.
Succinylcholine	Cholinesterase inhibitors	↑	Use extreme caution before or during general anesthesia to patients on cholinesterase inhibitors because of possible respiratory and cardiovascular collapse.
Anticholinesterases, systemic	Cholinesterase inhibitors	↑	Additive effects are possible; coadminister topical cholinesterase inhibitors cautiously, regardless of which therapy is added (see Warnings).

* ↑ = Object drug increased

Adverse Reactions:

Ophthalmic: Iris cysts (see Precautions); burning; lacrimation; lid muscle twitching; conjunctival and ciliary redness; browache; headache; activation of latent iritis or uveitis; induced myopia with visual blurring; retinal detatchment; lens opacities (see Precautions); conjunctival thickening and destruction of nasolacrimal canals (prolonged use).

Paradoxical increase in IOP by pupillary block may follow instillation.

Systemic: Nausea; vomiting; abdominal cramps; diarrhea; urinary incontinence; fainting; sweating; salivation; difficulty in breathing; cardiac irregularities.

Overdosage:

Treatment: Systemic effects can be reversed with atropine sulfate:

Adults – 0.4 to 0.6 mg.

Infants and children up to 12 years – 0.01 mg/kg repeated every 2 hours as needed until the desired effect is obtained, or adverse effects of atropine preclude further usage. The maximum single dose should not exceed 0.4 mg.

Much larger atropine doses for anticholinesterase intoxication in adults have been used. Initially, 2 to 6 mg followed by 2 mg every hour or more often, as long as muscarinic effects continue. Consider the greater possibility of atropinization with large doses, particularly in sensitive individuals.

Pralidoxime chloride (see Antidotes) has been useful in treating systemic effects due to cholinesterase inhibitors. However, use in addition to, not as a substitute for, atropine.

A short-acting barbiturate is indicated for convulsions not relieved by atropine. Promptly treat marked weakness or paralysis of respiratory muscles by maintaining a clear airway and by artificial respiration.

Patient Information:

Local irritation and headache may occur at initiation of therapy.

Notify physician if abdominal cramps, diarrhea or excessive salivation occurs.

Wash hands immediately after administration.

Use caution while driving at night or performing hazardous tasks in poor light.

Refer to the Dosage Forms and Routes of Administration chapter for more complete information.

Individual drug monographs are on the following pages.

PHYSOSTIGMINE

For complete prescribing information, refer to the Miotics, Cholinesterase Inhibitors group monograph.

Indications:

Glaucoma: Reduction of IOP.

Administration and Dosage:

Ointment: Apply small quantity to lower fornix, up to 3 times daily.

Storage: Keep tightly closed. Protect from heat.

Rx	**Eserine Sulfate** (Ciba Vision)	**Ointment**: 0.25% (as sulfate)	In 3.5 g.

DEMECARIUM BROMIDE

For complete prescribing information, refer to the Miotics, Cholinesterase Inhibitors group monograph. The following section is included here for completeness to show all of the clinical uses of this class of drug.

Indications:

Glaucoma: Treatment of open-angle glaucoma (use only when shorter-acting miotics have proved inadequate).

Aqueous outflow: Conditions affecting aqueous outflow (eg, synechial formation) that are amenable to miotic therapy.

Iridectomy: Following iridectomy procedure.

Accommodative esotropia: Treatment of accomodative esotripia (accomodative convergent stabismus).

Administration and Dosage:

Do not use more often than directed. Caution is necessary to avoid overdosage. Individualize dosage to use as little drug as possible to achieve the desired therapeutic effect.

Closely observe the patient during the initial period. If the response is not adequate within the first 24 hours, consider other measures. Keep frequency of use to a minimum in all patients, especially children, to reduce the chance of side effects.

Glaucoma:

Initial – Instill 1 drop into eye(s). A decrease in IOP should occur within a few hours. During this period, keep patient under supervision and perform tonometric examinations at least hourly for 3 or 4 hours to make sure no immediate rise in pressure occurs.

Usual dose – Instill 1 drop twice a week to 1 drop twice a day.

Accommodative esotropia: Essentially equal visual acuity of both eyes is a prerequisite to successful treatment.

Diagnosis – For initial evaluation, use as a diagnostic aid to determine if an accommodative factor exists. This is especially useful preoperatively in young children and in patients with normal hypermetropic refractive errors. Instill 1 drop daily for 2 weeks, then 1 drop every 2 days for 2 to 3 weeks. If the eyes become straighter, an accommodative factor is demonstrated. This technique may supplement or complement standard testing with atropine and trial with glasses for the accommodative factor.

Therapy – In esotropia uncomplicated by amblyopia or anisometropia, instill not more than 1 drop at a time in both eyes every day for 2 to 3 weeks; too severe a degree of miosis may interfere with vision. Then reduce dosage to 1 drop every other day for 3 to 4 weeks and reevaluate the patient's status. Continue with a dosage of 1 drop every 2 days to 1 drop twice a week (the latter dosage may be maintained for several months). Evaluate the patient's condition every 4 to 12 weeks. If improvement continues, reduce to 1 drop once a week and eventually to a trial without medication. However discontinue therapy after 4 months if control of the condition still requires 1 drop every 2 days.

Storage: Do not freeze. Protect from heat.

Rx	**Humorsol** (Merck)	**Solution**: 0.125%	In 5 ml Ocumeters.[1]
		0.25%	In 5 ml Ocumeters.[1]

[1] With 1:5000 benzalkonium chloride and sodium chloride.

ECHOTHIOPHATE IODIDE

For complete prescribing information, refer to the Miotics, Cholinesterase Inhibitors group monograph. The following section is included here for completeness to show all of the clinical uses of this class of drug.

Indications:

Glaucoma: Chronic open-angle glaucoma; if therapeutic goal is not achieved with direct-acting miotics, usually not useful in angle-closure glaucoma and most secondary glaucomas.

Accommodative esotropia: Concomitant esotropias with a significant accommodative component.

Administration and Dosage:

Tolerance may develop after prolonged use.

Glaucoma: 1 drop to eye(s) once or twice daily. Less frequent dosing can also produce the desired effect. Individualize dosage.

Concomitant therapy: May be coadministered with the other glaucomal medication classes.

Accommodative esotropia:

Diagnosis – Instill 1 drop of 0.125% solution once a day into both eyes at bedtime for 2 or 3 weeks. If the esotropia is accommodative, a favorable response may begin within a few hours.

Treatment – Use the lowest concentration and frequency that gives satisfactory results. After initial period of treatment for diagnostic purposes, reduce schedule to 0.125% every other day or 0.06% every day. Dosages can often be gradually lowered as treatment progresses. The 0.03% strength has proven effective in some cases. The maximum recommended dose is 0.125% once a day, although more intensive therapy has been used for short periods.

Duration of treatment – In diagnosis, only a short period is required and little time will be lost in instituting other procedures if the esotropia proves to be unresponsive. In therapy, there is no definite limit if the drug is well tolerated. However, if the eyedrops, with or without eyeglasses, are gradually withdrawn after a year or two and deviation recurs, consider surgery.

Storage/Stability: Store at room temperature 15° to 30°C (59° to 86°F). After reconstitution, keep eye drops in refrigerator to obtain maximum useful life of 6 months. Use within 1 month if stored at room temperature.

Rx	**Phospholine Iodide** (Wyeth-Ayerst)	**Powder for Reconstitution:** 1.5 mg to make 0.03%	With 5 ml diluent.[1]
		3 mg to make 0.06%	With 5 ml diluent.[1]
		6.25 mg to make 0.125%	With 5 ml diluent.[1]
		12.5 mg to make 0.25%	With 5 ml diluent.[1]

[1] With potassium acetate, 0.55% chlorobutanol and 1.2% mannitol.

PILOCARPINE AND EPINEPHRINE

Refer to the general discussion of Miotics, Cholinesterase Inhibitors for more information.

Ingredients:

Pilocarpine lowers IOP by a direct cholinergic action that improves outflow facility (see Agents for Glaucoma: Miotics, Direct-Acting).

Epinephrine reduces IOP by increasing outflow facility (see Agents for Glaucoma: Sympathomimetics).

The combination of pilocarpine and epinephrine provides additive effects in lowering IOP; opposing actions on the pupil may prevent marked miosis. These fixed combinations do not permit the flexibility necessary to adjust the dosage of each agent.

Administration and Dosage:

Instill 1 drop into the eye(s) 1 to 4 times daily. Determine concentration and frequency of instillation by patient response.

Storage: Store at 8° to 30°C (46° to 86°F). Keep tightly closed. Do not use solution if it is brown or contains a precipitate. Protect from light and heat.

Rx	**E-Pilo-1** (Ciba Vision)	**Solution:** 1% pilocarpine HCl, 1% epinephrine bitartrate	In 10 ml dropper bottles.[1]
Rx	**P_1E_1** (Alcon)		In 15 ml Drop-Tainers.[2]
Rx	**E-Pilo-2** (Ciba Vision)	**Solution:** 2% pilocarpine HCl, 1% epinephrine bitartrate	In 10 ml dropper bottles.[1]
Rx	**P_2E_1** (Alcon)		In 15 ml Drop-Tainers.[2]
Rx	**P_3E_1** (Alcon)	**Solution:** 3% pilocarpine HCl, 1% epinephrine bitartrate	In 15 ml Drop-Tainers.[2]
Rx	**E-Pilo-4** (Ciba Vision)	**Solution:** 4% pilocarpine HCl, 1% epinephrine bitartrate	In 10 ml dropper bottles.[1]
Rx	**P_4E_1** (Alcon)		In 15 ml Drop-Tainers.[2]
Rx	**E-Pilo-6** (Ciba Vision)	**Solution:** 6% pilocarpine HCl, 1% epinephrine bitartrate	In 10 ml dropper bottles.[1]
Rx	**P_6E_1** (Alcon)		In 15 ml Drop-Tainers.[2]

[1] With benzalkonium chloride, EDTA, mannitol and sodium bisulfite.

[2] With 0.01% benzalkonium chloride, methylcellulose, EDTA, chlorobutanol, polyethylene glycol and sodium bisulfite.

CARBONIC ANHYDRASE INHIBITORS

Actions:

Pharmacology: These agents are nonbacteriostatic sulfonamides that inhibit the enzyme carbonic anhydrase. This action reduces the rate of aqueous humor formation, resulting in decreased intraocular pressure (IOP).

Pharmacokinetics:

Pharmacokinetics of Oral Carbonic Anhydrase Inhibitors

Carbonic anhydrase inhibitor	IOP Lowering Effects: Onset (hours)	Peak effect (hours)	Duration (hours)	Relative inhibitor potency
Dichlorphenamide	within 1	2 to 4	6 to 12	30
Acetazolamide				
Tablets	1 to 1.5	1 to 4	8 to 12	1
Sustained release capsules	2	3 to 6	18 to 24	
Injection (IV)	2 min	15 min	4 to 5	
Methazolamide	2 to 4	6 to 8	10 to 18	†

† Quantitative data not available; reported to be more active than acetazolamide.

Methazolamide – Peak plasma concentrations for the 25, 50 and 100 mg twice daily regimens were 2.5, 5.1 and 10.7 mcg/ml, respectively. Approximately 55% is bound to plasma proteins. The mean steady-state plasma elimination half-life is approximately 14 hours. At steady state, approximately 25% of the dose is recovered unchanged in the urine. Renal clearance accounts for 20% to 25% of the total clearance of drug. After repeated dosing, methazolamide accumulates to steady-state concentrations in 7 days.

Dorzolamide – When topically applied, dorzolamide reaches the systemic circulation. It binds moderately to plasma proteins ($\approx$ 33%). The drug is primarily excreted unchanged in the urine, and the metabolite is also excreted in the urine.

After dosing is stopped, dorzolamide washes out of RBCs nonlinearly, resulting in a rapid decline of drug concentration initially, followed by a slower elimination phase with a half-life of about 4 months.

Indications:

The following section is included here for completeness to show all of the clinical uses of this class of drug.

Oral: For adjunctive treatment of glaucomas.

Ophthalmic: Treatment of elevated IOP in patients with ocular hypertension or open-angle glaucoma.

Dorzolamide: Only indicated to decrease IOP in patients with ocular hypertension or open-angle glaucoma.

Contraindications:

Hypersensitivity to these agents; depressed sodium or potassium serum levels; marked kidney and liver disease or dysfunction; suprarenal gland failure; hyperchloremic acidosis; adrenocortical insufficiency; severe pulmonary obstruction with inability to increase alveolar ventilation since acidosis may be increased (dichlorphenamide); cirrhosis (acetazolamide, methazolamide).

Warnings:

Renal function impairment: Dorzolamide has not been studied in patients with severe renal impairment (Ccr < 30 ml/min). However, because dorzolamide and its metabolite are excreted predominantly by the kidney, dorzolamide is not recommended in such patients.

Hepatic function impairment: Use of methazolamide in this condition could precipitate hepatic coma. Dorzolamide has not been studied in patients with hepatic impairment and should therefore be used with caution in such patients.

Carcinogenesis:

Dorzolamide – In a 2 year study of dorzolamide administered orally to rats, urinary bladder papillomas were seen in male rats in the highest dosage group of 20 mg/kg/day (250 times the recommended human ophthalmic dose). The increased incidence of urinary bladder papillomas is a class effect of carbonic anhydrase inhibitors in rats.

Pregnancy: Category C. Animal studies with some of these drugs have demonstrated teratogenicity (skeletal anomalies). Do not use during pregnancy, especially during the first trimester, unless the potential benefits outweigh the potential hazards.

Lactation: Safety for use in the nursing mother has not been established. It is not known whether all carbonic anhydrase inhibitors are excreted in breast milk. Acetazolamide appeared in breast milk of a patient taking 500 mg twice/day. However, the infant ingested only 0.06% of the dose, an amount unlikely to cause adverse effects.

Children: Safety and efficacy for use in children have not been established.

Precautions:

Monitoring: Monitor for hematologic reactions common to sulfonamides.

Hypokalemia may develop when severe cirrhosis is present, during concomitant use of steroids or ACTH, and with interference with adequate oral electrolyte intake. Hypokalemia can sensitize or exaggerate the response of the heart to the toxic effects of digitalis (eg, increased ventricular irritability). Hypokalemia may be avoided or treated with potassium supplements or foods with a high potassium content.

Pulmonary conditions: Use dichlorphenamide with caution in patients with severe degrees of respiratory acidosis. These drugs may precipitate or aggravate acidosis. Use with caution in patients with pulmonary obstruction or emphysema when alveolar ventilation may be impaired.

Cross-sensitivity between antibacterial sulfonamides and sulfonamide derivative diuretics, including acetazolamide and various thiazides, has occurred.

Corneal endothelium effects: The effect of continued administration of dorzolamide on the corneal endothelium has not been fully evaluated.

Ocular effects: Local ocular adverse effects, primarily conjunctivitis and lid reactions, occurred with chronic administration of dorzolamide. Many of these reactions had the clinical appearance and course of an allergic-type reaction that resolved upon discontinuation of drug therapy. If such reactions are observed, discontinue dorzolamide and evaluate the patient before considering restarting the drug.

Concomitant oral CA inhibitors: The concomitant administration of dorzolamide and oral CA inhibitors is not recommended.

Contact lenses: The preservative in dorzolamide solution, benzalkonium chloride, may be absorbed by soft contact lenses. Dorzolamide should be administered with this in mind.

Hazardous tasks: Carbonic anhydrase inhibitors may cause drowsiness in some patients. Observe caution while driving, operating machinery or performing other tasks requiring coordination or physical dexterity.

Drug Interactions:

Carbonic Anhydrase Inhibitor (CAI) Drug Interactions

Precipitant drug	Object drug*		Description
Acetazolamide	Cyclosporine	↑	Increased trough cyclosporine levels with possible nephrotoxicity and neurotoxicity may occur.
Acetazolamide	Primidone	↓	Primidone serum and urine concentrations may be decreased.
CAIs	Salicylates	↑	Concurrent use may result in accumulation and toxicity of the CAI, including CNS depression and metabolic acidosis. Also, CAI-induced acidosis may allow increased CNS penetration by salicylates.
Salicylates	CAIs	↑	
Diflunisal	CAIs	↑	Concurrent use may result in a significant decrease in intraocular pressure; the effect may be less pronounced with methazolamide. Increased side effects may also occur.

* ↑ = Object drug increased. ↓ = Object drug decreased

Adverse Reactions:

Sulfonamide-type adverse reactions may occur.

Dorzolamide: Ocular burning, stinging or discomfort immediately following administration (≈ 33%); bitter taste following administration (≈ 25%); superficial punctate keratitis (10% to 15%); signs and symptoms of ocular allergic reaction (≈ 10%); blurred vision, tearing, dryness, photophobia (≈ 1% to 5%); urolithiasis, iridocyclitis (rare).

GI: Melena; anorexia; nausea; vomiting; constipation; taste alteration; diarrhea.

Renal: Hematuria; glycosuria; urinary frequency; renal colic; renal calculi; crystalluria; polyuria; phosphaturia.

CNS: Convulsions; weakness; malaise; fatigue; nervousness; drowsiness; depression; dizziness; disorientation; confusion; ataxia; tremor; tinnitus; headache; lassitude; flaccid paralysis; paresthesias of the extremities.

Hematologic: Bone marrow depression; thrombocytopenia; thrombocytopenic purpura; hemolytic anemia; leukopenia; pancytopenia; agranulocytosis.

Dermatologic: Urticaria; pruritus; skin eruptions; rash (including erythema multiforme, Stevens-Johnson syndrome, toxic epidermal necrolysis); photosensitivity.

Miscellaneous: Weight loss; fever; acidosis (usually corrected with bicarbonate); decreased/absent libido; impotence; electrolyte imbalance; hepatic insufficiency; transient myopia.

Overdosage:

Symptoms of overdosage or toxicity may include drowsiness, anorexia, nausea, vomiting, dizziness, paresthesias, ataxia, tremor and tinnitus.

Treatment: In the event of overdosage, induce emesis or perform gastric lavage. The electrolyte disturbance most likely to be encountered from overdosage is hyperchloremic acidosis that may respond to bicarbonate administration. Potassium supplementation may be required. Observe carefully; give supportive treatment.

Patient Information:

Oral:

If GI upset occurs, take with food.

Avoid prolonged exposure to sunlight or sunlamps; may cause photosensitivity.

May cause drowsiness; observe caution while driving or performing other tasks requiring alertness, coordination or physical dexterity.

Notify physician if sore throat, fever, unusual bleeding or bruising, tingling or tremors in the hands or feet, flank or loin pain, skin rash or eye irritation occurs.

Bioavailability – Consult physician before switching brands of carbonic anhydrase inhibitors. Problems with bioavailability have been documented with products from different manufacturers.

Ophthalmic:

To avoid contamination, do not touch tip of container to any surface. Replace cap after use.

Advise patients that if they develop an intercurrent ocular condition (eg, trauma, ocular surgery, infection), they should immediately seek their physician's advice concerning the continued use of the present multidose container.

If more than one topical ophthalmic drug is being used, administer the drugs at least 10 minutes apart.

Dorzolamide should not be administered while wearing soft contact lenses.

Individual drug monographs are on the following pages.

ACETAZOLAMIDE

For complete prescribing information, see the Carbonic Anhydrase Inhibitors group monograph. The following section is included here for completeness to show all of the clinical uses of this class of drug.

Administration and Dosage:

To lower IOP:

Adults – 250 mg to 1 g/day, in divided doses every 6 to 12 hours. Dosage > 1 g daily does not usually increase the effect.

Secondary glaucoma and preoperative treatment of acute congestive (closed-angle) glaucoma:

Adults – Short-term therapy: 250 mg every 4 hours or 250 mg twice daily.

Acute cases: 500 mg followed by 125 or 250 mg every 4 hours.

IV therapy may be used for rapid decreases of intraocular pressure. A complementary effect occurs when used with miotics or beta blockers.

Children – Parenteral: 5 to 10 mg/kg/dose, IM or IV, every 6 hours.

Oral: 10 to 15 mg/kg/day in divided doses, every 6 to 8 hours.

Sustained release: 500 mg twice daily.

Parenteral: Direct IV administration is preferred; IM administration is painful because of the alkaline pH of the solution.

Preparation and storage of parenteral solution: Reconstitute each 500 mg vial with at least 5 ml of Sterile Water for Injection. Reconstituted solutions retain potency for 1 week if refrigerated. However, since this product contains no preservative, use within 24 hours of reconstitution.

Oral liquid dose form: If required, acetazolamide tablets may be crushed and suspended in a cherry, chocolate, raspberry or other sweet syrup. Do not use a vehicle with alcohol or glycerin. Alternatively, one tablet can be submerged in 10 ml of hot water and added to 10 ml of honey or syrup. When prepared in a 70% sorbitol solution with a pH of 4 to 5 and stored in amber glass bottles, the suspension is stable for at least 2 to 3 months at temperatures < 30°C (86°F).

Rx	**Acetazolamide** (Various, eg, Mutual, URL)	**Tablets**: 125 mg	In 50s, 100s, 250s, 500s and 1000s.
Rx	**Diamox** (Lederle)		In 100s.
Rx	**Acetazolamide** (Various, eg, Qualitest, Schein, URL)	**Tablets**: 250 mg	In 100s, 500s, 1000s and UD 100s.
Rx	**Dazamide** (Major)		In 100s, 250s, 1000s and UD 100s.
Rx	**Diamox** (Lederle)		In 100s, 1000s and UD 100s.
Rx	**Diamox Sequels** (Lederle)	**Capsules, sustained release**: 500 mg	In 30s and 100s.
Rx	**Acetazolamide** (Various, eg, Bedford Labs)	**Powder for injection, lyophilized**: 500 mg (as sodium)	In vials.

DICHLORPHENAMIDE

For complete prescribing information, refer to the Carbonic Anhydrase Inhibitors group monograph.

Administration and Dosage:

Glaucoma: Use adjunctively. In acute angle-closure glaucoma, dichlorphenamide may be used with miotics and osmotic agents to rapidly reduce intraocular tension.

Adults: Individualize dosage 25 to 50 mg 1 to 3 times daily.

Rx	**Daranide** (Merck)	**Tablets**: 50 mg	Lactose. In 100s.

METHAZOLAMIDE

For complete prescribing information, refer to the Carbonic Anhydrase Inhibitors group monograph.

Administration and Dosage:

Glaucoma: 25 to 100 mg 2 or 3 times daily. May be used with glaucoma agents from other classes.

Rx	**GlaucTabs** (Akorn)	**Tablets**: 25 mg	In 100s.
Rx	**Methazolamide** (Various, eg, Mikart)		In 100s.
Rx	**MZM Tablets** (Ciba Vision)		Lactose. In 100s.
Rx	**Neptazane** (Lederle)		In 100s.

GlaucTabs (Akorn)	**Tablets**: 50 mg	In 100s.
Methazolamide (Various, eg, Mikart)		In 100s.
MZM Tablets (Ciba Vision)		Lactose. In 100s.
Neptazane (Lederle)		In 100s.

DORZOLAMIDE HYDROCHLORIDE

Actions:

Pharmacology: Dorzolamide is a carbonic anhydrase inhibitor formulated for topical ophthalmic use. Carbonic anhydrase (CA) is an enzyme found in many tissues of the body, including the eye. It catalyzes the reversible reaction involving the hydration of carbon dioxide and the dehydration of carbonic acid. In humans, carbonic anhydrase exists as a number of isoenzymes, the most active being carbonic anhydrase II (CA-II), found primarily in red blood cells (RBCs), but also in other tissues. Inhibition of CA in the ciliary processes of the eye decreases aqueous humor secretion, presumably by slowing the formation of bicarbonate ions with subsequent reduction in sodium and fluid transport. The result is a reduction in intraocular pressure (IOP). Dorzolamide, by inhibiting CA-II, reduces elevated IOP. Elevated IOP is a major risk factor in the pathogenesis of optic nerve damage and glaucomatous visual field loss.

Pharmacokinetics: When topically applied, dorzolamide reaches the systemic circulation. To assess the potential for systemic CA inhibition following topical administration, drug and metabolite concentrations in RBCs and plasma and CA inhibition in RBCs were measured. Dorzolamide accumulates in RBCs during chronic dosing as a result of binding to CA-II. The parent drug forms a single N-desethyl metabolite that inhibits CA-II less potently than the parent drug but also inhibits CA-I. The metabolite also accumulates in RBCs, where it binds primarily to CA-I. Plasma concentrations of parent and metabolite are generally below the assay limit of quantitation. Dorzolamide binds moderately to plasma proteins (≈ 33%). The drug is primarily excreted unchanged in the urine, and the metabolite is also excreted in urine. After dosing is stopped, dorzolamide washes out of RBCs nonlinearly, resulting in a rapid decline of drug concentration initially, followed by a slower elimination phase with a half-life of about 4 months.

To simulate the systemic exposure after long-term topical ocular administration, dorzolamide was given orally to eight healthy subjects for up to 20 weeks. The oral dose of 2 mg twice daily closely approximates the amount of drug delivered by topical ocular administration of 2% three times daily. Steady state was reached within 8 weeks. The inhibition of CA-II and total CA activities was below the degree of inhibition anticipated to be necessary for a pharmacological effect on renal function and respiration in healthy individuals.

Clinical trials: The efficacy of dorzolamide was demonstrated in clinical studies in the treatment of elevated IOP in patients with glaucoma or ocular hypertension (baseline IOP ≥ 23 mm Hg). The IOP-lowering effect of dorzolamide was approximately 3 to 5 mm Hg throughout the day, and this was consistent in clinical studies with durations of up to 1 year.

Indications:

Elevated intraocular pressure (IOP): Treatment of elevated IOP in patients with ocular hypertension or open-angle glaucoma.

Contraindications:

Hypersensitivity to any component of this product.

Warnings:

Systemic effects: Dorzolamide is a sulfonamide and, although administered topically, is absorbed systemically. Therefore, the same types of adverse reactions attributable to sulfonamides may occur with topical administration of dorzolamide. Fatalities have occurred, although rarely, due to severe reactions to sulfonamides including Stevens-Johnson syndrome, toxic epidermal necrolysis, fulminant hepatic necrosis, agranulocytosis, aplastic anemia and other blood dyscrasias. Sensitization may recur when a sulfonamide is readministered regardless of the route of administration. If signs of serious reactions or hypersensitivity occur, discontinue the use of this preparation.

Renal/Hepatic function impairment: Dorzolamide has not been studied in patients with severe renal impairment (Ccr < 30 ml/min). However, because dorzolamide and its metabolite are excreted predominantly by the kidney, dorzolamide is not recommended in such patients.

Dorzolamide has not been studied in patients with hepatic impairment and should therefore be used with caution in such patients.

Carcinogenesis: In a 2 year study of dorzolamide administered orally to male and female Sprague-Dawley rats, urinary bladder papillomas were seen in male rats in the highest dosage group of 20 mg/kg/day (250 times the recommended human ophthalmic dose); papillomas were not seen in rats given oral doses equivalent to $\approx$ 12 times the recommended dose. The increased incidence of urinary bladder papillomas is a class effect of CA inhibitors in rats.

Elderly: Of all the patients in clinical studies, 44% were $\geq$ 65 years of age and 10% were $\geq$ 75 years of age. No overall differences in efficacy or safety were observed between these patients and younger patients, but greater sensitivity of some older individuals to the product cannot be ruled out.

Pregnancy: Category C. Studies in rabbits at oral doses of $\geq$ 2.5 mg/kg/day (31 times the recommended human ophthalmic dose) revealed malformations of the vertebral bodies. These malformations occurred at doses that caused metabolic acidosis with decreased body weight gain in dams and decreased fetal weights. There are no adequate and well controlled studies in pregnant women. Use during pregnancy only if the potential benefit justifies the risk to the fetus.

Lactation: In lactating rats, decreases in body weight gain of 5% to 7% were seen in offspring at an oral dose of 7.5 mg/kg/day (94 times the recommended human ophthalmic dose). A slight delay in postnatal development (incisor eruption, vaginal canalization and eye openings), secondary to lower fetal body weight, was noted.

It is not known whether this drug is excreted in breast milk. Because of the potential for serious adverse reactions in nursing infants, decide whether to discontinue nursing or to discontinue the drug, taking into account the importance of the drug to the mother.

Children: Safety and efficacy in children have not been established.

Precautions:

Corneal endothelium effects: The effect of continued administration of dorzolamide on the corneal endothelium has not been fully evaluated.

Ocular effects: Local ocular adverse effects, primarily conjunctivitis and lid reactions, were reported with chronic administration of dorzolamide. Many of these reactions had the clinical appearance and course of an allergic-type reaction that resolved upon discontinuation of drug therapy. If such reactions are observed, discontinue dorzolamide and evaluate the patient before considering restarting the drug.

Concomitant oral CA inhibitors: The concomitant administration of dorzolamide and oral CA inhibitors is not recommended.

Contact lenses: The preservative in dorzolamide solution, benzalkonium chloride, may be absorbed by soft contact lenses. Dorzolamide should not be administered while wearing soft contact lenses.

Drug Interactions:

Although acid-base and electrolyte disturbances were not reported in the clinical trials with dorzolamide, these disturbances have occurred with oral CA inhibitors and have, in some instances, resulted in drug interactions (eg, toxicity associated with high-dose salicylate therapy). Therefore, consider the potential for such drug interactions in patients receiving dorzolamide.

Adverse Reactions:

Ocular burning, stinging or discomfort immediately following administration (≈ 33%); bitter taste following administration (≈ 25%); superficial punctate keratitis (10% to 15%); signs and symptoms of ocular allergic reaction (≈ 10%); blurred vision, tearing, dryness, photophobia (≈ 1% to 5%); headache, nausea, asthenia/fatigue (infrequent); skin rashes, urolithiasis, iridocyclitis (rare).

Overdosage:

Electrolyte imbalance, development of an acidotic state and possible CNS effects may occur. Monitor serum electrolyte levels (particularly potassium) and blood pH levels. Significant lethality was observed in female rats and mice after single oral doses of 1927 and 1320 mg/kg, respectively.

Patient Information:

Dorzolamide is a sulfonamide and, although administered topically, it is absorbed systemically. Therefore, the same types of adverse reactions that are attributable to sulfonamides may occur with topical administration. Advise patients that if serious or unusual reactions or signs of hypersensitivity occur, they should discontinue use of the product.

Advise patients that if they develop any ocular reactions, particularly conjunctivitis and lid reactions, they should discontinue use and seek their physician's advice.

Instruct patients to avoid allowing the tip of the dispensing container to contact the eye or surrounding structures. Ocular solutions, if handled improperly or if the tip of the dispensing container contacts the eye or surrounding structures, can become contaminated by common bacteria known to cause ocular infections. Serious damage to the eye and subsequent loss of vision may result from using contaminated solutions.

Advise patients that if they develop an intercurrent ocular condition (eg, trauma, ocular surgery, infection), they should immediately seek their physician's advice concerning the continued use of the present multidose container.

If more than one topical ophthalmic drug is being used, administer the drugs 5 to 10 minutes apart with the drugs with sustained-release vehicles such as *Pilopine HS, Timoptic XE* and *Betoptic S* administered last.

Administration and Dosage:

Dosage: Instill 1 drop in the affected eye(s) 3 times daily; twice daily when used concomitantly with a beta blocker.

Concomitant therapy: Dorzolamide may be used concomitantly with other topical ophthalmic drug products to lower intraocular pressure. If more than one ophthalmic drug is being used, administer the drugs 5 minutes apart. Can be used twice daily with beta blocker or other aqueous-secretion inhibitor.

Rx	**Trusopt** (Merck)	**Solution:** 2%	In 5 and 10 ml.

PROSTAGLANDINS

LATANOPROST

Actions:

Pharmacology: Latanoprost is a prostanoid-selective FP receptor agonist for ophthalmic use. It is believed to reduce intraocular pressure by increasing the outflow of aqueous humor. Studies in animals and man suggest that increased uveoscleral outflow is the main mechanism of action.

Pharmacokinetics: Latanoprost is absorbed through the cornea where the isopropyl ester prodrug is hydrolyzed to the acid form to become biologically active. Studies in man indicate that peak concentration in the aqueous humor is reached approximately 2 hours after topical administration. The distribution volume in humans is 0.16 ± 0.02 L/kg. The acid of latanoprost could be measured in aqueous humor during the first 4 hours, and in plasma only during the first hour after local administration. Latanoprost is primarily metabolized by the liver with excretion by renal pathway. Approximately 88% and 98% of the dose is recovered in the urine after topical and intravenous dosing, respectively.

Animal studies – Latanoprost was shown to induce increased pigmentation of the iris in monkeys. The increased pigmentation is unlikely to be associated with proliferation of melanocytes and is believed to be caused by the stimulation of melanin production in melanocytes of the iris stroma. Doses of 4 times the daily human dose in cynomolgus monkeys demonstrated increased palpebral fissure. This effect has been reversible and occurred at doses above the standard clinical dose level.

Clinical trials: Patients with a mean baseline intraocular pressure of 24 to 25 treated with *Xalatan* 0.005% for 6 months demonstrated 6 to 8 mmHg reductions in intraocular pressure. This was equivalent to the effect of timolol 0.5% twice daily.

Indications:

To lower intraocular pressure in patients with open-angle glaucoma and ocular hypertension who are intolerant of other intraocular pressure lowering medications or who insufficiently responded (failed to achieve target IOP determined after multiple measurements over time) to another intraocular pressure lowering medication.

Contraindications:

Hypersensitivity to latanoprost, benzalkonium chloride or any other ingredient in the product.

Warnings:

Eye color change: Latanoprost may gradually change eye color by increasing the amount of brown pigmentation in the iris. This is caused by increasing the number of melanosomes (pigment granules) in melanocytes. The long term effects of this are currently unknown.

The color change occurs slowly and over a long period of time. Inform patients of the possibility of an increasing brown color in the eye. In patients receiving treatment in only one eye, heterochromia may occur between the eyes. The change in pigmentation may be permanent.

Renal/Hepatic function impairment: Use with caution in patients with renal or hepatic impairment as this drug has not been studied in these patients.

Carcinogenesis/Mutagenesis/Fertility impairment: Latanoprost was not carcinogenic in bacteria, mouse lymphoma or mouse micronucleus tests or when mice and rats were given doses up to 2800 times the recommended human dose for 20 and 24 months, respectively. Unscheduled DNA synthesis was negative in rats, both in vivo and in vitro. Additionally, latanoprost was not found to have any effect on fertility in animal studies. Chromosome aberrations were observed in vitro with human lymphocytes.

Pregnancy: Category C. In rabbits receiving 80 times the maximum human dose, 4 of 16 females had no viable fetuses, with the highest nonembryocidal dose approximately 15 times the maximum human dose. There are no adequate and well controlled studies in pregnant women. Use during pregnancy only if the potential benefit justifies the potential risk to the fetus.

Lactation: It is not known whether latanoprost or its metabolites is excreted in breast milk. Because many drugs are excreted in human milk, exercise caution when administering to a nursing woman.

Children: Safety and efficacy in children have not been established.

Precautions:

Cornea: Latanoprost is hydrolyzed in the cornea. The effect of continued administration of latanoprost on the corneal endothelium has not been fully evaluated.

Bacterial keratitis: There have been reports of bacterial keratitis with the use of multiple-dose containers or topical ophthalmic products due to the contamination of the containers by patients with concurrent corneal disease of a disruption of the ocular epithelial surface.

Brown pigmentation: Patients may develop increased brown pigmentation in the iris over several months to years. Usually, the brown pigmentation spreads toward the periphery of the affected eye, but the entire iris or parts of it may also become more brownish. Examine patients regularly. Treatment may be stopped if increased pigmentation occurs, depending upon the clinical situation. The increase in brown iris pigment did not progress further upon stopping treatment in clinical trials; however, the color change may be permament. Freckles and nevi of the iris did not appear to be affected by treatment.

Contact lenses: Do not administer latanoprost while wearing contact lenses.

Other conditions: There is no experience in the use of latanoprost for angle closure, inflammatory or neovascular glaucoma and only limited experience in pseudophakic patients.

Drug Interactions:

In vitro studies have shown that precipitation occurs when eye drops containing thimerosal are mixed with latanoprost. If using these drugs concurrently, allow at least 5 minutes between applications.

Adverse Reactions:

Ophthalmic: Blurred vision, burning and stinging, conjunctival hyperemia, foreign body sensation, itching, increased pigmentation of iris, punctate epithelial keratopathy (5% to 15%); dry eye, excessive tearing, eye pain, lid crusting, lid edema, lid erythema, lid discomfort/pain, photophobia (1% to 4%); conjunctivitis, diplopia, discharge from eye (<1%). The following events occurred extremely rarely: Retinal artery embolus, retinal detachment and vitreous hemorrhage from diabetic retinopathy.

Local conjunctival hyperemia occurred; however, less than 1% of patients discontinued therapy due to intolerance.

Systemic: Upper respiratory tract infection, cold, flu (≈ 4%); muscle, joint, back, chest pain, angina pectoris, rash, allergic skin reaction (1% to 2%).

Overdosage:

Symptoms: Ocular irritation and conjunctival or episcleral hyperemia are the only ocular side effects of a latanoprost overdose. Transient bronchoconstriction has occurred in monkeys receiving large doses intravenously. However, no bronchoconstriction was induced in 11 patients with bronchial asthma receiving latanoprost. No adverse reactions were observed in healthy volunteers receiving 3 mcg/kg infused intravenously, but mean plasma concentrations were 200 times higher than during clinical ocular topical treatment. IV dosages of 5.5 to 10 mcg/kg caused abdominal pain, dizziness, fatigue, hot flushes, nausea and sweating.

Treatment: Treat latanoprost overdosage symptomatically.

Patient Information:

The color of the iris can change due to an increase of the brown pigment. If only one eye is treated, a cosmetically different eye coloration may occur. Iris pigmentation changes may be more noticeable in patients with green-brown, blue/gray-brown, or yellow-brown irises.

Do not allow the dispensing container to touch the eye or surrounding structures to avoid contacting an eye infection from the resultant contamination of common bacteria. Serious damage to the eye and subsequent loss of vision can occur from using contaminated containers.

Patients should contact their physician concerning the continued use of the multidose container if they experience any eye trauma or infection or have ocular surgery.

Patients should contact their physician if they experience any ocular side effects, especially conjunctivitis and lid reactions.

Latanoprost contains benzalkonium chloride which may be absorbed by contact lenses. Remove contact lenses prior to administering the latanoprost solution. Lenses can be reinserted 15 minutes after latanoprost administration.

If using more than one topical ophthalmic drug, adminster drugs at least 5 minutes apart.

Administration and Dosage:

Administer 1 drop in the affected eye(s) once daily. Do not administer this medicine more frequently than once daily.

Reduction of intraocular pressure begins approximately 3 to 4 hours after administration, with the maximum effect reached after 8 to 12 hours. Preliminary data suggest that maximal effect is not achieved in some patients for weeks or months.

Latanoprost may be used with other topical ophthalmic products to lower intraocular pressure. If using more than one topical ophthalmic drug, administer the drugs at least 5 minutes apart.

Storage/Stability: Protect from light. Store unopened bottle in refrigerator at 2° to 8°C (36° to 46°F). Opened container may be stored at room temperature up to 25°C to (77°F) for 6 weeks.

Rx	**Xalatan** (Pharmacia & Upjohn)	**Solution:** 0.005%	In 2.5 ml plastic ophthalmic dispenser bottle with dropper tip.[1]

[1] With 0.02% benzalkonium chloride, sodium chloride, sodium dihydrogen phosphate monohydrate, disodium hydrogen phosphate anhydrous.

ODF

10

Hyperosmotic Agents

Hyperosmotic agents (also referred to as osmotic agents) can be administered topically, orally or intravenously to increase osmotic pressure of tears and plasma relative to that of the ocular structures. As a result of the osmotic gradient established, fluid moves from the eye to hyperosmotic tear fluid with topical instillation, or plasma of ocular blood vessels following oral or intravenous administration.

TOPICAL AGENTS

The clinical objective of topical osmotherapy is to enhance the rate of fluid movement from the edematous cornea. When these agents are applied to the eye, water is drawn from the cornea to the hyperosmolal tear film and eliminated through the usual tear flow mechanisms.

Sodium chloride, glycerol and glucose have proven useful for reducing corneal edema of various etiologies, including bullous keratopathy and Fuchs' endothelial dystrophy.

Hypertonic solutions of sodium chloride or glucose can be useful for prolonged treatment of corneal edema. Sodium chloride appears less effective when the corneal epithelium is traumatized due to its increased ability to penetrate the epithelial barrier. Both sodium chloride and glucose should be administered at regular intervals for maximum clinical effect. Since vision is usually worse upon awakening, more frequent application during the first waking hours can be helpful.

Glycerol can reduce corneal edema within 1 to 2 minutes following topical instillation to the eye. Since application is painful, a topical anesthetic must be instilled prior to its use. The osmotic action of glycerol is transient since the molecules mix readily with water. Therefore, for diagnostic purposes, its primary clinical use is to facilitate ophthalmoscopy and gonioscopy with edematous corneas.

SYSTEMIC AGENTS

Hyperosmotic agents administered by oral and intravenous routes are useful for initial management of acute angle-closure glaucoma and prior to intraocular surgery to reduce intraocular pressure (IOP).

Following systemic administration, a relatively rapid increase in serum osmolarity can occur. Transfer of fluid from the eye to the circulation results in a decrease in IOP. Factors that determine the difference in osmotic pressure between the ocular fluids and plasma include the following:

- Molecular weight and concentration
- Dose administered
- Rate of absorption
- Distribution in body water
- Ocular penetration
- Rate of excretion
- Nature of diuresis

The integrity of the ocular tissues can also influence the osmotic effect. Inflammation may enhance ocular penetration and decrease the osmotic gradient, resulting in a reduction in the pressure-lowering effect of these agents.

Systemic administration can result in a significant drop in IOP within 15 to 60 minutes, depending on the dosage given. The effect of systemic osmotherapy can last up to 8 hours. The primary use of these agents is to treat or prevent acute rises in IOP such as acute angle-closure glaucoma and postoperative spiking of IOP. Chronic administration is contraindicated.

Osmotic Diuretic Pharmacokinetics

Diuretic	Route	Onset (min)	Peak (hrs)	Duration (hrs)	Half-life	Metabolized (%)	Ocular penetration	Distribution
Glycerin	PO	10-30	1-1.5	4-5	30-45 minutes	80	poor	E[1]
Isosorbide	PO	10-30	1-1.5	5-6	5-9.5 hrs	0	good	TBW[2]
Mannitol	IV	30-60	1	6-8	15-100 minutes	7-10	very poor	E[1]
Urea	IV	30-45	1	5-6	–	–	good	TBW[2]

[1] E = extracellular water
[2] TBW = total body water

INTRAVENOUS ADMINISTRATION

Mannitol (*Osmitrol*) is currently the hyperosmotic of choice for intravenous use. It is not absorbed from the gastrointestinal tract and, therefore, is ineffective by the oral route. Intravenous administration can reduce IOP within 20 to 30 minutes. The effect can last 4 to 8 hours. Mannitol exhibits minimal cellular penetration, is not metabolized and is excreted in the urine. Therefore, it can be used in diabetic patients, but should be administered with caution in patients with renal disease. Since mannitol is confined to the extracellular fluid, dehydration and a profound diuresis can result following administration.

ORAL ADMINISTRATION

Glycerin (*Osmōglyn*) and isosorbide (*Ismotic*) are both readily absorbed from the gastrointestinal tract and are effective when administered by the oral route.

Glycerin is metabolized in the body analogous to other carbohydrates and produces 4.32 kcal/g. Use caution when administering glycerin to diabetic patients since hyperglycemia and glycosuria can result. Although reduction in IOP is somewhat less than with mannitol, administration of the recommended dosage reduces pressure within 30 to 60 minutes. The osmotic effect can last for several hours.

Isosorbide is not metabolized, and about 95% is excreted unchanged in the urine. Therefore, it provides no calories and, unlike glycerin, can be administered to diabetic patients. Isosorbide reduces IOP within 30 to 60 minutes. The effect can last as long as 5 to 6 hours.

Although oral administration simplifies osmotherapy, both glycerin and isosorbide exhibit characteristics limiting their use. Neither agent can be administered to patients who are nauseated or vomiting. Since both agents have a sweet taste, they may induce nausea or vomiting. In addition, the increase is serum osmolarity can cause dehydration, headache, confusion and disorientation.

Siret D. Jaanus, PhD
State University of New York

For More Information

Bartlett JD, Jaanus SD, eds. Clinical Ocular Pharmacology, ed. 3. Boston: Butterworth-Heinemann, 1995.

Becker B, et al. Hyperosmotic agents. In: Leopold IE, ed. Symposium in Ocular Therapy. St. Louis: C.V. Mosby Co., 1968.

Becker B, et al. Isosorbide: An oral hyperosmotic agent. *Arch Ophthalmol* 1967;78:147.

Galin MA, et al. Ophthalmological use of osmotic therapy. *Am J Ophthalmol* 1966;62:629.

Kolker AE. Hyperosmotic agents in glaucoma. *Invest Ophthalmol* 1970;9:418.

Lambert DW. Topical hyperosmotic agents and secretory stimulants. *Am J Ophthalmol* 1980;20:163.

Luxenberg MN, Green K. Reduction of corneal edema with topical hypertonic agents. *Am J Ophthalmol* 1970;9:418.

McCurdy DK, et al. Oral glycerol: The mechanism of intraocular hypotension. *Am J Ophthalmol* 1966;61:1244.

GLUCOSE, TOPICAL

Indications:

Corneal edema: Topical osmotherapy for reducing corneal edema.

Contraindications:

Hypersensitivity to any component of the product.

Precautions:

Irritation: If irritation develops, discontinue use.

Administration and Dosage:

May be used 2 to 6 times daily.

Depress lower lid with index finger while looking upward. Introduce a small amount of ointment behind depressed eyelid into conjunctival sac. Close and open eyes 2 times. Wipe off excess ointment. If eyelids are sticky, clean them before each application with a pledget of cotton and lukewarm boiled water.

Rx	**Glucose-40** (Ciba Vision)	**Ointment**: 40%	White petrolatum, anhydrous lanolin, parabens. In 3.5 g.

GLYCERIN, TOPICAL

Actions:

Pharmacology: Glycerin ophthalmic solution is used only for topical application to the cornea. By virtue of its osmotic action (attraction of water through the semipermeable corneal epithelium), it promptly reduces edema and causes clearing of corneal haze. The action is transient and therefore is used primarily for diagnostic purposes.

Indications:

Edematous cornea: To clear an edematous cornea in order to facilitate ophthalmoscopic and gonioscopic examination in acute glaucoma, bullous keratitis and Fuchs' endothelial dystrophy.

Contraindications:

Hypersensitivity to any component of the product.

Warnings:

Pregnancy: Category C. Safety for use during pregnancy has not been established. Use only when clearly needed.

Lactation: It is not known whether glycerin is excreted in breast milk. Exercise caution when administering to a nursing mother.

Children: Safety and efficacy for use in children have not been established.

Precautions:

Irritation: Because glycerin is an irritant and may cause pain, instill a local anesthetic before use.

Adverse Reactions:

Some pain or irritation may occur upon instillation.

Administration and Dosage:

Instill 1 or 2 drops prior to examination. In gonioscopy of an edematous cornea, additional glycerin may be used as a lubricant.

Storage: Keep bottle tightly closed. Store at room temperature 25°C (77°F). Discard product 6 months after dropper is first placed in the drug solution

Rx	**Ophthalgan** (Wyeth-Ayerst)	**Solution**: Glycerin	0.55% chlorobutanol. In 7.5 ml.

SODIUM CHLORIDE, HYPERTONIC

Actions:

Pharmacology: A hypertonic (hyperosmolar) solution exerts an osmotic gradient greater than that present in the body tissues and fluids, so that water is drawn from the body tissues and fluids across semipermeable membranes. Applied topically to the eye, a hypertonicity agent creates an osmotic gradient which draws water out of the cornea.

Indications:

Corneal edema: Temporary relief.

Contraindications:

Hypersensitivity to any component of the product.

Adverse Reactions:

May cause temporary burning and irritation upon instillation.

Patient Information:

To avoid contamination, do not touch tip of container to any surface. Replace cap after using.

Do not use this product except under the advice and supervision of a physician. If you experience eye pain, changes in vision, continued redness or irritation of the eye or if the condition worsens or persists, discontinue use and consult a physician.

Product may cause temporary burning and irritation when instilled into the eye.

If solution changes color or becomes cloudy, do not use.

Administration and Dosage:

Solution: Instill 1 or 2 drops in affected eye(s) every 3 or 4 hours, or as directed.

Ointment: Pull down lower eyelid of the affected eye(s) and apply a small amount (≈1/4 inch) of ointment to the inside of the affected eye(s) every 3 or 4 hours, or as directed.

Storage: Store at 8° to 30°C (46° to 86°F). Keep tightly closed. Protect from light.

otc	**Adsorbonac** (Alcon)	**Solution:** 2%	In 15 ml.[1]
otc	**Muro 128** (Bausch & Lomb)		In 15 ml.[2]
otc	**Adsorbonac** (Alcon)	**Solution:** 5%	In 15 ml.[1]
otc	**AK-NaCl** (Akorn)		In 15 ml.[3]
otc	**Muro 128** (Bausch & Lomb)		In 15 and 30 ml.[4]
otc	**Muroptic-5** (Optopics)		In 15 ml.[5]
otc	**AK-NaCl** (Akorn)	**Ointment:** 5%	Preservative free. In 3.5 g.[6]
otc	**Muro 128** (Bausch & Lomb)		In 3.5 g single and twin packs.[7]

[1] With povidone, hydroxyethylcellulose 2910, PEG-90M, poloxamer 188, 0.004% thimerosal, EDTA.
[2] With hydroxypropyl methylcellulose 2906, 0.046% methylparaben, 0.02% propylparaben, propylene glycol, boric acid.
[3] With hydroxypropyl methylcellulose, propylene glycol, 0.023% methylparaben, 0.01% propylparaben, boric acid.
[4] Boric acid, hydroxypropyl methylcellulose 2910, propylene glycol, 0.023% methylparaben, 0.01% propylparaben.
[5] With benzalkonium chloride, EDTA, polyvinyl alcohol, propylene glycol.
[6] With mineral oil, white petrolatum, lanolin oil.
[7] With mineral oil, white petrolatum, lanolin.

GLYCERIN (Glycerol)

Actions:

Pharmacology: An oral osmotic agent for reducing intraocular pressure. It adds to the tonicity of the blood until metabolized and eliminated by the kidneys.

Indications:

Glaucoma to interrupt acute attacks.

Prior to and after ocular surgery where reduction of intraocular pressure is indicated.

Off-labeled uses: Glycerin has also been given by the IV route (with proper preparation) to lower intraocular and intracranial pressure.

Contraindications:

Well established anuria; severe dehydration; frank or impending acute pulmonary edema; severe cardiac decompensation; hypersensitivity to any of the ingredients.

Warnings:

Route of administration: For oral use only; not for injection.

Pregnancy: Category C. Safety for use during pregnancy has not been established. Use only when clearly needed and when the potential benefits outweigh the potential hazards to the fetus.

Precautions:

Special risk patients: Use cautiously in hypervolemia, confused mental states, congestive heart disease, diabetic patients, severely dehydrated individuals and cardiac, renal or hepatic disease.

Urinary retention: Avoid acute urinary retention in the preoperative period. Continued use may result in weight gain.

Adverse Reactions:

Nausea, vomiting, headache, confusion and disorientation may occur. Severe dehydration, cardiac arrhythmias or hyperosmolar nonketotic coma which can result in death have occurred.

Administration and Dosage:

1 to 2 g/kg 1 to 1.5 hours prior to surgery.

Rx	**Osmōglyn** (Alcon)	**Solution**: 50% (0.6 g glycerin/ml)	Lime flavor. In 220 ml.

ISOSORBIDE

Actions:

Pharmacology: Isosorbide is rapidly absorbed after oral administration. It is essentially nonmetabolized, and in the circulation, it contributes to the tonicity of the blood until it is eliminated by the kidneys unchanged. While in the blood, isosorbide acts as an osmotic agent to promote redistribution of water toward the circulation with ultimate elimination in the urine. The physical action is similar to that of other osmotic agents.

Indications:

For the short-term reduction of intraocular pressure prior to and after intraocular surgery.

May be used to interrupt an acute attack of glaucoma. Use where less risk of nausea and vomiting than that posed by other oral hyperosmotic agents is needed.

Contraindications:

Well established anuria; severe dehydration; frank or impending acute pulmonary edema; severe cardiac decompensation; hypersensitivity to any component of this preparation.

Warnings:

Fluid/Electrolyte balance: With repeated doses, maintain adequate fluid and electrolyte balance.

Urinary output: If urinary output continues to decrease, closely review the patient's clinical status. Accumulation may result in overexpansion of the extracellular fluid.

Pregnancy: Category B. There is no adequate information on whether this drug affects fertility in humans or has a teratogenic potential or other adverse fetal effects. Use during pregnancy only if clearly needed.

Precautions:

Repetitive doses: Use repetitive doses with caution, particularly in patients with diseases associated with salt retention. Ensure that the patient's bladder has been emptied prior to surgery.

Adverse Reactions:

Nausea; vomiting; headache; confusion; disorientation; gastric discomfort; thirst; hiccoughs; hypernatremia; hyperosmolarity; rash; irritability; syncope; lethargy; vertigo; dizziness; lightheadedness.

Administration and Dosage:

For oral use only.

Initial dose: 1.5 g/kg (equivalent to 1.5 ml/lb).

Dose range: 1 to 3 g/kg 2 to 4 times a day as indicated.

Palatability may be improved if the medication is poured over cracked ice and sipped.

Rx	**Ismotic** (Alcon)	**Solution:** 45% (100 g per 220 ml)	With 4.6 mEq sodium and 0.9 mEq potassium per 220 ml. Alcohol, saccharin, sorbitol. Vanilla-mint flavor. In 220 ml.

MANNITOL

Actions:

Pharmacology: Mannitol is a nonelectrolyte osmotic diuretic that is pharmacologically inert.

IV mannitol is confined to the extracellular space. Only small amounts are metabolized. Mannitol is readily diffused through the glomeruli. Approximately 80% of a 100 g dose will appear in the urine in 3 hours, with lesser amounts thereafter. Even at peak concentrations, mannitol will exhibit less than 10% of tubular reabsorption and is not secreted by tubular cells. Mannitol will hinder tubular reabsorption of water and enhance excretion of sodium and chloride by elevating the osmolarity of the glomerular filtrate.

This increase in extracellular osmolarity affected by the IV administration of mannitol will induce the movement of intracellular water to the extracellular and vascular spaces. This action underlies the role of mannitol in reducing intracranial pressure, intracranial edema and elevated intraocular pressure (IOP).

Indications:

Reduction of elevated intraocular pressure when the pressure cannot be lowered by other means.

Contraindications:

Anuria due to severe renal disease; severe pulmonary congestion or frank pulmonary edema; active intracranial bleeding except during craniotomy; severe dehydration; progressive renal damage or dysfunction after instituting mannitol therapy, including increasing oliguria and azotemia; progressive heart failure or pulmonary congestion after mannitol therapy.

Warnings:

Fluid and electrolyte imbalance: By sustaining diuresis, mannitol may obscure and intensify inadequate hydration or hypovolemia. Excessive loss of water and electrolytes may lead to serious imbalances. Loss of water in excess of electrolytes can cause hypernatremia. Shift of sodium free intracellular fluid into the extracellular compartment following mannitol infusion may lower serum sodium concentration and aggravate preexisting hyponatremia. Also, movement of potassium ions from intracellular to extracellular space may cause hyperkalemia. Electrolyte measurements, including sodium and potassium, are therefore of vital importance in monitoring mannitol infusion.

Renal function impairment: Use a test dose (see Administration and Dosage); try a second test dose if there is an inadequate response, but do not attempt more than two test doses.

If urine output continues to decline during infusion, closely review the patient's clinical status and suspend mannitol infusion, if necessary. Accumulation of mannitol may result in overexpansion of the extracellular fluid which may intensify existing or latent CHF.

Osmotic nephrosis, a reversible vacuolization of the tubules of unknown clinical significance, may proceed to severe irreversible nephrosis; monitor renal function closely.

Pregnancy: Category C. It is not known whether mannitol can cause fetal harm when administered to a pregnant woman or can affect reproduction capacity. Give to a pregnant woman only if clearly needed.

Lactation: It is not known whether this drug is excreted in breast milk; exercise caution when administering to a nursing woman.

Children: Safety and efficacy for patients ≤ 12 years of age have not been established.

Precautions:

CHF: Carefully evaluate cardiovascular status before rapid administration of mannitol since sudden expansion of the extracellular fluid may lead to fulminating CHF.

Hypovolemia: By sustaining diuresis, mannitol may obscure and intensify inadequate hydration or hypovolemia.

Pseudoagglutination: Do not give electrolyte free mannitol solutions with blood. If blood is given simultaneously, add at least 20 mEq of sodium chloride to each liter of mannitol solution to avoid pseudoagglutination.

Hemoconcentration: The obligatory diuretic response following rapid infusion of 15%, 20% or 25% mannitol may further aggravate preexisting hemoconcentration.

Adverse Reactions:

Cardiovascular: Edema; thrombophlebitis; hypotension; hypertension; tachycardia; angina-like chest pains; CHF.

CNS: Headache; blurred vision; convulsions; dizziness.

GI: Nausea; vomiting; diarrhea.

Renal: Urinary retention; osmotic nephrosis.

Metabolic: Fluid and electrolyte imbalance; acidosis; electrolyte loss; dehydration.

Miscellaneous: Pulmonary congestion; dry mouth; thirst; rhinitis; local pain; skin necrosis; chills; urticaria; fever.

Overdosage:

Symptoms: Larger than recommended doses may result in increased electrolyte excretion, particularly sodium, chloride and potassium. Sodium depletion can result in orthostatic tachycardia or hypotension and decreased central venous pressure. Chloride metabolism closely follows that of sodium. Potassium deficit can impair neuromuscular function and cause intestinal dilation and ileus. If urine flow is inadequate, pulmonary edema or water intoxication may occur. Other symptoms include hypotension, polyuria that rapidly converts to oliguria, stupor, convulsions, hyperosmolality and hyponatremia.

Treatment: Discontinue infusion immediately. Institute supportive measures to correct fluid and electrolyte imbalances. Hemodialysis is beneficial to clear mannitol and reduce serum osmolality.

Administration and Dosage:

Reduction of intraocular pressure: 1.5 to 2 g/kg, as a 20% solution (7.5 to 10 ml/kg) or as a 15% solution (10 to 13 ml/kg) over a period as short as 30 minutes. When used preoperatively, administer 1 to 1.5 hours before surgery to achieve maximal effect.

Preparation of solution: When exposed to low temperatures, mannitol solution may crystallize. Concentrations > 15% have a greater tendency to crystallize. If crystals are observed, warm the bottle in a hot water bath, a dry heat oven or autoclave, then cool to at or below body temperature before administering.

When infusing concentrated mannitol, the administration set should include a filter.

Rx	**Osmitrol** (Baxter)	**Injection:** 5%	In 1000 ml.
		10%	In 500 and 1000 ml.
		15%	In 500 ml.
		20%	In 250 and 500 ml.
Rx	**Mannitol** (Various, eg, American Regent, Astra, IMS, Taylor Pharmaceuticals)	**Injection:** 25%	In 50 ml.

ODF

11

Surgical Adjuncts

Irrigating solutions, viscoelastic agents, botulinum toxin type A, absorbable gelatin film and proteolytic enzymes are adjuncts to a variety of ophthalmologic procedures and surgeries.

INTRAOCULAR IRRIGATING SOLUTIONS

Irrigating solutions are aqueous solutions used to cleanse and to maintain moisture of ocular tissue. Ideally these solutions are isotonic. The optimum pH is 7.4. A pH less than 7 or greater than 8 has caused cellular stress and death when the tissues have been exposed for a prolonged period of time.

The commercially available intraocular irrigating solutions (eg, *BSS* and *BSS Plus*) are used during ocular surgery to protect the lens and corneal endothelium. Unlike physiological saline and Lactated Ringer's solution, these balanced salt solutions provide the ions magnesium and calcium as cellular nutrients. These nutrients are required for intercellular and intracellular function during prolonged ocular surgery. In addition to magnesium and calcium, bicarbonate, glucose and glutathione are in these perfusion media (*BSS Plus*). These components help to maintain a deturgesced or thin cornea by avoiding corneal swelling.

For information on extraocular irrigating solutions, see the Nonsurgical Adjuncts chapter.

VISCOELASTIC AGENTS

Viscoelastic agents sodium hyaluronate and hydroxypropyl methylcellulose are used in many ophthalmic surgical procedures, including intraocular lens implantation and keratoplasty. In surgical procedures in the anterior segment of the eye, instillation maintains a deep anterior chamber, allowing for more efficient manipulation with less trauma to the corneal endothelium and surrounding tissues. The viscoelasticity of these agents helps push back the vitreous face and prevent formation of a postoperative flat chamber. The majority of the viscoelastic material is removed from the eye at the end of surgery to diminish the problems of glaucoma.

Viscoelastic agents are tissue-protective substances and do not interfere with normal wound healing. They are nonantigenic and do not contain proteins that may cause inflammation or foreign body reactions.

ABSORBABLE GELATIN FILM

In the dry state, absorbable gelatin film has the appearance and texture of cellophane. When moistened, it assumes a rubbery consistency and can be cut to desired size and shape and fitted to rounded or irregular surfaces.

It is used in many surgical procedures including glaucoma filtration operations (eg, iridencleisis and trephination), extraocular muscle surgery and diathermy or scleral "buckling" operations for retinal detachment to aid in preventing formation of adhesions between contiguous ocular structures.

Absence of undue tissue reaction incident to implantation and absorption of gelatin film, with consequent decreased likelihood of developing adhesions, has been found to be of particular value in dural and ocular implants.

BOTULINUM TOXIN TYPE A

Botulinum toxin is a form of purified botulinum toxin type A, produced from a culture of the Hall strain of *Clostridium botulinum*. Botulinum toxin type A blocks neuromuscular conduction by binding to receptor sites on motor nerve terminals, entering the nerve terminals and inhibiting the release of acetylcholine. When injected IM at therapeutic doses, the drug produces a localized chemical denervation muscle paralysis. When the muscle is chemically denervated, it atrophies and may develop extrajunctional acetylcholine receptors. There is evidence that the nerve can sprout and reinnervate the muscle, with the weakness thus being reversible. The paralytic effect on muscles injected with botulinum toxin type A is useful in reducing the excessive, abnormal contractions associated with blepharospasm.

SURGICAL ENZYMES

Alpha-chymotrypsin is a proteolytic surgical enzyme used to dissolve zonules of the lens during intracapsular cataract surgery. Destruction of the equatorial pericapsular membrane of the lens occurs in 5 minutes. Zonular fibers are lysed within 10 to 15 minutes of application; complete lysis of the entire zonular membrane may take up to 30 minutes.

Many chemicals and natural body fluids are capable of inactivating alpha-chymotrypsin. Examples of products that may cause zonulysis to fail include: Serum, blood, detergents, alkali, acids, antiseptics and epinephrine 1:100. These products may be used to inactivate alpha-chymotrypsin after zonulysis is complete. Pilocarpine (eg, *Isopto Carpine*), tetracaine (eg, *Pontocaine HCl*), acetylcholine *(Miochol)* and epinephrine 1:1000 will not inactivate this surgical enzyme.

Two other enzymes have been used during ocular surgery: Hyaluronidase and urokinase. *Hyaluronidase* is added to local anesthetic solutions to increase drug absorption and dispersion. This enzyme hydrolyzes hyaluronic acid in the connective tissue, which increases tissue permeability.

Urokinase has been used to irrigate hyphemas and to treat acute retinal artery and vein occlusions. The conversion of plasminogen to the proteolytic enzyme plasmin by urokinase causes degradation of plasma proteins, fibrinogen and fibrin clots.

Tissue plasminogen activator (*tPA*) is an enzyme that has the property of fibrin-enhanced conversion of plasminogen to plasmin. It produces limited conversion of plasminogen in the absence of fibrin. When introduced into the systemic circulation of pharmacologic concentration, it binds to fibrin in a thrombus and converts the entrapped plasminogen to plasmin. This initiates local fibrinolysis with limited systemic proteolysis.

J. James Rowsey, MD
University of South Florida

For More Information

Duane TD, ed. Clinical Ophthalmology. Philadelphia: Lippincott-Raven, 1987.

Ellis PP. Ocular Therapeutics and Pharmacology, ed. 7. St. Louis: C.V. Mosby, 1985.

Goodman LS, Gilman A. The Pharmacological Basis of Therapeutics, ed. 7. New York: MacMillan, 1985.

Havener WH. Ocular Pharmacology, ed. 5. St Louis: C.V. Mosby, 1983.

Whikehart Dr. Irrigating Solutions. In: Bartlett JD, Jaanus SD, eds. Clinical Ocular Pharmacology, ed. 3. Boston: Butterworth-Heinemann, 1995.

INTRAOCULAR IRRIGATING SOLUTIONS

Actions:

Pharmacology: Sterile irrigating solution is a sterile physiological balanced salt solution, each ml containing sodium chloride 0.64%, potassium chloride 0.075%, calcium chloride dihydrate 0.048%, magnesium chloride hexahydrate 0.03%, sodium acetate trihydrate 0.39%, sodium citrate dihydrate 0.17%, sodium hydroxide or hydrochloric acid (to adjust pH) and water. This solution is isotonic to ocular tissue and contains electrolytes required for normal cellular metabolic functions.

Indications:

Irrigation: For irrigation during various ocular surgical procedures. Some products may also be used for ears, nose and throat (consult specific product labeling).

Warnings:

Route of administration: Not for injection or IV infusion. Use aseptic technique only.

Precautions:

Preservative free solutions: Do not use for more than one patient.

Corneal clouding and edema have occurred following ocular surgery in which balanced salt solution was used as an irrigating solution. Take appropriate measures to minimize trauma to the cornea and other ocular tissues.

Concomitant medication: Addition of any medication to balanced salt solution may result in damage to intraocular tissue.

Diabetics: Studies suggest that intraocular irrigating solutions which are iso-osmotic with normal aqueous fluids should be used with caution in diabetic patients undergoing vitrectomy as intraoperative lens changes have been observed.

Adverse Reactions:

When corneal endothelium is abnormal, irrigation or any other trauma may result in bullous keratopathy. Postoperative inflammatory reactions and corneal edema and decompensation have occurred. Relationship to balanced salt solution is not established.

Administration and Dosage:

Use balanced salt solution according to the established practices for each surgical procedure. Follow the manufacturer directions for the particular administration set to be used. For products with separate solutions for reconstitution, never use either Part I or Part II alone; this could result in damage to the eye.

Storage/Stability: Store at 8° to 30°C (46° to 86°F). Avoid excessive heat. Do not freeze. Discard prepared solution after 6 hours. Do not use if cloudy or if seal or packaging is damaged. Do not use reconstituted solution if it is discolored or contains a precipitate.

Rx	**Balanced Salt Solution** (Various, eg, Akorn)	**Solution:** 0.64% NaCl, 0.075% KCl, 0.03% magnesium chloride, 0.048% calcium chloride, 0.39% sodium acetate, 0.17% sodium citrate and sodium hydroxide or hydrochloric acid	In 18 and 500 ml.
Rx	**AMO Endosol** (Allergan)		Preservative free. In 500 ml.
Rx	**BSS** (Alcon)		Preservative free. In 15, 30, 250 and 500 ml.
Rx	**Iocare Balanced Salt** (Ciba Vision)		Preservative free. In 15 ml.
Rx	**AMO Endosol Extra** (Allergan)	**Solution:** Mix aseptically just prior to use. **Part** I: 7.14 mg NaCl, 0.38 mg KCl, 0.154 mg calcium chloride dihydrate, 0.2 mg magnesium chloride hexahydrate, 0.92 mg dextrose, hydrochloric acid or sodium hydroxide/ml	Preservative free. In 515 ml.
		Part II: 1081 mg sodium bicarbonate, 216 mg dibasic sodium phosphate (anhydrous) and 95 mg glutathione disulfide (oxidized glutathione)/vial	Preservative free. In 60 ml.
Rx	**BSS Plus** (Alcon)	**Solution:** Mix aseptically just prior to use. **Part** I: 7.44 mg NaCl, 0.395 mg KCl, 0.433 mg dibasic sodium phosphate, 2.19 mg sodium bicarbonate, hydrochloric acid or sodium hydroxide/ml	Preservative free. In 240 ml.
		Part II: 3.85 mg calcium chloride dihydrate, 5 mg magnesium chloride hexahydrate, 23 mg dextrose, 4.6 mg glutathione disulfide/ml	Preservative free. In 10 ml.
Rx	**B-Salt Forte** (Akorn)	**Solution:** Mix aseptically just prior to use. **Part** I: 7.14 mg NaCl, 0.38 mg KCl, 0.154 mg calcium chloride dihydrate, 0.2 mg magnesium chloride hexahydrate, 0.92 mg dextrose, hydrochloric acid or sodium hydroxide/ml	Preservative free. In 515 ml.
		Part II: 1081 mg sodium bicarbonate, 216 mg dibasic sodium phosphate (anhydrous) and 95 mg glutathione disulfide (oxidized glutathione)/vial	Preservative free. In 60 ml.

POVIDONE IODINE

Actions:

Pharmacology: Povidone iodine has broad-spectrum antimicrobial action.

Indications:

Ophthalmic preoperative prep: Used prior to eye surgery to prep the periocular region (lids, brow and cheek) and irrigate the ocular surface (cornea, conjunctiva and palpebral fornices).

Contraindications:

Hypersensitivity to iodine.

Warnings:

For external use only: Not for intraocular injection or irrigation.

Pregnancy: Category C. Safety for use during pregnancy has not been established. Use only when clearly needed.

Lactation: Because of the potential for adverse reactions in nursing infants, decide whether to discontinue nursing or discontinue the drug, taking into account the importance of the drug to the mother.

Children: Safety and efficacy have not been established.

Precautions:

Thyroid disorders: Use caution in patients with thyroid disorders due to the possibility of iodine absorption.

Adverse Reactions:

Local sensitivity has been exhibited by some individuals.

Administration and Dosage:

Do not use in an open globe, as endothelial toxicity may ensue.

Transfer solution to a sterile prep cup. Apply to lashes and lid margins with sterile applicator, repeat once. Apply to lids, brow and cheek in a circular ever-expanding fashion with sterile applicator, repeat 3 times. While separating the lids, irrigate cornea, conjunctiva and palpebral fornices with solution and leave in for 2 minutes; flush with sterile saline solution.

Rx	**Betadine 5% Sterile Ophthalmic Prep Solution** (Akorn)	**Solution:** 5% povidone iodine	In 50 ml.[1]

[1] Glycerin, sodium chloride, sodium hydroxide and sodium phosphate.

SODIUM HYALURONATE

Actions:

Pharmacology: Sodium hyaluronate and sodium chondroitin sulfate are widely distributed in extracellular matrix of connective tissues. They are found in synovial fluid, skin, umbilical cord and vitreous and aqueous humor. The cornea is the ocular tissue having the greatest concentration of sodium chondroitin sulfate; the vitreous and aqueous humor contain the greatest concentration of sodium hyaluronate.

This preparation is a specific fraction of sodium hyaluronate developed for use in anterior segment and vitreous procedures as a viscoelastic agent. It has high molecular weight, is nonantigenic, does not cause inflammatory or foreign body reactions and has a high viscosity. The 1% solution is transparent and remains in the anterior chamber for < 6 days. It protects corneal endothelial cells and other ocular structures. It does not interfere with epithelialization and normal wound healing.

Indications:

Surgical aid: As a surgical aid in cataract extraction (intra- and extracapsular), intraocular lens implantation (IOL), corneal transplant, glaucoma filtration, retinal attachment surgery and posterior segment surgery to gently separate, maneuver and hold tissues.

To maintain a deep anterior chamber in surgical procedures in the anterior segment of the eye, allowing for efficient manipulation with less trauma to the corneal endothelium and other surrounding tissues.

To push back the vitreous face and prevent formation of a postoperative flat chamber.

To create a clear field of vision, facilitating intra- and postoperative inspection of the retina and photocoagulation.

Off-labeled uses: Sodium hyaluronate has been used in the treatment of refractory dry eye syndrome.

Warnings:

Hypersensitivity: Because this preparation is extracted from avian tissues and contains minute amounts of protein, risks of hypersensitivity may exist.

Precautions:

For intraocular use: Use only if solution is clear. Do not reuse cannulas.

Postoperative intraocular pressure (IOP) may be elevated as a result of preexisting glaucoma, compromised outflow and by operative procedures and sequelae, including enzymatic zonulysis, absence of an iridectomy, trauma to filtration structures and by blood and lenticular remnants in the anterior chamber. Because the exact role of these factors is difficult to predict in any individual case, the following precautions are recommended:

> *Do not overfill the anterior chamber* (except in glaucoma surgery). (See Administration and Dosage.)
>
> *Carefully monitor IOP,* especially during the immediate postoperative period. Treat significant increases appropriately.
>
> *In posterior segment surgery,* in aphakic diabetics, exercise special care to avoid using large amounts of the drug. Remove some of the preparation by irrigation or aspiration at the close of surgery (except in glaucoma surgery). (See Administration and Dosage.)
>
> Avoid trapping air bubbles behind the drug.

Cloudiness/Precipitate: Reports indicate that the drug may become cloudy or form a slight precipitate after instillation. The clinical significance is not known because the majority do not indicate any harmful effects on ocular tissues. Be aware of this phenomenon and remove cloudy or precipitated material by irrigation or aspiration. In vitro studies suggest that this phenomenon may be related to interactions with certain concomitantly administered ophthalmic medications.

ProVisc: The device used to obtain *ProVisc* material may cause an allergic reaction in susceptible persons.

Adverse Reactions:

Although well tolerated, a transient postoperative increase of IOP has been reported (see Precautions).

Other reactions that have occurred include postoperative inflammatory reactions (iritis, hypopyon); corneal edema; corneal decompensation.

Administration and Dosage:

Cataract surgery - IOL implantation: Slowly introduce a sufficient amount (using cannula or needle) into anterior chamber. Inject either before or after delivery of lens. Injection before lens delivery protects corneal endothelium from possible damage from removal of the cataractous lens. May use to coat surgical instruments and the IOL prior to insertion. May inject additional amounts during surgery to replace any of the drug lost.

Glaucoma filtration surgery: In conjunction with the performance of the trabeculectomy, inject slowly and carefully through a corneal paracentesis to reconstitute the anterior chamber. Further injection can be continued to allow it to extrude into the subconjunctival filtration site through and around the sutured outer scleral flap.

Corneal transplant surgery: After removal of the corneal button, fill the anterior chamber with the drug. Then, suture the donor graft in place. An additional amount may be injected to replace the lost amount as a result of surgical manipulation.

Sodium hyaluronate has also been used in the anterior chamber of the donor eye prior to trepanation to protect the corneal endothelial cells of the graft.

Retinal attachment surgery: Slowly introduce into the vitreous cavity. The injection may be directed to separate membranes from retina for safe excision and release of traction. Also serves to maneuver tissues into desired position (eg, to gently push back a detached retina or unroll a retinal flap); aids in holding retina against the sclera for reattachment.

Storage: Amvisc/Amvisc Plus, Healon/Healon GV: Store at 2° to 8°C (36° to 46°F).

AMO Vitrax – Store at room temperature (15° to 30°C; 59° to 86°F). Do not freeze. Protect from light.

ProVisc – Drug should reach room temperature before use (approximately 20–40 minutes depending on quantity). Store in refrigerator 2° to 8°C (36° to 46°F).

Rx	**Healon** (Kabi Pharmacia)	**Injection:** 10 mg/ml[1]	In 0.4, 0.55, 0.85 and 2 ml disp. syringes.
Rx	**ProVisc** (Alcon)		In 0.4, 0.55 and 0.85 ml disposable glass syringes.
Rx	**Amvisc** (Chiron)	**Injection:** 12 mg/ml[2]	In 0.5 or 0.8 ml disp. syringes.
Rx	**Healon GV** (Kabi Pharmacia)	**Injection:** 14 mg/ml[1]	In 0.55 and 0.85 ml disp. syringes.
Rx	**Amvisc Plus** (Chiron)	**Injection:** 16 mg/ml[2]	In 0.5 or 8 ml disp. syringes.
Rx	**AMO Vitrax** (Allergan)	**Injection:** 30 mg/ml[3]	In 0.65 ml disp. syringe.

[1] With 8.5 mg NaCl per ml.
[2] With 9 mg NaCl per ml.
[3] With 3.2 mg NaCl, 0.75 mg KCl, 0.48 mg calcium chloride, 0.3 mg magnesium chloride, 3.9 mg sodium acetate and 1.7 mg sodium citrate per ml.

SODIUM HYALURONATE AND CHONDROITIN SULFATE

Refer to the Sodium Hyaluronate monograph for more complete information.

Indications:

Surgical aid: A surgical aid in anterior segment procedures including cataract extraction and intraocular lens implantation.

Off-labeled uses: Topical treatment of severe dry eye disorders.

Administration and Dosage:

Carefully introduce (using a 27-gauge cannula) into the anterior chamber. May inject prior to or following delivery of the crystalline lens. Instillation prior to lens delivery provides additional protection to corneal endothelium, protecting it from possible damage arising from surgical instrumentation. May also be used to coat intraocular lens and tips of surgical instruments prior to implantation surgery. May inject additional solution during anterior segment surgery to fully maintain the chamber or to replace solution lost during surgery. At the end of surgery, remove solution by thoroughly irrigating the eye with a balanced salt solution. Alternatively, the solution may be left in the eye when used as directed.

Storage: Store at 2° to 8°C (36° to 46°F). Do not freeze.

Rx	**Viscoat** (Alcon)	**Solution:** ≤ 40 mg sodium chondroitin sulfate, 30 mg sodium hyaluronate per ml	0.45 mg sodium dihydrogen phosphate hydrate, 2 mg disodium hydrogen phosphate, 4.3 mg sodium chloride per ml. In 0.5 ml disposable syringes.

SODIUM HYALURONATE AND FLUORESCEIN SODIUM

Refer to the Sodium Hyaluronate and Fluorescein Sodium monographs for more complete information.

Indications:

Surgical aid: A surgical aid in anterior segment procedures including cataract extraction, intraocular lens (IOL) implantation and corneal transplant surgery. The fluorescein sodium facilitates visualization of the product during the surgical procedure.

Precautions:

IOP: Do not overfill the anterior segment as it may result in increased intraocular pressure, glaucoma or other ocular damage.

Administration and Dosage:

Cataract surgery/IOL implantation: Carefully introduce (using a 27–gauge cannula) into the anterior chamber. May inject prior to or following delivery of the lens. Instillation prior to lens delivery provides additional protection to corneal endothelium, protecting it from possible damage arising from removal of the cataractous lens. May also be used to coat the intraocular lens and surgical instruments prior to insertion. May inject additional solution during surgery to replace solution lost during surgical manipulation. Remove solution by irrigation or aspiration at the close of surgery.

Corneal transplant surgery: After removal of the corneal button, fill the anterior chamber with the solution. Then, suture the donor graft in place. May inject additional solution to replace solution lost during surgical manipulation. Remove solution by irrigation or aspiration at the close of surgery.

Storage: Store at 2° to 8°C (36° to 46°F). Allow to attain room temperature (approximately 30 min) prior to use. Do not freeze. Protect from light.

Rx	**Healon Yellow** (Pharmacia & Upjohn)	**Solution:** 10 mg sodium hyaluronate, 0.005 mg fluorescein sodium per ml	8.5 mg NaCl, 0.28 mg disodium hydrogen phosphate dihydrate, 0.04 mg sodium dihydrogen phosphate hydrate per ml. In 0.55 or 0.85 ml disposable syringes with cannula.

HYDROXYPROPYL METHYLCELLULOSE

Actions:

Pharmacology: Hydroxypropyl methylcellulose is an isotonic, nonpyrogenic viscoelastic solution with a high molecular weight (> 80,000 daltons). It maintains a deep chamber during anterior segment surgery and allows for more efficient manipulation with less trauma to the corneal endothelium and other ocular tissues. The viscoelasticity helps the vitreous face to be pushed back, preventing formation of a postoperative flat chamber. It is also used as a demulcent agent.

Indications:

Surgical aid:

2% solution – An ophthalmic surgical aid in anterior segment surgical procedures including cataract extraction and intraocular lens implantation.

2.5% solution – For professional use in gonioscopic examinations.

Precautions:

Intraocular pressure (IOP): Transient increased IOP may occur following surgery because of preexisting glaucoma or due to the surgery itself. If the postoperative IOP increases above expected values, administer appropriate therapy.

Adverse Reactions:

Although well tolerated, a transient, postoperative increase in IOP has been reported (see Precautions). Other reactions that have occurred include postoperative inflammatory reactions (iritis, hypopyon), corneal edema and corneal decompensation.

Administration and Dosage:

Anterior segment surgery: Carefully introduce into the anterior chamber using a 20–gauge or smaller cannula. The 2% solution may be used prior to or following delivery of the crystalline lens. Injection of 2% solution prior to lens delivery will provide additional protection to the corneal endothelium and other ocular tissues.

The 2% solution may also be used to coat an intraocular lens and tips of surgical instruments prior to implantation surgery. May inject during anterior segment surgery to fully maintain the chamber, or to replace fluid lost during the surgical procedure. Remove solution from the anterior chamber at the end of surgery.

Gonioscopic examinations: Fill gonioscopic prism with 2.5% solution, as necessary.

Storage/Stability: If this solution dries on optical surfaces, let them stand in cool water before cleansing. If solution changes color or becomes cloudy, do not use. Not for use with hot laser treatment as solution clouding will occur.

To avoid contamination, do not touch tip of container to any surface. Replace cap after using. Keep container tightly closed. Store at room temperature 15° to 30°C (59° to 86°F). Avoid excessive heat over 60°C (140°F). Protect from light.

Rx	**OcuCoat** (Storz)	**Solution**: 2%	In a balanced salt solution. In 1 ml syringe with cannula.
otc	**Gonak** (Akorn)	**Solution**: 2.5%	In 15 ml.[1]
otc	**Goniosol** (Ciba Vision)		In 15 ml.[1]

[1] With 0.01% benzalkonium chloride and EDTA.

HYDROXYETHYLCELLULOSE

Indications:

Gonioscopic bonding: For use in bonding gonioscopic prisms to the eye.

Administration and Dosage:

Storage: Store at room temperature 15° to 30°C (59° to 86°F).

Rx	**Gonioscopic** (Alcon)	**Solution**: Hydroxyethylcellulose	0.004% thimerosal, 0.1% EDTA. In 15 ml Drop-Tainers.

ABSORBABLE GELATIN FILM, STERILE

Actions:

Pharmacology: A sterile, absorbable gelatin film for use in ocular surgery.

In the dry state, it has the appearance and texture of cellophane of equivalent thickness; when moistened, it assumes a rubbery consistency and can then be cut to desired size and fitted to rounded or irregular surfaces. The rate of absorption after implantation ranges from 1 to 6 months, depending upon the size of the implant and the site of implantation. Pleural and muscle implants are completely absorbed in 8 to 14 days; dural and ocular implants usually require at least 2 to 5 months for complete absorption. The absence of undue tissue reactions, with the consequent decreased likelihood of developing adhesions, has been of particular value in the case of dural and ocular implants.

Indications:

Ocular surgery: In glaucoma filtration operations (ie, iridencleisis and trephination), extraocular muscle surgery and diathermy or scleral "buckling" operations for retinal detachment. There is a remarkable lack of cellular reaction to the film implanted subconjunctivally or used as a seton into the anterior chamber. Evidence shows that implants help prevent formation of adhesions between contiguous ocular structures.

Contraindications:

Since the rate of absorption is likely to be increased in the presence of purulent exudation, do not implant in grossly contaminated or infected surgical wounds.

Administration and Dosage:

Preparation: Immerse in sterile saline solution; soak until quite pliable; cut to the desired size and shape; apply as follows:

As a seton in iridencleisis: Place a small piece (≈ 4 mm x 10 mm) over the prolapsed iris pillar parallel to the limbus; Tenon's capsule and the conjunctiva are then closed with continuous absorbable sutures closely spaced to ensure tight wound closure.

Diathermy or scleral "buckling" operations: Place film over the sclera, then suture the muscle and the conjunctiva over the underlying film.

Extraocular muscle surgery: Place film over and beneath the muscle before Tenon's capsule and the conjunctiva are closed in layers.

Storage: Store at room temperature 15° to 30°C (59° to 86°F). To insure sterility, use immediately after withdrawal from the envelope.

Rx	**Gelfilm** (Pharmacia & Upjohn)	100 mm x 125 mm	In 1s.
Rx	**Gelfilm Ophthalmic** (Pharmacia & Upjohn)	25 mm x 50 mm	In 6s.

MIOTICS, DIRECT-ACTING

For complete prescribing information, see the Miotics, Direct-Acting monograph in the Agents for Glaucoma chapter.

Actions:

Pharmacology: The direct-acting miotics are parasympathomimetic (cholinergic) drugs which duplicate the muscarinic effects of acetylcholine. When applied topically, these drugs produce pupillary constriction, stimulate the ciliary muscles and increase aqueous humor outflow facility.

ACETYLCHOLINE CHLORIDE, INTRAOCULAR

Indications:

To produce complete miosis in seconds after delivery of the lens in cataract surgery. In penetrating keratoplasty, iridectomy and other anterior segment surgery where rapid, complete miosis may be required.

Administration and Dosage:

Solution: Instill the solution into the anterior chamber before or after securing one or more sutures. The pupil is rapidly constricted and the peripheral iris drawn away from the angle of the anterior chamber if there are no mechanical hindrances. Any anatomical hindrance to miosis may require surgery to permit desired effect of drug.

0.5 to 2 ml produces satisfactory miosis. Solution need not be flushed from the chamber after miosis occurs. Since acetylcholine has a short duration of action, pilocarpine may be applied topically before dressing to maintain miosis.

Preparation of solution: The aqueous solution of acetylcholine chloride is unstable. Prepare solution immediately before use. Do not use solution which is not clear and colorless. Discard any solution that has not been used. Do not gas sterilize.

Storage: Store at room temperature 15° to 30°C (59° to 86°F). Do not freeze.

Rx	**Miochol-E** (Ciba Vision)	**Solution**: 1:100 acetylcholine chloride when reconstituted	In 2 ml dual chamber univial (lower chamber 20 mg lyophilized acetylcholine chloride and 56 mg mannitol; upper chamber 2 ml electrolyte diluent[1] and sterile water for injection).

[1] Sodium chloride, potassium chloride, magnesium chloride hexahydrate, calcium chloride dihydrate.

CARBACHOL, INTRAOCULAR

For complete prescribing information, refer to the Miotics, Direct-Acting group monograph in the Agents for Glaucoma chapter. The following section is included here for completeness to show all of the clinical uses of this class of drug.

Ingredients:

Miosis: Intraocular use for miosis during surgery.

Administration and Dosage:

For single-dose intraocular use only. Discard unused portion.

Open under aseptic conditions only.

Gently instill no more than 0.5 ml into the anterior chamber before or after securing sutures. Miosis is usually maximal 2 to 5 minutes after application.

Storage: Store at room temperature 15° to 30°C (59° to 86°F).

Rx	**Carbastat** (Ciba Vision)	**Solution**: 0.01%	In 1.5 ml vials.[1]
Rx	**Miostat** (Alcon)		In 1.5 ml vials.[1]

[1] With 0.64% sodium chloride, 0.075% potassium chloride, 0.048% calcium chloride dihydrate, 0.03% magnesium chloride hexahydrate, 0.39% sodium acetate trihydrate, 0.17% sodium citrate dihydrate, sodium hydroxide, hydrochloric acid.

POLYDIMETHYLSILOXANE (Silicone Oil)

Actions:

Pharmacology: Polydimethylsiloxane, an oil that is injected into the vitreous space of the eye, is used as a prolonged retinal tamponade in select cases of retinal detachment.

Clinical trials:

Anatomic reattachment rates – Successful reattachment of the retina occurred in 64% to 75% of the patients who were treated with polydimethylsiloxane. This rate varied depending on the specific etiology of the disease and the severity of the condition. In AIDS CMV retinitis patients receiving silicone oil as a primary means for reattaching the retina, attachment rates were as high as 90% within an average 6 month follow-up period.

Visual acuity outcomes – From 45% to 70% of patients showed improvements in visual acuity at 6 months. In about 15% to 26% of patients, visual acuity did not change and in about 15% to 30%, worsening of visual acuity occurred. Deterioration of visual acuity in treated patients appeared to be related to redetachment of the retina, further progression of retinal disease, or to keratopathy and cataract complications. In AIDS CMV retinitis patients, improvement or maintenance of visual acuity was documented in 57% of the patients within an average 6 month follow-up period. In AIDS patients, further decline in visual acuity was seen due to continuing progression of retinal and optic nerve disease and development of oil related cataracts in 33% of patients within 4 to 5 months of oil instillation.

Indications:

Retinal detachments: Prolonged retinal tamponade in selected cases of complicated retinal detachments where other interventions are not appropriate for patient management. Complicated retinal detachments or recurrent retinal detachments occur most commonly in eyes with proliferative vitreoretinopathy (PVR), proliferative diabetic retinopathy (PDR), cytomegalovirus (CMV) retinitis, giant tears and following perforating injuries.

For primary use in detachments due to AIDS-related CMV retinitis and other viral infections.

Contraindications:

Pseudophakic patients with silicone intraocular lens (silicone oil can chemically interact and opacify silicone elastomers).

Warnings:

Cataract: Approximately 50% to 70% of phakic patients developed a cataract within 12 months of oil instillation. Approximately 33% of phakic AIDS CMV retinitis patients developed some degree of cataract within an average 4 to 5 month time frame from oil instillation.

Anterior chamber oil migration: In 17% to 20% of patients, oil emulsification or migration into the anterior chamber was observed. Migration into the anterior chamber occurred in both phakic and aphakic patients.

Keratopathy: From 8% to 20% of patients developed keratopathy (0.6%, AIDS patients). This complication occurred most frequently in aphakic patients (18% to 21%) and in the patients in whom oil had migrated into the anterior chamber (30%); the keratopathy in these cases was attributed to prolonged physical contact between the corneal endothelium and the silicone oil.

Glaucoma: Approximately 19% to 20% (0.06%, AIDS patients) of patients developed a persistent elevation in intraocular pressure (> 23 to 25 mm Hg). The neovascular glaucoma rate was about 8%. Moderate temporary postoperative increases occurred within the first 3 weeks of treatment. Thereafter, secondary ocular hypertension occurred by several mechanisms. Glaucoma complications occurred in approximately 30% of patients in which anterior chamber oil is noted. Patients with proliferative diabetic retinopathy were at highest risk for development of glaucoma following silicone oil instillation into the vitreous space.

Precautions:

Long-term use: The safety and efficacy of long-term use have not been established.

Adverse Reactions:

Most common: The most common adverse reactions include: Cataract (50% to 70%); anterior chamber oil migration (17% to 20%); keratopathy (8% to 20%); glaucoma (19% to 20%). See Warnings.

Miscellaneous: Other adverse reactions ranked by frequency of occurrence: Redetachment, optic nerve atrophy, rubeosis iritis, temporary IOP increase, macular pucker, vitreous hemorrhage, phthisis, traction detachment, angle block (> 2%); subretinal strands, retinal rupture, endophthalmitis, subretinal silicone oil, choroidal detachment, aniridia, PVR reproliferation, cystoid macular edema, enucleation (< 2%).

Administration and Dosage:

Polydimethylsiloxane can be used in conjunction with or following standard retinal surgical procedures including scleral buckle surgery, vitrectomy, membrane peeling and retinotomy or relaxing retinectomy.

Avoid introduction of air bubbles into the oil by careful withdrawal or decanting of the oil into the syringe. The oil can be injected into the vitreous from the syringe via a single use cannulated infusion line or syringe needle. Subretinal fluid can be drained with a flute needle concurrent with polydimethylsiloxane infusion. The vitreous space can be filled with the oil to between 80% and 100% while exchanging for fluid or air, taking necessary precautions to avoid high intraocular pressure from developing during the exchange. Because the polydimethylsiloxane is less dense than the eye aqueous fluid, a basal iridectomy at the 6 o'clock meridian (Ando iridectomy) is recommended to minimize oil-induced pupillary block and early angle-closure glaucoma. Upon choice of the physician, it may be desirable to have the patient assume a face-down posture during the first 24 hours following surgery.

Monitor the patient closely for development of glaucoma, cataract and keratopathy complications and schedule for follow-up reexamination at regular intervals.

It is recommended that polydimethylsiloxane be removed at an appropriate interval within 1 year following instillation if the retina is stable, attached and without significant remnants of proliferation. Although there is insufficient clinical evidence to support justification for longer term tamponade, whether or not the oil should be removed in patients at high risk for redetachment or the development of phthisis and shrinkage due to hypotony must be determined individually by the physician. In order to minimize the number of invasive traumatic experiences for patients with AIDS and CMV retinitis at high risk for redetachment and who have a shortened expected lifespan, avoid silicone oil removal procedures if the patient concurs.

Polydimethylsiloxane can be removed from the posterior chamber by withdrawal with a normal 10 ml syringe and a wide bore 1 mm cannula. By repeated oil-fluid exchange most of the remaining small silicone oil droplets can subsequently be mobilized and removed from the eye. Alternatively, oil may be passively removed by infusion of an appropriate aqueous solution under the oil bubble, while allowing the oil to effuse out of a sclerotomy incision, or limbal incision in aphakic patients.

As there is a possible correlation between the migration of polydimethylsiloxane into the anterior chamber and the appearance of corneal changes such as edema, hazing or opacification, Descemet folds or decompensation, perform regular monitoring of the patient's corneal status and take early corrective action if necessary, including extraction of the oil from the anterior chamber. Large bubbles or droplets of oil in the anterior chamber can be removed manually by syringe. Further standard practice for medical treatment of the keratopathy is recommended.

Temporary pressure increases > 3 weeks after surgery that can normalize either spontaneously or that can be corrected by surgical treatment are those in which the polydimethylsiloxane causes a mechanical blockage of the pupil or inferior iridectomy or causes chamber angle closure by forcing its way anteriorly. In these situations some of the oil may be withdrawn to relieve the mechanical force of the oil interface. Presence of polydimethylsiloxane droplets in the anterior chamber may also cause a chronic outflow obstruction of the trabecular meshwork. In such situations elevated intraocular pressure can be managed with anti-glaucoma medication in the majority of outflow obstruction patients.

Admixture incompatibility: Do not admix with any other substances prior to injection.

Storage/Stability: Store at room or cool temperature 8° to 24°C (46° to 75°F). Polydimethylsiloxane is supplied in a sterile vial intended for single use only and contains no preservative. Do not resterilize. Discard unused portions. Product should be discarded following expiration date.

Rx	**AdatoSil 5000** (Escalon Ophthalmics)	**Injection**: Polydimethylsiloxane oil	In single-use 10 and 15 ml vials.

BOTULINUM TOXIN TYPE A

Actions:

Pharmacology: Botulinum toxin is a sterile, lyophilized form of purified botulinum toxin type A, produced from a culture of the Hall strain of *Clostridium botulinum* grown in a medium containing N-Z amine and yeast extract. Botulinum toxin type A blocks neuromuscular conduction by binding to receptor sites on motor nerve terminals, entering the nerve terminals, and inhibiting the release of acetylcholine. When injected IM at therapeutic doses, botulinum toxin type A produces a localized chemical denervation muscle paralysis. When the muscle is chemically denervated, it atrophies and may develop extrajunctional acetylcholine receptors. There is evidence that the nerve can sprout and reinnervate the muscle, with the weakness thus being reversible.

The paralytic effect on muscles injected with botulinum toxin type A is useful in reducing the excessive, abnormal contractions associated with blepharospasm.

When used for the treatment of strabismus, the administration of botulinum toxin type A may affect muscle pairs by inducing an atrophic lengthening of the injected muscle and a corresponding shortening of the muscle's antagonist. Following periocular injection of botulinum toxin type A, distant muscles show electrophysiologic changes, but no clinical weakness or other clinical change for a period of several weeks or months, parallel to the duration of local clinical paralysis.

Clinical trials: In one study, botulinum toxin was evaluated in 27 patients with essential blepharospasm; 26 had previously undergone drug treatment utilizing benztropine mesylate, clonazepam or baclofen without adequate clinical results. Three of these patients then underwent muscle stripping surgery still without an adequate outcome. Upon using botulinum toxin, 25 of the 27 patients reported improvement within 48 hours. One of the other patients was later controlled with a higher dosage. The remaining patient reported only mild improvement but remained functionally impaired.

In another study, 12 patients with blepharospasm were evaluated in a double-blind, placebo controlled study. All patients receiving botulinum toxin (n = 8) were improved compared with no improvements in the placebo group (n = 4). The mean dystonia score improved by 72%, the self-assessment score rating improved by 61%, and a videotape evaluation rating improved by 39%. The effects of the treatment lasted a mean of 12.5 weeks.

Patients with blepharospasm (n = 1684) evaluated in an open trial showed clinical improvement lasting an average of 12.5 weeks prior to need for retreatment.

Patients with strabismus (n = 677) treated with one or more injections of botulinum toxin type A were evaluated in an open trial; 55% were improved to an alignment of 10 prism diopters when evaluated ≥ 6 months following injection. These results are consistent with results from additional open label trials.

Indications:

Treatment of strabismus and blepharospasm associated with dystonia, including benign essential blepharospasm or VII nerve disorders in patients ≥ 12 years of age.

Contraindications:

Hypersensitivity to any ingredient in the formulation.

Warnings:

Strabismus: The efficacy of botulinum toxin type A in deviations > 50 prism diopters, in restrictive strabismus, in Duane's syndrome with lateral rectus weakness, and in secondary strabismus caused by prior surgical over-recession of the antagonist is doubtful, or multiple injections over time may be required. Botulinum toxin type A is ineffective in chronic paralytic strabismus except to reduce antagonist contracture in conjunction with surgical repair.

Dosage: Do not exceed the recommended dosages and frequencies of administration. There have been no reported instances of systemic toxicity resulting from accidental injection or oral ingestion of botulinum toxin type A. Should accidental injection or oral ingestion occur, medically supervise the person for several days on an outpatient basis for signs or symptoms of systemic weakness or muscle paralysis. The entire contents of a vial is below the estimated dose for systemic toxicity in humans weighing ≥ 6 kg.

Hypersensitivity: As with all biologic products, epinephrine and other precautions should be available should an anaphylactic reaction occur.

Pregnancy: Category C. It is not known whether botulinum toxin type A can cause fetal harm when administered to a pregnant woman or can affect reproduction capacity. Administer to pregnant women only if clearly needed.

Lactation: It is not known whether this drug is excreted in breast milk. Exercise caution when botulinum toxin type A is administered to a nursing woman.

Children: Safety and efficacy in children < 12 years of age have not been established.

Precautions:

Safe and effective use of botulinum toxin type A depends upon proper storage of the product, selection of the correct dose and proper reconstitution and administration techniques. Physicians administering botulinum toxin type A must understand the relevant neuromuscular and orbital anatomy and any alterations to the anatomy due to prior surgical procedures, and standard electromyographic techniques.

Retrobulbar hemorrhages: During the administration of botulinum toxin type A for the treatment of strabismus, retrobulbar hemorrhages sufficient to compromise retinal circulation have occurred from needle penetrations into the orbit. Have appropriate instruments to decompress the orbit accessible. Ocular (globe) penetrations by needles have also occurred. An ophthalmoscope to diagnose this condition should be available.

Reduced blinking from botulinum toxin type A injection of the orbicularis muscle can lead to corneal exposure, persistent epithelial defect and corneal ulceration, especially in patients with VII nerve disorders. One case of corneal perforation in an aphakic eye requiring corneal grafting has occurred because of this effect. Carefully test corneal sensation in eyes previously operated upon, avoid injection into the lower lid area to avoid ectropion and vigorously treat any epithelial defect. This may require protective drops, ointment, therapeutic soft contact lenses, or closure of the eye by patching or other means.

Antibodies: Presence of antibodies to botulinum toxin type A may reduce the effectiveness of therapy. In clinical studies, reduction in effectiveness due to antibody production has occurred in one patient with blepharospasm receiving 3 doses over a 6 week period totaling 92 U and in several patients with torticollis who received multiple doses experimentally, totaling over 300 U in 1 month. For this reason, keep the dose of botulinum toxin type A for strabismus and blepharospasm as low as possible, in any case < 200 U in a 1 month period.

Drug Interactions:

Aminoglycosides: The effect of botulinum toxin may be potentiated by aminoglycoside antibiotics or any other drug that interferes with neuromuscular transmission. Exercise caution when botulinum toxin type A is used in patients taking these drugs.

Adverse Reactions:

Ophthalmic:

Strabismus – Inducing paralysis in one or more extraocular muscles may produce spatial disorientation, double vision or past-pointing. Covering the affected eye may alleviate these symptoms. Extraocular muscles adjacent to the injection site are often affected, causing ptosis or vertical deviation, especially with higher doses. Side effects in 2058 adults who received 3650 injections for horizontal strabismus included ptosis (15.7%) and vertical deviation (16.9%). The incidence of ptosis was much less after inferior rectus injection (0.9%) and much greater after superior rectus injection (37.7%).

Side effects persisting for > 6 months in an enlarged series of 5587 injections of horizontal muscles in 3104 patients included ptosis lasting over 180 days (0.3%) and vertical deviation > 2 prism diopters lasting over 180 days (2.1%).

In these patients, the injection procedure itself caused 9 scleral perforations. A vitreous hemorrhage occurred and later cleared in one case. No retinal detachment or visual loss occurred in any case; 16 retrobulbar hemorrhages occurred. Decompression of the orbit after 5 minutes was done to restore retinal circulation in one case. No eye lost vision from retrobulbar hemorrhage. Five eyes had pupillary change consistent with ciliary ganglion damage (Adies pupil).

Blepharospasm – In 1684 patients who received 4258 treatments (involving multiple injections) for blepharospasm, incidence of adverse reactions per treated eye was: Ptosis (11%); irritation/tearing, includes dry eye, lagophthalmos, and photophobia (10%); ectropion, keratitis, diplopia and entropion occurred rarely (< 1%).

Ecchymosis occurs easily in the soft eyelid tissues. This can be prevented by applying pressure at the injection site immediately after the injection. In two cases of VII nerve disorder (one case of an aphakic eye), reduced blinking from botulinum toxin type A injection of the orbicularis muscle led to serious corneal exposure, persistent epithelial defect and corneal ulceration. Perforation requiring corneal grafting occurred in one case, an aphakic eye (see Precautions).

Two patients previously incapacitated by blepharospasm experienced cardiac collapse attributed to over-exertion within 3 weeks following botulinum toxin type A therapy. Caution sedentary patients to resume activity slowly and carefully following the administration of botulinum toxin type A.

Local: Diffuse skin rash (n = 7) and local swelling of the eyelid skin (n = 2) lasting for several days following eyelid injection have occurred.

Overdosage:

In the event of overdosage or injection into the wrong muscle, additional information may be obtained by contacting Allergan Pharmaceuticals at (800) 347-5063 from 8 am to 4 pm Pacific Time, or at (714) 724-5954 for a recorded message at other times.

Patient Information:

Patients with blepharospasm may have been extremely sedentary for a long time. Caution these patients to resume activity slowly and carefully follow administration.

Administration and Dosage:

Strabismus: Botulinum toxin type A is intended for injection into extraocular muscles utilizing the electrical activity recorded from the tip of the injection needle as a guide to placement within the target muscle. Injection without surgical exposure or electromyographic guidance should not be attempted. Physicians should be familiar with electromyographic technique.

Preparation: An injection of botulinum toxin type A is prepared by drawing into a sterile 1 ml tuberculin syringe an amount of the properly diluted toxin (see Dilution Table) slightly greater than the intended dose. Air bubbles in the syringe barrel are expelled and the syringe is attached to the electromyographic injection needle, preferably a 1½ inch, 27 gauge needle. Injection volume in excess of the intended dose is expelled through the needle into an appropriate waste container to ensure patency of the needle and to confirm that there is no syringe-needle leakage. Use a new, sterile needle and syringe to enter the vial on each occasion for dilution or removal of botulinum toxin type A.

To prepare the eye for botulinum toxin type A injection, give several drops of a local anesthetic and an ocular decongestant several minutes prior to injection.

Strabismus: The volume of botulinum toxin type A injected for treatment of strabismus should be between 0.05 to 0.15 ml per muscle.

The initial listed doses of the diluted botulinum toxin type A (see Dilution table) typically create paralysis of injected muscles beginning 1 to 2 days after injection and increasing in intensity during the first week. The paralysis lasts for 2 to 6 weeks and gradually resolves over a similar time period. Overcorrections lasting > 6 months have been rare. About one half of patients will require subsequent doses because of inadequate paralytic response of the muscle to the initial dose, or because of mechanical factors such as large deviations or restrictions, or because of the lack of binocular motor fusion to stabilize the alignment.

1. Initial doses in units (U). Use the lower listed doses for treatment of small deviations. Use the larger doses only for large deviations.
   a. For vertical muscles, and for horizontal strabismus of < 20 prism diopters: 1.25 to 2.5 U in any one muscle.
   b. For horizontal strabismus of 20 prism diopters to 50 prism diopters: 2.5 to 5 U in any one muscle.
   c. For persistent VI nerve palsy of ≥ 1 month duration: 1.25 to 2.5 U in the medial rectus muscle.

2. Subsequent doses for residual or recurrent strabismus.
   a. Re-examine patients 7 to 14 days after each injection to assess the effect of that dose.
   b. Patients experiencing adequate paralysis of the target muscle who require subsequent injections should receive a dose comparable to the initial dose.
   c. Subsequent doses for patients experiencing incomplete paralysis of the target muscle may be increased up to twofold the previously administered dose.
   d. Subsequent injections should not be administered until the effects of the previous dose have dissipated as evidenced by substantial function in the injected and adjacent muscles.
   e. Maximum recommended dose as a single injection for any one muscle is 25 U.

Blepharospasm: Diluted botulinum toxin type A (see Dilution table) is injected using a sterile, 27 to 30 gauge needle without electromyographic guidance. Initially, 1.25 to 2.5 U (0.05 to 0.1 ml volume at each site) injected into the medial and lateral pre-tarsal orbicularis oculi of the upper lid and into the lateral pre-tarsal orbicularis oculi of the lower lid is the initial recommended dose.

In general, the initial effect of the injections is seen within 3 days and reaches a peak at 1 to 2 weeks post-treatment. Each treatment lasts approximately 3 months, following which the procedure can be repeated indefinitely. At repeat treatment sessions, the dose may be increased up to twofold if the response from the initial treatment is considered insufficient (usually defined as an effect that does not last > 2 months). However, there appears to be little benefit obtainable from injecting > 5 U per site. Some tolerance may be found when botulinum toxin type A is used in treating blepharospasm if treatments are given any more frequently than every 3 months, and it is rare to have the effect be permanent.

The cumulative dose of botulinum toxin type A in a 30 day period should not exceed 200 U.

Dilution technique: To reconstitute lyophilized botulinum toxin type A, use sterile normal saline without a preservative; 0.9% sodium chloride injection is the recommended diluent. Draw up the proper amount of diluent in the appropriate size syringe. Since botulinum toxin type A is denatured by bubbling or similar violent agitation, inject the diluent into the vial gently. Discard the vial if a vacuum does not pull the diluent into the vial. Record the date and time of reconstitution on the space on the label. Administer within 4 hours after reconstitution.

During this time period, store reconstituted botulinum toxin type A in a refrigerator 2° to 8°C (36° to 46°F). Reconstituted botulinum toxin type A should be clear, colorless and free of particulate matter. The use of one vial for more than one patient is not recommended because the product and diluent do not contain a preservative.

Dilution of Botulinum Toxin Type A

Diluent added (0.9% sodium chloride injection)	Resulting dose
1 ml	10 units
2 ml	5 units
4 ml	2.5 units
8 ml	1.25 units

These dilutions are calculated for an injection volume of 0.1 ml. A decrease or increase in the botulinum toxin type A dose is also possible by administering a smaller or larger injection volume – from 0.05 ml (50% decrease in dose) to 0.15 ml (50% increase in dose).

Storage: Store the lyophilized product in a freezer at or below -5°C (23°F). Administer within 4 hours after the vial is removed from the freezer and reconstituted. During these 4 hours, store reconstituted botulinum toxin type A in a refrigerator 2° to 8°C (36° to 46°F). Reconstituted botulinum toxin type A should be clear, colorless and free of particulate matter.

Rx	**Botox** (Allergan)	**Powder for Injection (lyophilized):** 100 units of lyophilized *Clostridium botulinum* toxin type A[1]	Preservative free. 0.05 mg albumin (human), 0.9 mg sodium chloride. In vials.

[1] One unit corresponds to the calculated median lethal intraperitoneal dose (LD/50) in mice of the reconstituted drug injected.

ODF

12

Nonsurgical Adjuncts

Dapiprazole HCl, extraocular irrigating solutions, lid scrubs and vitamins and minerals are adjuncts to a variety of ophthalmic procedures and conditions.

DAPIPRAZOLE HYDROCHLORIDE

Dapiprazole is classified pharmacologically as an alpha-adrenergic antagonist. This drug demonstrates rapid reversal of mydriasis produced by phenylephrine and, to a lesser extent, tropicamide. The miosis produced by dapiprazole 0.5% begins 10 minutes following instillation and results in a significant reduction in pupil size. About half of the pupils of treated eyes will achieve their premydriatic diameter within 2 hours of dilation with phenylephrine 2.5% and tropicamide 1%. In patients with brown irides, the rate of pupillary constriction may be slightly slower than in individuals with blue or green irides. The most significant side effect is conjunctival hyperemia associated with the alpha-receptor blockade of the conjunctival vasculature. The conjunctival injection lasts about 20 minutes in more than 80% of patients, and burning or stinging on instillation of the drug is reported in about half the patients.

EXTRAOCULAR IRRIGATING SOLUTIONS

Extraocular irrigating solutions are sterile isotonic solutions for general ophthalmic use. Office uses include irrigating procedures following tonometry, gonioscopy, foreign body removal or use of fluorescein. They are also used to soothe and cleanse the eye, and in conjunction with hard contact lenses. Because these solutions have a short contact time with the eye, they do not need to provide nutrients to cells. Unlike intraocular irrigants, irrigants for extraocular use contain preservatives that prevent bacterial contamination. However, the preservatives are exceedingly toxic to the corneal endothelium, and intraocular use of extraocular irrigating fluids is contraindicated.

LID SCRUBS

The mainstay of therapy for blepharitis is generally careful eyelid hygiene. This is easily accomplished at home by the patient. Although baby shampoo is frequently used for this purpose, commercially available eyelid cleansers are now available and are known to be effective with potentially less ocular stinging, burning and toxicity. Commercial lid scrub products are designed to aid in the removal of oils, debris or desquamated skin associated with the inflamed eyelid. The lid scrubs can also be used for hygienic eyelid cleansing in contact lens wearers. These products are designed to be used full strength on eyelid tissues but must not be instilled directly into the eyes.

Some of the commercial products are packaged with gauze or cotton pads, which provide an abrasive action to augment the cleansing properties of the detergent solution.

VITAMINS AND MINERALS

Deficiencies of vitamin A and zinc have sometimes been associated with certain adverse ocular effects. Beyond replacement of documented deficiencies, however, treatment or prevention of ophthalmic diseases using vitamins and minerals is not clearly established. Recently, various investigators have explored the use of vitamins A, C and E, as well as zinc, as preventative measures for degenerative ophthalmic conditions often associated with the aging process. The primary mechanisms of action offered to explain the effectiveness of such therapy include antioxidation and free radical scavenging. Several products are now commercially available for the prevention and treatment of macular degeneration, but considerably more data will be required before the efficacy of these products becomes well established.

Jimmy D. Bartlett, OD, DOS
University of Alabama at Birmingham

For More Information

Blaho K. Adjunctive agents. In: Bartlett JD, Jaanus SD, eds. Clinical Ocular Pharmacology, ed. 3. Boston: Butterworth-Heinemann, 1995.

Doughty MJ, Lyle WM. A review of the clinical pharmacokinetics of pilocarpine, moxisylyte (thymoxamine), dapiprazole in the reversal of diagnostic pupillary dilation. *Optom Vis Sci* 1992;69:358-68.

Allison RW, et al. Reversal of mydriasis by dapiprazole. *Ann Ophthalmol* 1990;92:131-38.

Bartlett JD, Classe JG. Dapiprazole: Will it affect the standard of care for pupillary dilation? *Optom Clin* 1992;2(3):65-75.

Whikehart DR. Irrigating solutions. In: Bartlett JD, Jaanus SD, eds. Clinical Ocular Pharmacology, ed. 3. Boston: Butterworth-Heinemann, 1995.

Polack FM, Goodman DF. Experience with a new detergent lid scrub in the management of chronic blepharitis. *Arch Ophthalmol* 1988;106:719-20.

Sperduto RD. Do we have a nutritional treatment for age-related cataract or macular degeneration? *Arch Ophthalmol* 1990;108:1403-5.

DAPIPRAZOLE HYDROCHLORIDE

Actions:

Pharmacology: Dapiprazole acts through blocking the alpha-adrenergic receptors in smooth muscle and produces miosis through an effect on the dilator muscle of the iris.

The drug does not have any significant activity on ciliary muscle contraction and, therefore, does not induce a significant change in the anterior chamber depth or the thickness of the lens.

Dapiprazole has demonstrated safe and rapid reversal of mydriasis produced by phenylephrine and, to a lesser degree, tropicamide. In patients with decreased accommodative amplitude due to treatment with tropicamide, the miotic effect of dapiprazole may partially increase the accommodative amplitude.

Eye color affects the rate of pupillary constriction. In individuals with brown irides, the rate of pupillary constriction may be slightly slower than in individuals with blue or green irides. Eye color does not appear to affect the final pupil size.

Dapiprazole does not significantly alter intraocular pressure (IOP) in normotensive eyes or in eyes with elevated IOP.

Indications:

Mydriasis: Treatment of iatrogenically induced mydriasis produced by adrenergic (phenylephrine) or parasympatholytic (tropicamide) agents.

Contraindications:

When constriction is undesirable, such as in acute iritis; hypersensitivity to any component of this preparation.

Warnings:

For topical ophthalmic use only. Not for injection.

Frequency of use: Do not use more frequently than once a week.

IOP reduction: Not indicated for the reduction of IOP or in the treatment of open-angle glaucoma.

Vision reduction: May cause difficulty in dark adaptation and may reduce field of vision. Patients should exercise caution in night driving or when performing other activities in poor illumination.

Pregnancy: Category B. There are no adequate and well controlled studies in pregnant women. Use during pregnancy only when clearly needed and when potential benefits outweigh the potential hazards to the fetus.

Lactation: It is not known whether this drug is excreted in breast milk. Exercise caution when dapiprazole is administered to a nursing woman.

Children: Safety and efficacy for use in children have not been established.

Adverse Reactions:

Conjunctival injection lasting 20 minutes (> 80%); burning on instillation (≈ 50%); ptosis, lid erythema, lid edema, chemosis, itching, punctate keratitis, corneal edema, browache, photophobia, headaches (10% to 40%); dryness of the eye, tearing, blurring of vision (less frequent).

Patient Information:

May cause difficulty in dark adaptation and may reduce field of vision. Exercise caution when driving at night or performing other activities in poor illumination.

To avoid contamination, do not touch tip of container to any surface.

Do not use more frequently than once a week.

Discard any solution that is not clear and colorless.

Administration and Dosage:

Instill 2 drops into the conjunctiva of each eye followed 5 minutes later by an additional 2 drops. Administer after the ophthalmic examination to reverse the diagnostic mydriasis.

Shake container for several minutes to ensure mixing.

Storage/Stability: Store at room temperature 15° to 30°C (59° to 86°F) for 21 days after reconstitution.

Rx	**Rēv-Eyes** (Storz/Lederle)	**Powder, lyophilized:** 25 mg (0.5% solution when reconstituted)	In vial with 5 ml diluent and dropper.[1]

[1] With 2% mannitol, 0.4% hydroxypropyl methylcellulose, 0.01% EDTA, 0.01% benzalkonium chloride and sodium chloride.

EXTRAOCULAR IRRIGATING SOLUTIONS

Actions:

Pharmacology: These sterile isotonic solutions are for general ophthalmic use. Office uses include irrigating procedures following tonometry, gonioscopy, foreign body removal or use of fluorescein; they are also used to soothe and cleanse the eye. Because these solutions have a short contact time with the eye, they do not need to provide nutrients to cells. Unlike intraocular irrigants, irrigants for extraocular use contain preservatives which prevent bacteriostatic contamination. However, the preservatives are exceedingly toxic to the corneal endothelium and intraocular use of extraocular irrigating fluids is contraindicated.

Indications:

Irrigation: For irrigating the eye to help relieve irritation by removing loose foreign material, air pollutants (smog or pollen) or chlorinated water.

Contraindications:

Hypersensitivity to any component of the formulation; as a saline solution for rinsing and soaking contact lenses; injection or intraocular surgery.

Patient Information:

If you experience eye pain, changes in vision, continued redness or irritation of the eye, or if the condition worsens or persists, consult a doctor.

Obtain immediate medical treatment for all open wounds in or near the eyes.

If solution changes color or becomes cloudy, do not use.

Do not use these products with contact lenses.

To avoid contamination, do not touch tip of the container to any surface. Replace cap after using.

Administration and Dosage:

Solution: Flush the affected eye(s) as needed, controlling the rate of flow of solution by pressure on the bottle.

Eyecup: Fill the sterile eyecup halfway with eye wash. Apply the cup tightly to the affected eye and tilt the head backward. Open eyes wide, rotate eye and blink several times to ensure that the solution completely floods the eye. Discard the wash. Rinse the cup with clean water and repeat the procedure with the other eye, if necessary.

Rinse the eyecup before and after every use. Avoid contamination of the rim or inside surfaces of the cup.

Storage: If solution changes color or becomes cloudy, do not use.

otc	**AK-Rinse** (Akorn)	**Solution:** Sodium carbonate, KCl, boric acid, EDTA, 0.01% benzalkonium Cl	In 30 and 118 ml.
otc	**Blinx** (Akorn)	**Solution:** NaCl, KCl, sodium phosphate, 0.005% benzalkonium Cl, 0.02% EDTA	In 120 ml.
otc	**Collyrium for Fresh Eyes Wash** (Wyeth-Ayerst)	**Solution:** Boric acid, sodium borate, benzalkonium Cl	In 120 ml.
otc	**Dacriose** (Ciba Vision)	**Solution:** NaCl, KCl, sodium phosphate, sodium hydroxide, 0.01% benzalkonium Cl, EDTA	In 15 and 120 ml.
otc	**Eye Stream** (Alcon)	**Solution:** 0.64% NaCl, 0.075% KCl, 0.03% magnesium Cl hexahydrate, 0.048% calcium Cl dihydrate, 0.39% sodium acetate trihydrate, 0.17% sodium citrate dihydrate, 0.013% benzalkonium Cl	In 30 and 118 ml.
otc	**Eye Wash** (Bausch & Lomb)	**Solution:** Boric acid, KCl, EDTA, sodium carbonate, 0.01% benzalkonium Cl	In 118 ml.
otc	**Eye Wash** (Zenith-Goldline)	**Solution:** Boric acid, KCl, EDTA, anhydrous sodium carbonate, 0.01% benzalkonium Cl	In 118 ml.

otc	**Eye Wash** (Lavoptik)	**Solution:** 0.49% NaCl, 0.4% sodium biphosphate, 0.45% sodium phosphate, 0.005% benzalkonium Cl	In 180 ml with eyecup.
otc	**Eye Irrigating Wash** (Roberts Hauck)	**Solution:** Boric acid, KCl, sodium carbonate, EDTA, 0.01% benzalkonium Cl	In 120 ml.
otc	**Eye Irrigating Solution** (Rugby)	**Solution:** NaCl, mono- and dibasic sodium phosphate, benzalkonium Cl, EDTA	In 118 ml.
otc	**Irrigate Eye Wash** (Optopics)	**Solution:** NaCl, mono- and dibasic sodium phosphate, benzalkonium Cl, EDTA	In 118 ml.
otc	**Optigene** (Pfeiffer)	**Solution:** NaCl, mono- and dibasic sodium phosphate, EDTA, benzalkonium Cl	In 118 ml.
otc	**Visual-Eyes** (Optopics)	**Solution:** NaCl, mono- and dibasic sodium phosphate, benzalkonium Cl, EDTA	In 120 ml.

LID SCRUBS

Indications:

Eyelid cleansing: To aid in the removal of oils, debris or desquamated skin.

Precautions:

For external use only. Do not instill directly into eye.

Administration and Dosage:

Close eye(s) and gently scrub on eyelid(s) and lashes using lateral side-to-side strokes; rinse thoroughly.

otc	**Eye•Scrub** (Ciba Vision)	**Solution:** PEG-200 glyceryl tallowate, disodium laureth sulfosuccinate, cocoamidopropylamine oxide, PEG-78 glyceryl cocoate, benzyl alcohol, EDTA	In UD 30s (pads) and kit (120 ml and 60 pads).
otc	**Lid Wipes-SPF** (Akorn)	**Solution:** PEG-200 glyceryl tallowate, PEG-80 glyceryl cocoate, laureth-23, cocoamidopropylamine oxide, NaCl, glycerin, sodium phosphate, sodium hydroxide	Preservative free. In UD 30s (pads).
otc	**OCuSOFT** (OCuSOFT)	**Solution:** PEG-80 sorbitan laurate, sodium trideceth sulfate, PEG-150 distearate, cocoamidopropyl hydroxysultaine, lauroamphocarboxyglycinate, sodium laureth-13 carboxylate, PEG-15 tallow polyamine, quaternium-15	Alcohol and dye free. In UD 30s (pads), 30, 120 and 240 ml and compliance kit (120 ml and 100 pads).

TEAR TEST STRIPS

Indications:

Schirmer Tear Test:

Test I – To diagnose dry eye syndrome, to evaluate lacrimal gland function in contact lens wearers, to check tear production prior to eyelid surgery and prior to corneal transplantation and cataract surgery.

Test II – To assess the adequacy of reflex lacrimation.

Sno-Strips: Perform test on eye before any topical medication (especially anesthetic) is administered or other procedures are carried out (eg, manipulation of eyelids).

Zone-Quick: To indicate tear volume. No anesthesia required. If eyedrops have been used, perform test at least 5 minutes later. Test may be performed during contact lens wear.

Precautions:

Zone-Quick: Tear volume may vary. Repeat testing on different days will give a more accurate volume representation.

Zone-Quick may induce a slight mechanical irritation leading to lacrimination in some patients (rarely). In those patients it may be necessary to use another tear test in addition to *Zone-Quick*.

Administration and Dosage:

Schirmer Tear Test: Strips are placed at the junction of the middle and temporal one-third of the eyelid margin. To avoid increased reflex lacrimation and pain, do not touch the cornea.

Sno-Strips: Apply to lower temporal lid margin of eye. The distance between notch and shoulder of strip is 10 mm, which should be wetted in approximately 3 minutes. Repeat if > 5 minutes; > 10 minutes indicates reduced tear secretion.

Zone-Quick: Test eyes one at a time. Thread is placed on the palpebral conjunctiva. Patient should look straight ahead and blink normally for 15 seconds. After 15 seconds, gently pull the lower eyelid down and remove thread with upward motion. Measure entire length of red portion of thread in millimeters.

Storage/Stability: Store in dark place at room temperature.

otc	**Sno-Strips** (Akorn)	**Strips:** Sterile tear flow test strips	In 100s.
otc	**Schirmer Tear Test** (Various, eg, Alcon)	**Strips:** Sterile test strips	In 250s.
otc	**Zone-Quick** (Menicon USA)	**Threads:** Phenol red threads (PRT)	In 50 aluminum pkg sets (100 threads).

HAMAMELIS WATER

Indications:

Optic opacity: The manufacturer claims usefulness for the treatment of "optic opacity caused by cataract." Not intended for use in glaucoma. Efficacy has not been demonstrated in controlled clinical studies.

Administration and Dosage:

Instill 2 drops morning and night into affected eye(s).

Rx	**Succus Cineraria Maritima** (Walker Pharm)	**Solution:** Aqueous and glycerin solution of senecio compositae, hamamelis water, boric acid	In 7 ml.

ZINC SULFATE SOLUTION

Indications:

Astringent: A mild astringent for temporary relief of minor eye irritation.

Warnings:

Irritation/Eye pain: If irritation persists or increases, or if eye pain or a change in vision occurs, discontinue use and consult physician.

Administration and Dosage:

Instill 1 to 2 drops into eye(s) up to 4 times daily. If solution discolors or becomes cloudy, do not use.

otc	**Eye-Sed** (Scherer)	**Solution:** 0.25%	In 15 ml.[1]

[1] With 0.05% tetrahydrozoline HCl, EDTA, benzalkonium Cl and NaCl.

VITAMINS AND MINERALS

Actions:

Pharmacology: Certain vitamin and mineral deficiencies have been associated with adverse ocular effects, most notably vitamin A and zinc. Beyond replacement of documented deficiency, treatment or prevention of ophthalmic diseases with vitamins and minerals is not well established.

However, investigators are beginning to explore this area. Some claims are being made for vitamins A, C and E, as well as zinc as preventatives for degenerative ophthalmic changes often associated with aging. The principal mechanisms of action are offered as antioxidation and free radical scavenging.

Much more data are required before actual recommendations can be made. However, products are available, labeled with such claims.

Administration and Dosage:

Take with meals.

Adults: 1 to 2 tablets 1 or 2 times daily or as directed by a physician.

Storage: Store at room temperature 15° to 30°C (59° to 86°F) .

otc	**Vitamin A Palmitate** (Freeda)	**Tablets**: 10,000 IU	In 100s and 250s.
		15,000 IU	In 100s and 250s.
		25,000 IU	In 100s and 250s.
otc	**Beta Carotene** (Freeda)	**Tablets**: 10,000 IU	In 100s, 250s and 500s.
otc	**Palmitate-A** (Akorn)	**Tablets**: 15,000 IU vitamin A palmitate	In 100s.
otc	**Palmitate-A 5000** (Akorn)	**Tablets**: 5000 IU vitamin A palmitate	In 100s.
otc	**Icaps Plus** (Ciba Vision)	**Tablets**: 6000 IU vitamin A[1], 200 mg C, 20 mg B_2, 60 IU E, 40 mg Zn[2], 2 mg Cu, 5 mg Mn, 20 mcg Se	In 60s, 120s and 180s.
otc	**Icaps Time Release** (Ciba Vision)	**Tablets**: 7000 IU vitamin A[1], 200 mg C, 20 mg B_2, 100 IU E, 40 mg Zn[2], 2 mg Cu, 20 mcg Se	In 60s and 120s.
otc	**AntiOxidants** (Akorn)	**Caplets**: 5000 IU vitamin A[1], 400 mg C[3], 200 IU E[4], 40 mg Zn[5], 5 mg L-glutathione, 3 mg sodium pyruvate, 2 mg Cu[6], 40 mcg Se[7]	In 60s.
otc	**Oxi-Freeda** (Freeda)	**Tablets**: 5000 IU beta carotene, 150 IU E, 20 mg B_1, 20 mg B_2, 20 mg B_6, 10 mcg B_{12}, 15 mg elemental Zn, 50 mcg Se, 20 mg calcium pantothenate, 40 mg glutathione, 40 mg B_3, 100 mg C, 75 mg L-cysteine	In 100s and 250s.
otc	**One-A-Day Extras Anti-oxidant** (Bayer)	**Capsules, softgel**: 5000 IU vitamin A[1], 200 IU E, 250 mg C, 7.5 mg Zn, 1 mg Cu, 15 mcg Se, 1.5 mg Mn	(One-A-Day). Tartrazine. In 50s.
otc	**OCuSoft VMS** (OCu-Soft)	**Tablets**: 5000 IU vitamin A, 30 IU E, 60 mg C, 40 mg Zn, 2 mg Cu, 40 mcg Se	Film coated. In 60s.
otc	**Ocuvite** (Storz/Lederle)	**Tablets**: 40 mg elemental Zn[8], 2 mg elemental Cu[9], 40 mcg elemental Se[10], 5000 IU vitamin A[1], 30 IU E[4] and 60 mg C[3]	In 60s and 120s.
otc	**Ocuvite Extra** (Storz/Lederle)	**Tablets**: 40 mg elemental Zn[8], 2 mg elemental Cu[9], 200 mg C, 50 IU E, 6000 IU vitamin A[1], 40 mcg elemental Se, 3 mg B_2, 40 mg B_3, 5 mg elemental Mn, 5 mg L-glutathione	In 50s.

[1] As beta carotene.
[2] As zinc acetate.
[3] As ascorbic acid.
[4] As dl-alpha tocopheryl acetate.
[5] As zinc ascorbate.
[6] As copper ascorbate.
[7] As L-selenomethionine.
[8] As zinc oxide.
[9] As cupric oxide.
[10] As sodium selenate.

ODF

13

Contact Lens Care

Over 25 million Americans wear contact lenses. Contact lenses can offer patients a natural appearance, increased visual performance and convenience. They can successfully correct most refractive errors such as myopia, hyperopia and astigmatism. Bifocal contact lenses are available for the presbyopic patient. Tinted contact lenses can enhance or completely change the color of a patient's eyes. Research and development by major ophthalmic corporations have produced a variety of new lens materials and designs. With new contact lens products and patient education, contact lens use should continue to grow.

The number of contact lens care products has also increased dramatically. Patients may become confused because there are over 125 different products sold for contact lens care.

COMPLIANCE

Successful contact lens wear includes good vision, lens comfort and normal ocular health. Contact lens success is dependent upon patient compliance in caring for their contact lenses. Several studies indicate that between 40% and 74% of soft contact lens patients are not following the care regimen prescribed by their doctor. In another study, it was found that 50% of the patients harbored potentially pathogenic microorganisms in their care systems. Noncompliance among contact lens wearers can have many consequences. Inadequate cleaning can lead to lens discoloration and lens surface buildup of protein, lipids, minerals and other environmental contaminants, which can contribute to giant papillary conjunctivitis (GPC), superficial punctate keratitis and corneal abrasion. Irregular contact lens disinfection can cause severe ocular infection.

Doctors, pharmacists and opticians must have a thorough understanding of all contact lens materials and care systems. With this knowledge, they can educate the patient, increase compliance and therefore decrease lens-related complications. Compliance has been defined by the Food and Drug Administration (FDA) as the use of an approved contact lens care regimen in a manner both in agreement with the manufacturer's instructions and consistent with good general hygiene. Compliance must meet four criteria:

1. The patient should always wash his or her hands before lens manipulation;

2. The patient should use an FDA-approved care system in an appropriate manner;

3. The patient should wear lenses only on a daily wear schedule unless the lenses are approved by the FDA for extended wear;

4. All solutions should be free of bacterial contamination.

CONTACT LENS GUIDELINES
♦ Proper contact lens care will increase success and decrease complications.
♦ Cleaning does not disinfect lenses.
♦ Disinfecting does not clean lenses.
♦ Enzyme solutions are not a substitute for disinfection.
♦ Wash and rinse hands thoroughly before handling contact lenses.
♦ Do not insert contact lenses if eyes are red or irritated. If eyes become painful or vision worsens while wearing lenses, remove lenses and consult an eye-care practitioner immediately.
♦ Do not wear contact lenses while sleeping unless they have been prescribed for extended wear.
♦ For soft lens care, use only products designed for soft lenses.
♦ For rigid lens care, use only products designed for rigid lenses.
♦ Do not change or substitute products from a different manufacturer without consulting a doctor.
♦ Always follow label directions or doctor's recommendations.
♦ Do not store lenses in tap water.
♦ Never use saliva to wet contact lenses.
♦ Keep lens care products out of the reach of children.
♦ Do not instill topical medications while contact lenses are being worn unless directed by a doctor.
♦ Do not get cosmetic lotions, creams or sprays in your eyes or on lenses. It is best to put on lenses before putting on makeup and remove them before removing makeup. Water-base cosmetics are less likely to damage lenses than oil-based products.
♦ Schedule and keep follow-up appointments with your eye-care practitioner (approximately every 6 to 12 months or as recommended).
♦ Contact lenses wear out with time and should be replaced regularly. Throw away disposable lenses after the recommended wearing period.

CONTACT LENS MATERIALS

Three types of contact lenses are manufactured: Hard, rigid gas permeable (RGP) and soft.

Hard Contact Lenses

Hard contact lenses are made from polymethylmethacrylate (PMMA). PMMA does not transmit the oxygen needed for normal corneal integrity. Hard contact lenses have caused chronic corneal edema, corneal distortion, edematous corneal formations, spectacle blur, polymegathism and corneal abrasions. Because of these ocular complications, hard lenses are seldom the lens of choice for a new contact lens patient. Less than 1% of the contact lens population wear hard contact lenses.

Rigid Gas Permeable Lenses (RGP)

Approximately 20% of contact lens patients wear rigid gas permeable (RGP) lenses. These lenses are oxygen permeable; therefore, the RGP patient does not have the severe physiological complications of the hard lens patient. Several lens polymers with a high degree of oxygen permeability have been approved by the FDA for extended wear. RGP lenses provide the patient with good vision, durability and easy care.

Soft Contact Lenses

Soft contact lenses were invented in the early 1960s by Otto Wichterle, a Czechoslovakian scientist. The first soft lens marketed in the US was in 1971. A soft lens is manufactured from a hydrophilic polymer. Today, soft lenses are manufactured from polymers which contain 38% to 79% water.

Daily wear soft contact lenses are designed to be worn all day (12 to 14 hours), but must be removed nightly to be cleaned and disinfected. Extended wear soft lenses can be worn for ≥ 24 hours. The FDA and most eye care practitioners recommend a maximum wearing period of 7 days. The lenses must then be removed overnight for cleaning and disinfection. The major advantage of extended wear lenses is convenience. Daily wear soft lenses provide the same level of comfort and vision as extended wear soft lenses. The popularity of extended wear soft lenses has decreased in the last few years, due to the reported risk of infection.

Disposable soft lenses are designed to eliminate the complications of lens deposits by replacing lenses at frequent intervals. Lens deposits can interfere with vision, cause corneal irritation and contribute to ocular infection. In addition, disposable lenses offer the patient the convenience of reduced lens care.

Some disposable lenses are approved for daily wear and others for extended wear. It is recommended that conventional soft lenses be discarded after 12 weeks of wear. Disposable lenses should be replaced every 1 to 2 weeks. Planned replacement lenses are replaced every 1, 3 or 6 months. The doctor will prescribe the replacement schedule for each patient. If a disposable lens is not discarded immediately after lens removal, it should be cleaned with a surfactant cleaner and stored in a disinfection solution.

Recently, two companies have introduced a 1 day single use soft lens. This lens is designed to be worn one time and then thrown away. The patient will apply a fresh, clean, sterile lens each day of lens wear. Contact lens care products (ie, lens case, cleaning solution and disinfection solution) are not needed with these new soft lenses.

CONTACT LENS CARE PRODUCTS

Products for use with contact lenses possess the same general characteristics of all ophthalmic products; they are sterile, isotonic and free of particulate matter. Additionally, product formulations contain various components to achieve specific goals of contact lens care.

Although all contact lenses serve similar functions in correcting visual defects, each distinct type of lens material requires a unique lens care program. In selecting appropriate lens care solutions, it is essential to correctly identify the type of lens the patient is using.

Hard and Rigid Gas Permeable (RGP) Lenses

Similar lens care is used for the hard and RGP lenses. Products include wetting/soaking/disinfection solutions, cleaning agents, lubricants and rewetting solutions.

When a rigid contact lens is removed from the eye, it may be covered with lipids, proteins, eye makeup and other debris. After removal, immediately clean the lens with a *surfactant cleaner*. Improper cleaning can contribute to a lens surface buildup that can interfere with vision and potentially cause corneal irritation.

Soak rigid lenses overnight in a *wetting/soaking/disinfecting solution*. This solution has four major functions:

1. To enhance the lens surface wettability;
2. To maintain the lens hydration similar to that achieved during daily contact lens wear;
3. To disinfect the lens;
4. To act as a mechanical buffer between the lens and the cornea.

It is not uncommon for a rigid lens patient to experience dryness after several hours of wear. This is especially true with RGP lens patients because of the hydrophobic nature of some lens materials. *Rewetting drops* can provide temporary relief by rinsing debris off the lens surface and rewetting the eye and the lens.

Many clinicians routinely recommend the weekly use of an enzyme (papain) cleaner with RGP lenses. This weekly cleaning process is very effective in removing protein deposits from the lens surface. A protein film on an RGP lens can decrease vision and cause giant papillary conjunctivitis.

Soft Contact Lenses

Soft contact lens care systems are designed to clean, disinfect and re-wet the lenses. The first step is proper cleaning. Cleaning the lens gently in the palm of the hand with a *daily surfactant cleaner* will remove fresh lipids, oils and other environmental debris. Clean soft lenses thoroughly with a surfactant cleaner each time a lens is removed. After cleaning the lens, thoroughly rinse with a soft lens *rinsing/storage solution*. All rinsing/storage solutions contain 0.9% saline. Some are available with no preservatives in unit-dose vials or aerosol containers. Other saline solutions contain preservatives to decrease microorganism growth. Discourage use of saline made with salt tablets because of the risk of contamination and infection (see Precautions).

Enzymatic cleaners are generally used on a weekly basis. They are more effective in removing protein deposits than surfactant cleaners because they contain proteolytic enzymes (papain, pancreatin or subtilisin). Most enzymes are dissolved directly in saline, but the subtilisin enzyme tablet can be dissolved in a hydrogen peroxide disinfection solution.

Soft lens *disinfection* is the most important step in soft lens care. Disinfection is achieved by using a thermal (heat) or chemical (cold) system.

Thermal disinfection was the first system approved for soft contact lenses. A heat unit specially designed for soft lenses is used for 10 minutes at 80°C (176°F). This procedure will kill most microorganisms that are dangerous to the eye. Recently, *Acanthamoeba* keratitis has become a concern of many clinicians. Heat disinfection is the most effective procedure to successfully kill *Acanthamoeba*; however, heat disinfection cannot be used with all soft lens materials. Also, continued use of heat can shorten the life of a soft lens.

Recommended Chemical Disinfection Times for Soft Lenses			
System	Manufacturer	Disinfection Time (minimum)	Neutralization Time (minimum)
AOSEPT	Ciba Vision	6 hours[1]	6 hours[1]
Complete All-in-One	Allergan	4 hours	none
Disinfecting Solution	Bausch & Lomb	4 hours	none
Flex-Care Especially for Sensitive Eyes	Alcon	4 hours	none
Hydrocare Cleaning and Disinfecting	Allergan	4 hours	none
MiraSept	Alcon	10 minutes	10 minutes
Opti-Free	Alcon	4 hours	none
Opti-One	Alcon	4 hours	none
Oxysept	Allergan	10 minutes	10 minutes
Quick CARE	Ciba Vision	5 minutes	none
ReNu Multi-Purpose	Bausch & Lomb	4 hours	none
Soft Mate Disinfecting for Sensitive Eyes	PBH Wesley Jessen	4 hours	none
Soft Mate Consept	PBH Wesley Jessen	10 minutes	10 minutes
Ultra-Care	Allergan	2 hours[2]	2 hours[2]

[1] One-step method: Disinfection and neutralization occur together for a total of 6 hours.
[2] One-step method: Disinfection and neutralization occur together for a total of 2 hours.

The original chemical soft lens disinfection systems used thimerosal with either chlorhexidine or a quaternary ammonium compound. These systems had a high incidence of sensitivity reactions. But, in the last few years, *Opti-Free* by Alcon, *ReNu* by Bausch & Lomb and *Complete* by Allergan have gained a large share of the chemical disinfection market. The disinfection agents utilized in these three care systems (*OptiFree-Polyquad, ReNu-Dymed, Complete-Trischem*) have caused a minimum of sensitivity reactions.

In addition, *Opti-One* by Alcon and *Quick CARE* by Ciba Vision are approved chemical disinfection systems.

Opti-One is a multi-purpose solution used for the cleaning, rinsing, disinfection and storage of disposable soft lenses prescribed to be replaced within a 2 week period. *Opti-One* uses *Polyguard* as a disinfection agent. If lenses are to be worn longer than 2 weeks, Alcon recommends that patients use the *Opti-Free* system.

Quick CARE is a unique system that cleans, disinfects and conditions soft lenses so they are ready to wear in about 5 minutes. The *Quick CARE* system contains a starting solution, a disposable lens case and a finishing solution. One of the major advantages of this system is that it provides total lens care in about 5 minutes. In today's busy society this factor should enhance lens care compliance.

Hydrogen peroxide is an excellent disinfecting agent for soft lenses, and with proper neutralization a sensitivity reaction is very rare. Various hydrogen peroxide care systems are currently available in the US. Most systems require two steps to achieve disinfection and hydrogen peroxide neutralization; one system combines disinfection and neutralization in a single step. Hydrogen peroxide (3%) is a very effective disinfection agent and can be used with all soft lens polymers. However, hydrogen peroxide care systems can be complex and expensive. Generic peroxide solutions should not be substituted for solutions that have been formulated for contact lenses. They may be contaminated with heavy metals, have different concentrations of hydrogen peroxide or use stabilizers that may discolor soft lenses.

Soft lens rewetting solutions permit the lubrication of the soft lens while it is on the eye. Most patients find these rewetting drops minimally effective in reducing dryness. Maximum relief can be achieved by removing the lens, cleaning it with a daily surfactant cleaner and thoroughly rinsing it with a rinsing/storage saline solution.

PRECAUTIONS FOR CONTACT LENS USE

Acanthamoeba Keratitis

Soft contact lens wearers who use homemade saline solution are at risk of developing *Acanthamoeba* keratitis, a serious and painful corneal infection that may cause blindness or impaired vision. Homemade saline solutions (nonsterile) may be used during the thermal disinfection phase but NOT after disinfection.

Drug Interference with Contact Lens Use

Systemic medications may affect the physiology of the cornea, lids and tear system. In addition, some drugs may discolor soft contact lenses. Pharmacists and eye-care practitioners should be aware of the interaction of systemic medications and contact lenses.

Drug Interference With Contact Lens Use		
Drug	RGP[1]/Hard/Soft Lens	Action
Anticholinergics (eg, *Isopto Atropine*)	RGP, hard, soft	Tear volume decreased
Antihistamines, sympathomimetics	RGP, hard, soft	Tear volume decreased, blink rate decreased
Chlorthalidone (eg, *Hygroton*)	RGP, hard, soft	Causes lid or corneal edema
Clomiphene (eg, *Clomid)*	RGP, hard, soft	Causes lid or corneal edema
Diuretics, Thiazide (eg, *HydroDIURIL*)	RGP, hard, soft	Tear volume decreased
Dopamine (eg, *Intropin*)	soft	Discoloration of contact lenses
Epinephrine, topical (eg, *Epifrin*)	soft	Discoloration of contact lenses
Fluorescein, topical (eg, *Ful-Glo*)	soft	Lens absorbs the yellow dye
Hypnotics, sedatives, muscle relaxants (eg, *Amytal)*	RGP, hard, soft	Blink rate decreased
Iodine Groups (eg, *Phospholine Iodide*)	soft	Discoloration of contact lenses
Nitrofurantoin (eg, *Furadantin*)	soft	Discoloration of contact lenses
Oral contraceptives (eg, *Ortho-Novum*)	RGP, hard, soft	Increased stickiness of mucus; corneal lid edema due to fluid retention properties of estrogens
Phenazopyridine (eg, *Pyridium*)	soft	Discoloration of contact lenses
Phenolphthalein (eg, *Modane*)	soft	Discoloration of contact lenses
Phenylephrine (eg, *Neo-Synephrine*)	soft	Discoloration of contact lenses
Primidone (eg, *Mysoline*)	RGP, hard, soft	Causes lid or corneal edema
Rifampin (eg, *Rifadin*)	soft	Lens absorbs drug, causing orange discoloration
Sulfasalazine (eg, *Azulfidine*)	soft	Yellow staining
Tricyclic antidepressants (eg, *Elavil)*	RGP, hard, soft	Tear volume decreased

[1] Rigid gas permeable.

Products listed on the following pages are grouped as follows:

Contact Lens Solution	
Type of Lens	Type of Solution
Hard	Wetting Cleaning/Soaking/Wetting Wetting/Soaking Rewetting Cleaning Cleaning/Soaking
Rigid Gas Permeable	Disinfecting/Wetting/Soaking Cleaning/Disinfecting/Soaking Cleaning Enzymatic Cleaning Rewetting
Soft	Surfactant Cleaning Rinsing/Storage Enzymatic Cleaning Chemical Disinfection Rewetting

N. Rex Ghormley, OD, FAAO
Contact Lens and Vision Care Consultants, St. Louis, MO

For More Information

Aquavella JV, Rao GN. Contact Lenses. Philadelphia: J.B. Lippincott Co., 1987.

Barr JT, ed. Contact Lens Pocket Guide. Irvine, CA: Allergan Optical Corporation, 1987.

Bennett ES, Grone RM, eds. Rigid Gas-Permeable Contact Lenses. New York: Professional Press Books, Fairchild Publications, 1986.

Chun MW, Weissmann BA. Compliance in contact lens care. *Am J Optom Physiol Opt* 1987; 64:274-76.

Collins MJ, Carney LG. Patient compliance and its influence on contact lens wearing problems. *Am J Optom Physiol Opt* 1986;63:952-56.

Duane TD, ed.. Clinical Ophthalmology. Philadelphia: Lippincott-Raven, 1997.

Lowther GE, et al. The Pharmacist's Guide to Contact Lenses and Lens Care. Atlanta: CIBAVision Corporation, 1988.

Mondino BJ, et al. Corneal ulcers associated with daily wear and extended wear contact lenses. *Am J Ophthalmol* 1986;102:58-65.

Smith MB. Contact lens care systems. *Contact, The Eye Care Journal for Pharmacists* 1988;1:14-22.

HARD (PMMA) CONTACT LENS PRODUCTS

Conventional hard lenses are made of a rigid hydrophobic polymer, polymethylmethacrylate (PMMA). For optimum comfort, these lenses require care with separate wetting, cleaning and soaking solutions. Refer to the general discussion of these products.

WETTING SOLUTIONS, HARD LENSES

Wetting solutions contain surfactants to facilitate hydration of the hydrophobic hard lens surface. These solutions include methylcellulose and derivatives, polyvinyl alcohol, povidone, some newer polymers, preservatives and buffers. These agents increase solution viscosity and act as a physical cushioning agent between lens and cornea.

otc	**Liquifilm Wetting** (Allergan)	**Solution:** 0.004% benzalkonium chloride, EDTA, hydroxypropyl methylcellulose, NaCl, KCl, polyvinyl alcohol	In 60 ml.
otc	**Sereine** (Optikem)	**Solution:** Buffered. 0.1% EDTA, 0.01% benzalkonium chloride	In 60 and 120 ml.

CLEANING/SOAKING/WETTING SOLUTIONS, HARD LENSES

otc	**Total** (Allergan)	**Solution:** Buffered, isotonic. Polyvinyl alcohol, benzalkonium chloride, EDTA	In 60 and 120 ml.

WETTING/SOAKING SOLUTIONS, HARD LENSES

otc	**Sereine** (Optikem)	**Solution:** Buffered, isotonic. 0.1% EDTA, 0.01% benzalkonium chloride	In 120 ml.
otc	**Soac-Lens** (Alcon)	**Solution:** Buffered. 0.004% thimerosal, 0.1% EDTA, wetting agents	In 118 ml.
otc	**Wet-N-Soak Plus** (Allergan)	**Solution:** Buffered, isotonic. 0.003% benzalkonium chloride, polyvinyl alcohol, EDTA	In 120 and 180 ml.

REWETTING SOLUTIONS, HARD LENSES

Rewetting solutions are intended for use directly in the eye in conjunction with a contact lens. These products improve wearing time by rehydrating the lens, which may become dry and contaminated during wear, although more benefit is obtained by actually removing and rewetting the lens. The principle components of these solutions are wetting agents.

otc	**Adapettes** (Alcon)	**Solution:** Buffered, isotonic. Povidone and other water-soluble polymers, sorbic acid, EDTA	Thimerosal free. In 15 ml.
otc	**Clerz 2** (Alcon)	**Solution:** Isotonic. Hydroxyethylcellulose, poloxamer 407, NaCl, KCl, sodium borate, boric acid, sorbic acid, EDTA	Thimerosal free. In 5, 15 and 30 ml.

otc	**Lens Lubricant** (Bausch & Lomb)	**Solution:** Buffered, isotonic. 0.004% thimerosal, 0.1% EDTA, povidone, polyoxyethylene	In 15 ml.
otc	**Opti-Tears** (Alcon)	**Solution:** Isotonic. 0.1% EDTA, 0.001% polyquaternium-1, dextran, NaCl, KCl, hydroxymethylcellulose	Thimerosal and sorbic acid free. In 15 ml.
otc	**Lens Drops** (Ciba Vision)	**Solution:** Buffered, isotonic. NaCl, carbamide, poloxamer 407, 0.2% EDTA, 0.15% sorbic acid	Thimerosal free. In 15 ml.

CLEANING SOLUTIONS, HARD LENSES

Cleaning solutions contain surfactant cleaners to facilitate removal of oleaginous, proteinaceous and other types of debris from the lens surface. To adequately clean, physically rub lens in the palm of the hand or between thumb and finger with solution for about 20 seconds and rinse with water or sterile saline solution.

otc	**LC-65** (Allergan)	**Solution:** Buffered. 0.001% thimerosal, EDTA	In 15 and 60 ml.
otc	**MiraFlow Extra Strength** (Ciba Vision)	**Solution:** 15.7% isopropyl alcohol, poloxamer 407, amphoteric 10	Preservative free. In 12 ml.
otc	**Opti-Clean** (Alcon)	**Solution:** Buffered, isotonic. Tween 21, hydroxyethylcellulose, polymeric cleaners, 0.004% thimerosal, 0.1% EDTA	In 12 and 20 ml.
otc	**Opti-Clean** II (Alcon)	**Solution:** Buffered, isotonic. Tween 21, polymeric cleaners, 0.1% EDTA, 0.001% polyquaternium-1	Thimerosal free. In 12 and 20 ml.
otc	**Resolve/GP** (Allergan)	**Solution:** Buffered. Cocoamphocarboxyglycinate, sodium lauryl sulfate, hexylene glycol, alkyl ether sulfate, fatty acid amide surfactants	Preservative free. In 30 ml.
otc	**Sereine** (Optikem)	**Solution:** Cocoamphodiacetate and glycols, 0.1% EDTA, 0.01% benzalkonium chloride	In 60 ml.

CLEANING AND SOAKING SOLUTIONS, HARD LENSES

otc	**Clean-N-Soak** (Allergan)	**Solution:** Buffered. Surfactant cleaning agent with 0.004% phenylmercuric nitrate	In 120 ml.

RIGID GAS PERMEABLE CONTACT LENS PRODUCTS

Refer to the general discussion of these products.

Actions:

Pharmacology:

Gas permeable hard lenses – Silicone/acrylate and fluoropolymers are used in rigid gas permeable (RGP) contact lenses. Lens care regimens include the use of a surfactant cleaner, enzyme cleaner and storage in a chemical disinfecting solution. Advise patients to follow the lens care protocol provided by the lens manufacturer or the instructions of their doctor.

DISINFECTING/WETTING/SOAKING SOLUTIONS, RGP LENSES

otc	**Boston Advance Comfort Formula** (Polymer Tech)	**Solution:** Buffered, slightly hypertonic. 0.00015% polyaminopropyl biguanide, 0.05% EDTA, cationic cellulose derivative polymer (wetting agent)	In 120 ml.
otc	**Boston Conditioning Solution** (Polymer Tech)	**Solution:** Buffered, slightly hypertonic, low viscosity. 0.05% EDTA, 0.006% chlorhexidine gluconate, cationic cellulose derivative polymer as wetting agent	In 120 ml.
otc	**Claris Rewetting Drops** (Allergan)	**Solution:** Buffered, isotonic. Hydroxyethyl cellulose, 0.006% polixetonium chloride (as preservative)	Thimerosal free. In ½ fl oz.
otc	**ComfortCare GP Wetting & Soaking** (Allergan)	**Solution:** Buffered, isotonic. 0.005% chlorhexidine gluconate, 0.02% EDTA, octylphenoxy (oxyethylene) ethanol, povidone, polyvinyl alcohol, propylene glycol, hydroxyethylcellulose, NaCl	In 120 and 240 ml.
otc	**Flex-Care Especially for Sensitive Eyes** (Alcon)	**Solution:** Buffered, isotonic. 0.1% EDTA, 0.005% chlorhexidine gluconate, NaCl, sodium borate, boric acid	Thimerosal free. In 118, 237 and 355 ml.
otc	**Wetting and Soaking Solution** (Bausch & Lomb)	**Solution:** Buffered, hypertonic. 0.006% chlorhexidine gluconate, 0.05% EDTA, cationic cellulose derivative polymer	Thimerosal free. In 118 ml.
otc	**Wet-N-Soak Plus** (Allergan)	**Solution:** Buffered, isotonic. 0.003% benzalkonium chloride, polyvinyl alcohol, EDTA	In 120 and 180 ml.

CLEANING SOLUTIONS, RGP LENSES

otc	**Boston Advance Cleaner** (Polymer Tech)	**Solution:** Concentrated homogenous surfactant. Alkyl ether sulfate, ethoxylated alkyl phenol, tri-quaternary cocoa-based phospholipid, silica gel	In 30 ml.
otc	**Boston Cleaner** (Polymer Tech)	**Solution:** Concentrated homogenous surfactant. Alkyl ether sulfate, silica gel, titanium dioxide	In 30 ml.
otc	**Claris Cleaning and Soaking Solution** (Allergan)	**Solution:** Lauryl sulfate salt of imidazoline, octylphenoxypolyethoxyethanol, 0.3% benzyl alcohol, 0.5% trisodium EDTA	Thimerosol free. In 4 fl oz.
otc	**Concentrated Cleaner** (Bausch & Lomb)	**Solution:** Surfactant solution with alkyl ether sulfate and silica gel	Preservative free. In 30 ml.
otc	**Gas Permeable Daily Cleaner** (Allergan)	**Solution:** 0.13% potassium sorbate, 2% EDTA, ethoxylated polyoxypropylene glycol, tris (hydroxymethyl) amino methane, hydroxyethylcellulose	Thimerosal free. In 30 ml.
otc	**LC-65** (Allergan)	**Solution:** Buffered cleaning agent. 0.001% thimerosal and EDTA	In 15 and 60 ml.

otc	**Opti-Clean** (Alcon)	**Solution:** Buffered, isotonic. 0.004% thimerosal, 0.1% EDTA, Tween 21, hydroxyethylcellulose, *Microclens* polymeric cleaners	In 12 and 20 ml.
otc	**Opti-Clean** II **Especially for Sensitive Eyes** (Alcon)	**Solution:** Buffered, isotonic. 0.1% EDTA, 0.001% polyquaternium-1, *Microclens* polymeric cleaners, Tween 21	Thimerosal free. In 12 and 20 ml.
otc	**Resolve/GP** (Allergan)	**Solution:** Buffered. Cocoamphocarboxyglycinate, sodium lauryl sulfate, hexylene glycol, alkyl ether sulfate, fatty acid amide surfactants	Preservative free. In 30 ml.

ENZYMATIC CLEANERS, RGP LENSES

otc	**Opti-Zyme Enzymatic Cleaner Especially for Sensitive Eyes** (Alcon)	**Tablets:** Highly purified pork pancreatin. *To make solution for soaking, dilute in preserved saline or sterile unpreserved saline solution*	Preservative free. In 8s, 24s, 36s and 56s.
otc	**ProFree/GP Weekly Enzymatic Cleaner** (Allergan)	**Tablets:** Papain, NaCl, sodium carbonate, sodium borate, EDTA	In 16s and 24s with vials.

REWETTING SOLUTIONS, RGP LENSES

otc	**Boston Rewetting Drops** (Polymer Tech)	**Solution:** Buffered, slightly hypertonic. 0.006% chlorhexidine gluconate, 0.05% EDTA, cationic cellulose derivative polymer as wetting agent	In 10 ml.
otc	**Wet-N-Soak** (Allergan)	**Solution:** Borate buffered, isotonic. 0.006% WSCP, hydroxyethylcellulose	In 15 ml.

SOFT (HYDROGEL) CONTACT LENS PRODUCTS

Refer to the general discussion of these products.

Warning:

Do NOT use conventional (hard) lens solutions on soft contact lenses. Use caution in product selection. Not all products are intended for use on all types of soft lenses.

Actions:

Pharmacology: Soft (hydrogel) contact lenses are made of hydrophilic polymers. Hydrogel lenses must be maintained in a hydrated state in physiological saline to prevent them from becoming brittle. Hydrogel lenses will absorb many substances; therefore, use only solutions specifically formulated for hydrogel lenses. In addition, these lenses must be disinfected either by heating in saline solution or by soaking in a chemical solution. Heating a lens in solutions used for chemical disinfection only may cause the lens to become opaque.

Soft lens solutions are especially formulated to be compatible with, and to meet the particular needs of, soft contact lenses. Of particular importance to soft lens care is the need for thorough cleaning to remove deposits which coat and may discolor the lens, especially when subjected to asepticizing by heating.

SURFACTANT CLEANING SOLUTIONS, SOFT CONTACT LENSES

Indications:

Cleaning solutions are used for daily prophylactic cleaning to prevent the accumulation of proteinaceous (mucus) deposits and to remove other debris.

otc	**Preflex Daily Cleaning Especially for Sensitive Eyes** (Alcon)	**Solution**: Buffered, isotonic. NaCl, sodium phosphates, tyloxapol, hydroxyethylcellulose, polyvinyl alcohol, EDTA, sorbic acid	In 30 ml.
otc	**DURAcare** II (Blairex)	**Solution**: Buffered, hypertonic. 0.1% sodium bisulfite, 0.1% sorbic acid, 0.25% EDTA, salt buffers, ethylene/propylene oxide, octylphenoxypolyethoxyethanol, lauryl sulfate salt of imidazoline	Thimerosal free. In 30 ml.
otc	**LC-65** (Allergan)	**Solution**: Buffered. 0.001% thimerosal, EDTA	In 15 and 60 ml.
otc	**Ciba Vision Cleaner for Sensitive Eyes** (Ciba Vision)	**Solution**: Cocoamphorcarboxyglycinate, sodium lauryl sulfate, hexylene glycol, 0.1% sorbic acid, 0.2% EDTA	In 15 ml.
otc	**Lens Plus Daily Cleaner** (Allergan)	**Solution**: Buffered. Cocoamphocarboxyglycinate, sodium lauryl sulfate, hexylene glycol, NaCl, sodium phosphate	Preservative free. In 15 and 30 ml.
otc	**MiraFlow Extra Strength** (Ciba Vision)	**Solution**: 15.7% isopropyl alcohol, poloxamer 407, amphoteric 10	Thimerosal free. In 12 and 20 ml.
otc	**Opti-Clean** (Alcon)	**Solution**: Buffered, isotonic. 0.004% thimerosal, 0.1% EDTA, Tween 21, hydroxyethylcellulose, *Microclens* polymeric cleaners	In 12 and 20 ml.
otc	**Opti-Clean** II (Alcon)	**Solution**: Buffered, isotonic. 0.1% EDTA, 0.001% polyquaternium-1, *Microclens* polymeric cleaners, Tween 21	Thimerosal free. In 12 and 20 ml.
otc	**Opti-Free** (Alcon)	**Solution**: Buffered, isotonic. 0.01% EDTA, 0.001% polyquaternium-1, *Microclens* polymeric cleaners, Tween 21	Thimerosal free. In 12 and 20 ml.
otc	**Pliagel** (Alcon)	**Solution**: 0.25% sorbic acid, 0.5% EDTA, NaCl, KCl, poloxamer 407	In 25 ml.
otc	**Sensitive Eyes Daily Cleaner** (Bausch & Lomb)	**Solution**: Buffered, isotonic. 0.25% sorbic acid, 0.5% EDTA, NaCl, hydroxypropyl methylcellulose, poloxamine, sodium borate	In 20 ml.
otc	**Sensitive Eyes Saline/ Cleaning** (Bausch & Lomb)	**Solution**: Buffered, isotonic. 0.15% sorbic acid, 0.1% EDTA, boric acid, poloxamine, sodium borate, NaCl	In 237 ml.
otc	**Soft Mate Hands Off Daily Cleaner** (PBH Wesley Jessen)	**Solution**: Isotonic. Octylphenoxy ethanol, hydroxyethylcellulose, NaCl, 0.13% potassium sorbate, 0.2% EDTA	In 240 ml.

RINSING/STORAGE SOLUTIONS, SOFT CONTACT LENSES

Use these solutions for rinsing and storage of hydrogel lenses in conjunction with heat disinfection. Prepared saline solutions may contain chelating agents (EDTA) which prevent calcium deposits from forming. Thimerosal-free preserved saline solutions may be used by patients sensitive to thimerosal or mercury-containing compounds. Preservative-free solutions are for patients intolerant to preservatives. Salt tablets are available to make saline solution; however, these solutions are nonsterile and contain no preservatives; use only with heat disinfection methods. Because cases of *Acanthamoeba* keratitis (a serious eye infection) have occurred in patients using homemade saline solutions, the use of salt tablets for soft contact lens storage/rinsing solution is not recommended.

Individual drug monographs are on the following pages.

PRESERVED SALINE SOLUTIONS, SOFT CONTACT LENSES

otc	**Hydrocare Preserved Saline** (Allergan)	**Solution:** Buffered, isotonic. 0.01% EDTA, 0.001% thimerosal, NaCl, sodium hexametaphosphate, boric acid, sodium borate	In 240 and 360 ml.
otc	**Opti-Soft** (Alcon)	**Solution:** Buffered, isotonic. 0.1% EDTA, 0.001% polyquaternium-1, NaCl, borate buffer system. For lenses with ≤ 45% water content.	Thimerosal free. In 355 ml.
otc	**ReNu** (Bausch & Lomb)	**Solution:** Buffered, isotonic. 0.00003% polyaminopropyl biguanide, NaCl, boric acid, EDTA	In 355 ml.
otc	**Saline** (Bausch & Lomb)	**Solution:** Buffered, isotonic. 0.001% thimerosal, boric acid, NaCl, EDTA	In 355 ml.
otc	**Sensitive Eyes** (Bausch & Lomb)	**Solution:** Buffered, isotonic. 0.1% sorbic acid, 0.025% EDTA, NaCl, boric acid, sodium borate	Thimerosal free. In 118, 237 and 355 ml.
otc	**Sensitive Eyes Plus** (Bausch & Lomb)	**Solution:** Boric acid, sodium borate, KCl, NaCl, 0.00003% polyaminopropyl biguanide, 0.025% EDTA	In 118 and 355 ml.
otc	**BarnesHind Saline for Sensitive Eyes** (PBH Wesley Jessen)	**Solution:** Isotonic. 0.13% potassium sorbate, 0.025% EDTA	In 360 ml (2s).
otc	**Your Choice Sterile Preserved Saline Solution** (Amcon)	**Solution:** Isotonic. 0.1% sorbic acid, boric buffer, EDTA, NaCl	In 60 and 360 ml.
otc	**Alcon Saline Especially for Sensitive Eyes** (Alcon)	**Solution:** Buffered, isotonic. NaCl, borate buffer system, sorbic acid, EDTA	Thimerosal free. In 360 ml.
otc	**SoftWear** (Ciba Vision)	**Solution:** Isotonic. NaCl, boric acid, sodium borate, sodium perborate (generating up to 0.006% hydrogen peroxide stabilized with phosphonic acid)	Thimerosal free. In 120, 240 and 360 ml.

PRESERVATIVE FREE SALINE SOLUTIONS, SOFT CONTACT LENSES

otc	**Blairex Sterile Saline** (Blairex)	**Solution:** Buffered, isotonic. NaCl, boric acid, sodium borate	In 90, 240 and 360 ml aerosol.
otc	**Unisol** (Alcon)		Thimerosal free. In 15 ml (25s) and 120 ml (2s, 3s).
otc	**Unisol 4** (Alcon)		Thimerosal free. In 120 ml.
otc	**Unisol Plus** (Alcon)		In 240 and 360 ml aerosol.
otc	**Your Choice Non-Preserved Saline Solution** (Amcon)		In 360 ml.
otc	**Ciba Vision Saline** (Ciba Vision)	**Solution:** Buffered, isotonic. NaCl, boric acid, sodium borate	In 240 and 360 ml aerosol.
otc	**Lens Plus Sterile Saline** (Allergan)	**Solution:** Buffered, isotonic. NaCl, boric acid, nitrogen	In 90, 240 and 360 ml aerosol.

otc	**Oxysept 2** (Allergan)	**Solution:** Buffered, isotonic. NaCl, catalytic neutralizing agent, EDTA, mono- and dibasic sodium phosphates	In 15 ml single-use containers (25s).

SALT TABLETS FOR NORMAL SALINE, SOFT CONTACT LENSES

Actions:

Pharmacology: Reconstitute tablets in container provided with distilled, deionized or purified water; do not use mineral or tap water. These solutions are not sterile and are intended only for use in conjunction with heat disinfection regimens. Use only as a rinse *prior* to heat disinfection and as storage *during* heat disinfection. Not for use as a rinse *after* disinfection (ie, before lens placement in the eye). Not for use in the eye. See Precautions in the Contact Lens Products monograph/introduction.

otc	**Marlin Salt System** (Marlin)	**Tablets:** 250 mg NaCl	In 200s with 27.7 ml bottle.

ENZYMATIC CLEANERS, SOFT CONTACT LENSES

Actions:

Pharmacology: Enzymatic cleaning, by soaking in a solution prepared from enzyme tablets, is recommended once weekly to remove protein and other lens deposits.

otc	**Allergan Enzymatic** (Allergan)	**Tablets:** Papain, NaCl, sodium carbonate, sodium borate, EDTA. *To make solution for soaking, dilute in sterile saline.*	In 12s, 24s, 36s and 48s.
otc	**Enzymatic Cleaner for Extended Wear** (Alcon)	**Tablets:** Highly purified pork pancreatin. *To make solution for soaking, dilute in preserved saline or sterile unpreserved saline.*	In 12s.
otc	**Opti-zyme Enzymatic Cleaner Especially for Sensitive Eyes** (Alcon)		Preservative free. In 8s, 24s, 36s and 56s.
otc	**Vision Care Enzymatic Cleaner** (Alcon)		In 24s.
otc	**Opti-Free** (Alcon)	**Tablets:** Highly purified pork pancreatin. *To make solution for soaking, dilute in* **Opti-Free** disinfecting solution.	In 10s, 20s and 30s.
otc	**ReNu Thermal Enzymatic Cleaner** (Bausch & Lomb)	**Tablets:** Subtilisin, sodium carbonate, NaCl, boric acid. *To make solution for heat disinfection directly in lens carrying case.*	In 16s.
otc	**Ultrazyme Enzymatic Cleaner** (Allergan)	**Tablets:** Effervescing, buffering and tableting agents. Subtilisin A. *To make solution for soaking, dilute in 3% hydrogen peroxide disinfecting solution.*	In 5s, 10s, 15s and 20s.
otc	**Complete Weekly Enzymatic Cleaner** (Allergan)	**Tablets:** Effervescing, buffering and tableting agents. Subtilisin A. *To make solution for soaking, dilute in sterile saline.*	In 8s.

otc	**Opti-Free Supra Clens** (Alcon)	**Solution**: Propylene glycol, sodium borate, highly purified porcine pancreatin enzymes	Preservative free. In 5 ml.[1]

[1] Developed for use with Opti-Free Rinsing, Disinfecting and Storage Solution and Opti-Free Express Multi-Purpose Solution. Its effectiveness has not been demonstrated with other products.

CHEMICAL DISINFECTION SYSTEMS

Actions:

Pharmacology: Two-solution systems use separate disinfecting and rinsing solutions. One-solution systems use the same solution for rinsing and storage.

Warnings:

Heat disinfection: Do NOT disinfect lenses by heating when using these solutions.

HYDROGEN PEROXIDE-CONTAINING SYSTEMS, SOFT LENSES

otc	**MiraSept** (Alcon)	**Disinfecting Solution**: 3% hydrogen peroxide, sodium stannate, sodium nitrate	In 120 ml.
		Rinse and Neutralizer: Isotonic. Boric acid, sodium borate, NaCl, sodium pyruvate, EDTA	In 120 ml (2s).
otc	**Oxysept** (Allergan)	**Disinfecting Solution**: 3% hydrogen peroxide, sodium stannate, sodium nitrate, phosphate buffer	In 240 and 360 ml.
		Neutralizer Tablets: Catalase, buffering agents	In 12s (with Oxy-Tab cup) and 36s.
otc	**Soft Mate Consept** (PBH Wesley Jessen)	**Consept 1 Cleaning and Disinfecting Solution**: 3% hydrogen peroxide, polyoxyl 40 stearate, sodium stannate, sodium nitrate, phosphate buffer	In 240 ml.
		Consept 2 Neutralizing and Rinsing Spray: Isotonic. 0.5% sodium thiosulfate, borate buffers	Aerosol. In 360 ml.
		Consept 2 Neutralizing and Rinsing Solution: Isotonic. 0.5% sodium thiosulfate, borate buffers, 0.001% chlorhexidine gluconate	In 360 ml.
otc	**Ultra-Care** (Allergan)	**Disinfecting Solution**: 3% hydrogen peroxide, sodium stannate, sodium nitrate, phosphate buffer	In 120 and 360 ml.
		Neutralizer Tablets: Catalase, hydroxypropyl methylcellulose, buffering agents	In 12s and 36s with cup.
otc	**AOSEPT** (Ciba Vision)	**Disinfecting Solution**: 3% hydrogen peroxide, 0.85% NaCl, phosphoric acid, phosphate buffers	In 120, 240 and 360 ml.
		AODISC Neutralizer: Platinum-coated tablet	Tablet good for 100 uses or 3 months of daily use.[1]

[1] For use only with the AOSEPT system.

NON-HYDROGEN PEROXIDE-CONTAINING SYSTEMS, SOFT LENSES

otc	**Complete All-in-One** (Allergan)	**Solution**: Buffered, isotonic. NaCl, 0.0001% polyhexamethylene biguanide, tromethamine, tyloxapol, EDTA	Thimerosal free. In 120 and 360 ml.
otc	**Disinfecting Solution** (Bausch & Lomb)	**Solution**: Buffered, isotonic. 0.005% chlorhexidine, 0.1% EDTA, 0.001% thimerosal, NaCl, sodium borate, boric acid	In 355 ml.
otc	**Flex-Care Especially for Sensitive Eyes** (Alcon)	**Solution**: Buffered, isotonic. 0.1% EDTA, 0.005% chlorhexidine gluconate, NaCl, sodium borate, boric acid	In 360 ml.
otc	**Hydrocare Cleaning and Disinfecting** (Allergan)	**Solution**: Buffered, isotonic. 0.002% thimerosal, Tris (2-hydroxyethyl) and bis (2-hydroxyethyl) tallow ammonium Cl, sodium bicarbonate, sodium phosphates, hydrochloric acid, propylene glycol, polysorbate 80, polyhema	In 240 and 360 ml.
otc	**Opti-Free** (Alcon)	**Solution**: Isotonic. 0.05% EDTA, 0.001% polyquaternium-1, citrate buffer, NaCl	Thimerosal free. In 118, 237 and 355 ml.
otc	**Opti-Free Express Multipurpose Solution** (Alcon)	**Solution**: Buffered, isotonic. 0.05% EDTA, sodium citrate, NaCl, 0.001% polyquaternium as preservative	In 118 and 355 ml.
otc	**Opti-One** (Alcon)	**Solution**: Buffered, isotonic. 0.05% EDTA, 0.001% polyquaternium-1, sodium citrate, NaCl	In 120 ml.
otc	**Quick CARE** (Ciba Vision)	**Disinfecting Solution**: Isopropanol, NaCl, polyoxypropylenepolyoxyethylene block copolymer, disodium lauroamphodiacetate	In 15 ml.
		Rinse and Neutralizer: Isotonic. Sodium borate, boric acid, sodium perborate (generating up to 0.006% hydrogen peroxide), phosphonic acid	In 360 ml.
otc	**ReNu Multi-Purpose** (Bausch & Lomb)	**Solution**: Isotonic. 0.00005% polyaminopropyl biguanide, 0.01% EDTA, NaCl, sodium borate, boric acid, poloxamine	In 118, 237 and 355 ml.
otc	**Soft Mate Disinfecting for Sensitive Eyes** (PBH Wesley Jessen)	**Solution**: Isotonic. 0.1% EDTA, 0.005% chlorhexidine gluconate, NaCl, povidone, octylphenoxy (oxyethylene) ethanol, borate buffer	Thimerosal free. In 240 ml.
otc	**SOLO-care Multi-Purpose Solution** (Ciba Vision)	**Solution**: Isotonic. NaCl, polyoxyethylene polyoxpropylene block copolymer, sodium phosphate dibasic, sodium phosphate monobasic, 0.025% edetate disodium dihydrate, 0.0001% polyhexanide.	Thimerosal free. In 118 ml and 355 ml.

REWETTING SOLUTIONS, SOFT CONTACT LENSES

otc	**Adapettes Especially For Sensitive Eyes** (Alcon)	**Solution:** Buffered, isotonic. Povidone and other water-soluble polymers, sorbic acid, EDTA	Thimerosal free. In 15 ml.

otc	**Blairex Lens Lubricant** (Blairex)	**Solution**: Isotonic. 0.25% sorbic acid, 0.1% EDTA, borate buffer, NaCl, hydroxypropyl methylcellulose, glycerin	Thimerosal free. In 15 ml.
otc	**Clerz 2** (Alcon)	**Solution**: Isotonic. NaCl, KCl, hydroxyethylcellulose, poloxamer 407, sodium borate, boric acid, sorbic acid, EDTA	Thimerosal free. In 5 (2s), 15 and 30 ml.
otc	**Lens Lubricant** (Bausch & Lomb)	**Solution**: Buffered, isotonic. 0.004% thimerosal, 0.1% EDTA, povidone, polyoxyethylene	In 15 ml.
otc	**Lens Plus Rewetting Drops** (Allergan)	**Solution**: Buffered, isotonic. NaCl, boric acid	Preservative free. In 0.35 ml (30s).
otc	**Opti-Tears** (Alcon)	**Solution**: Isotonic. 0.1% EDTA, 0.001% polyquaternium-1, dextran, NaCl, KCl, hydroxypropyl methylcellulose	Thimerosal free. In 15 ml.
otc	**Opti-Free** (Alcon)	**Solution**: Isotonic. Citrate buffer, NaCl, 0.05% EDTA, 0.001% polyquaternium-1	In 10 and 20 ml.
otc	**Opti-One** (Alcon)		In 10 ml.
otc	**Sensitive Eyes Drops** (Bausch & Lomb)	**Solution**: Buffered. 0.1% sorbic acid, 0.025% EDTA, NaCl, boric acid, sodium borate	In 30 ml.
otc	**Soft Mate Comfort Drops** (PBH Wesley Jessen)	**Solution**: Borate buffered. 0.13% potassium sorbate, 0.1% EDTA, NaCl, hydroxyethylcellulose, octylphenoxy-ethanol	In 15 ml.
otc	**Lens Drops** (Ciba Vision)	**Solution**: Buffered, isotonic. NaCl, borate buffer, poloxamer 407, 0.2% EDTA, 0.15% sorbic acid, carbamide	In 15 ml.
otc	**Complete** (Allergan)	**Solution**: Buffered, isotonic. NaCl, 0.0001% polyhexamethylene biguanide, tromethamine, tyloxapol, EDTA	In 15 ml.

ODF

14

EXTEMPORANEOUS PREPARATIONS

Extemporaneous compounding of ophthalmic solutions may include the preparation of topical, periocular or intraocular injections. Many topical ophthalmic solutions or suspensions are commercially available. However, certain topical ophthalmic solutions and all periocular and intraocular solutions are neither FDA-approved nor commercially available for ophthalmic administration. When these preparations are required, injectable sources are frequently used. In many cases, this may be limited to dilution of injectable products or the addition of injectable products to commercial ophthalmic preparations to increase their concentration, or "fortify" them. These extemporaneously prepared products are considered the community standard based upon clinical research and ethical practice, and as such, may be required to effectively treat a patient with ophthalmic conditions.[1–2] Considerations for ophthalmic compounding must include topical (usually topical solutions), periocular (subconjunctival or sub-Tenon's; retrobulbar) or intraocular (intravitreal or intracameral) products.

GUIDELINES

Requirements for the preparation of topical ophthalmic preparations are published in the United States Pharmacopoeia.[3] The USP guidelines describe the requirements for the preparation of ophthalmic ointments, solutions, suspensions and strips. Isotonicity, buffering, sterilization, preservation and thickening agents are specifically addressed.

Because of concerns for possible eye infections, guidelines for the preparation of all sterile ophthalmic products were published by the American Society of Health-Systems Pharmacists (ASHP).[4] These guidelines state that all extemporaneous ophthalmic products be prepared in an approved and certified laminar airflow or biohazard hood. Proper aseptic technique is essential, as is required for any sterile product. Accuracy is stressed to prevent any miscalculation, especially a concern with preparation of intravitreal injections. The use of a 5 micron filter is recommended when a drug is reconstituted or if it is supplied in a glass ampule. When a drug product is not available in a sterile dosage form, a 0.22 micron filter should be used. The use of a preservative-free product is recommended when feasible. Such guidelines are particularly helpful for healthcare personnel who are not familiar with preparing ophthalmic extemporaneous products. Information on more than 50 ophthalmic medications including topical, subconjunctival and intraocular formulations, is available in a "cookbook" format by Reynolds.[5] The uses, concentrations, dosing and references also are included.

References found in the literature for the ocular administration of non-commercial ophthalmic products (eg, acetylcysteine, ceftazidime, disodium EDTA) only provide some assurance that the medication is tolerated in the eye without obvious ocular side effects. Most of these references do not contain which vehicles were used, expirations or other essential information required to properly prepare the product.

STABILITY

Stability data must be based upon concerns for maintaining sterility rather than just the stability of the product itself. Obviously, if sterility cannot be maintained, then stability of the product is secondary. There is little published information available on stability dating of extemporaneously prepared topical ophthalmic solutions. Many institutions have extrapolated from published intravenous product stability, even though this may not always be appropriate. Gentamicin and tobramycin fortified ophthalmic solutions are stable at 4° to 8°C for 3 months.[6] The stability of several antibiotics, including vancomycin, gentamicin, bacitracin and cephalothin, in commercially available 0.5% hydroxypropyl methylcellulose artificial tear solution,[7] demonstrated no significant loss of potency at room temperature for 7 days. However, the use of different vehicles, antibiotic concentrations, storage conditions, etc may influence product stability. Frozen and refrigerated stability may be useful if multiple bottles are prepared. Stability must be established if the product is dispensed for outpatient use or if it is utilized in a hospital setting. Extemporaneously prepared ophthalmic solutions should be refrigerated after dispensing to reduce the risk of microbial growth or to ensure minimal loss of potency. A 7 day in-use storage life is acceptable for unpreserved eye drops containing alkaloids or antibiotics if they are stored in the refrigerator after opening.[8]

The stability of periocular or intraocular preparations is usually restricted to 6 to 24 hours expirations because information is limited and these expiration times are commonly used for other extemporaneously prepared injectable products.

Stability and sterility appear to be maintained with some preparations that are aseptically prepared, sealed and frozen. Frozen stability of products such as periocular mitomycin,[9] intraocular ganciclovir[10] and topical cefazolin[11] and vancomycin[11] has provided extended dating for these products.

STERILITY

Sterility must be maintained with any extemporaneously prepared ophthalmic product. The USP and ASHP recommend that sterile membrane filtration (0.22 micron filter) be utilized under aseptic conditions whenever possible.[3-4] Many institutions prepare extemporaneous ophthalmic products and employ a 0.22 micron filter for the final step to ensure sterilization. Some medications should not be filtered with a 0.22 micron filter. Amphotericin B, a colloidal suspension, should be filtered with nothing smaller than a 5 micron filter to prevent loss of drug. Suspensions and other formulations such as liposomal products should be researched to determine if membrane filtration is acceptable.

PH/BUFFERING

The pH of an extemporaneously prepared topical ophthalmic product is most often considered because of the concern for ocular irritation associated with eyedrops. The eye can tolerate a rather wide range of pH (between 3.5 and 10) for a single drop administration. If the pH is too high or too low, reflex tearing will dilute the drug concentration more quickly than if the pH is in the physiologic range of 7.4 for lacrimal fluid. Some medications require lower pH values to maintain longer shelf lives since they may be chemically unstable at higher pH levels. Buffering systems are not commonly employed in the current practice of preparing extemporaneous ophthalmic preprations. It is important that if a buffer system is used, that it is chosen close to pH 7.4, but does not hasten deterioration or precipitation of the drug.[3]

The pH of the eyedrop may influence absorption of a drug into the intraocular fluids and tissues. Generally, the unionized form of a drug will penetrate the lipophilic corneal epithelium, the first significant barrier to intraocular penetration, better than will a hydrophilic form. The cornea contains tight epithelial and endothelial cell junctions that slow or prevent the passage of a drug through the cornea. A drug must penetrate the three layers of the cornea, including the epithelium (lipophilic barrier), stroma (water soluble) and endothelium (lipid soluble). Increasing the pH of a solution increases the amount of the unionized form, thereby increasing initial epithelial penetration of the drug.

ISOTONICITY

Isotonicity is not essential even for topical ophthalmic solutions. An acceptable range is from 0.7% to 2.0% (0.9% sodium chloride is considered isotonic). In fact, some ophthalmic products are produced as hypertonic (sodium chloride 5%) or hypotonic (*Hypotears*) solutions for their desired pharmacologic effects.

VEHICLES

Vehicles utilized for topical ophthalmic solutions vary and are usually either normal saline, water, various biocompatible polymers used in artifical tears or occasionally balanced salt solution. Artificial tear polymer may provide comfort, prolonged contact time with the eye, the presence of a preservative system and a neutral pH. However, potential problems include incompatibilities between the active or inactive ingredients, and a reduction in preservative effectiveness caused by dilution from the active drug. Some of the artificial tear preparations contain methylcellulose, which is an acceptable thickening agent to increase the viscosity and contact time of the ophthalmic solution.[3] Sterile water or normal saline is often used, but they contain no preservatives. The concern for potential contamination associated with the repeated administration of unpreserved solutions must be considered. If the active component has an initial low pH, the lower pH of water and normal saline may further contribute to irritation of the ophthalmic solution. Balanced salt solutions (bss) contain no preservatives, and potential incompatibilities with the various components of the bss should be considered.

Intraocular or periocular preparations most often use sterile water or normal saline as the preferred diluent. Caution must be used if balanced salt solutions are employed as vehicles because potential incompatibilities, especially with magnesium and calcium salts, may exist with the active ingredient or its inactive components. Balanced salt solution should not be used as a diluent for cromolyn sodium or tissue plasminogen activator.[5,12]

TOPICAL PREPARATIONS

Topical forms of administration include drops, ointments, gels, contact lenses and collagen shields. The most common extemporaneously prepared product is the topical ophthalmic solution. Topical formulations provide the drug to the site of action and therefore reduce the risk of systemic side effects, but do not totally alleviate them.

Extemporaneously prepared topical eye solutions are prepared most often in the treatment of bacterial keratitis. Until the recent approval of the fluoroquinolone antibiotics ciprofloxacin and ofloxacin for bacterial keratitis, standard regimens consisted of an alternating aminoglycoside (usually gentamicin or tobramycin fortified solutions) with a cephalosporin, most often cefazolin.[1,2,13-14] Some of the most common concentrations of antibiotic drops are gentamicin 13.6 mg/ml, tobramycin 13.6 mg/ml, cefazolin 50 mg/ml and vancomycin 50 mg/ml.[15]

The aminoglycoside products (usually gentamicin or tobramycin) are fortified to a concentration of 9 to 14 mg/ml from the commerically available strength of 3 mg/ml. An injectable form of the active drug is added under aseptic conditions, in a lamellar flow hood, to an ophthalmic dropper bottle to "fortify" the commercial strength. Cefazolin ophthalmic solution (25 to 100 mg/ml) is made from the injectable product and is reconstituted in water and further diluted in water, normal saline or artificial tear solution.

Polyhexamethylene biguanide (PHMB 20%) is an environmental biocide for swimming pools. PHMB 0.02% is useful in *Acanthamoeba* keratitis as an extemporaneously prepared topical ophthalmic product.[17] Because the initial concentration is 20%, an intermediate dilution is suggested to ensure an accurate final concentration of 0.02%, since this is a 1000 fold difference.[16]

Ophthalmic ointments usually consist of a petrolatum and mineral oil base (added to reduce the temperature at which the ointment melts). Some ointments contain lanolin (emulsifier to incorporate water-soluble drugs into the ointment). Allergies to ophthalmic ointments are most often related to the incorporated lanolin. Most drugs are very stable in ointments and do not ionize. Ophthalmic ointments provide longer ocular contact time and comfort. However, contact time may not increase bioavailability since only the drug at the ointment-tear interface will be absorbed. Ointments also are associated with blurred vision and provide poor patient acceptance. Although ointments occasionally are extemporaneously prepared, this is uncommon because of the time required to prepare them, the rare instances of a clinical indication and the special ophthalmic ointment tubes are required.

Antibiotic-soaked collagen shields provide for prolonged topical drug levels. However, potential drug incompatibility problems, loss of the shield from the eye, requirements for rehydration with the antibiotic and cost have limited their use.

PERIOCULAR

Periocular administration includes injections below the conjunctiva or Tenon's capsule. They are given either to prolong administration or to increase penetration of the drug into the eye. Advantages include increased local concentration of the drug, thereby avoiding potential systemic toxicity, and higher intraocular tissue concentrations. Because no FDA-approved formulations are available for periocular administration, injectable preparations are often used. In many cases, the concentration required is drawn directly from a commercial strength vial. An example of this is gentamicin, which is given in a safe subconjunctival dose of 20 mg per 0.5 ml. Direct use from the vial, or sometimes after a single dilution, is often employed with antibiotics, anesthetics and corticosteroid preparations for use as subconjunctival or sub-Tenon's injections. A common peribulbar or retrobulbar anesthetic combination utilizes a 50:50 mixture of lidocaine and bupivacaine, often supplemented with hyaluronidase for increased tissue penetration.

INTRAOCULAR

Intraocular injections are often used in serious eye infections and inflammatory conditions such as endophthalmitis, retinal necrosis, and cytomegalovirus retinitis. Intraocular injections provide immediate therapeutic drug levels. It is essential to ensure that the correct dose is prepared to prevent retinal toxicity. The half-life of the drug in the vitreous cavity is a consideration especially if reinjection may be required. The volume of drug administered is usually in the 0.05 to 0.1 ml range. Proper injection technique is critical to prevent damage to any intraocular structures. Commonly used intraocular medications include vancomycin, ceftazidime, amikacin, ganciclovir, foscarnet, dexamethasone and amphotericin B.[1,5]

Intraocular doses are often in the microgram to milligram range. The proper dose must be established before the medication is prepared. In some instances, multiple dilutions are required to obtain an accurate concentration for intravitreal injection. Amphotericin B is administered as a 5 microgram injection and must be prepared from a commercial vial of 50 milligrams.[5] Amikacin is administered in a 400 mcg dose or less and must be diluted from a 500 mg or 100 mg (pediatric) vial.[5] Vancomycin is injected intravitreally in a dose of 1 mg after being diluted from a vial containing 500 mg. These concentrations may reflect a 10 or even 1000 fold dilution from the commercial strength product. Careful calculation and validation from others is appropriate. Syringes must be able to precisely measure low concentrations. An adequate initial volume must be drawn up so that a reasonable volume can be transferred for further dilution.[4,5] To ensure no loss of drug in the needle hub of a tuberculin syringe, it is more accurate to deliver 0.3 ml from the 0.6 ml to 0.3 ml gradations on the syringe barrel than from the 0.3 mark to zero. To prevent any miscalculation, no air bubbles should be left in the syringe or needle when preparing the injection. It is prudent to add both drug and diluent to a single sterile vial to prevent any misclaculation in volume.[5] A larger volume of the final concentration of drug should be dispensed (eg, draw up 0.4 ml of a 1 mg/0.1 ml vancomycin) and labeled appropriately. The larger volume will allow for easy transfer of the final concentration of drug to another syringe, should this be required.

Richard G. Fiscella, RPh, MPH
University of Illinois

For More Information

1. Glasser DB and Baum J. Antibacterial Agents in Infections of the Eye, 2nd ed. Tabbara KF and Hyndiuk RA. Eds. Little, Brown and Company, Boston MA. 1996;207-31.

2. Liesegang TJ. Bacterial keratitis. *Infec Dis Clin NA* 1992;6:815-30.

3. United States Pharmacopoeia XXIII 1995;1945-46.

4. Reynolds LA. Guidelines for the preparation of sterile ophthalmic products. *Am J Hosp Pharm* 1991;48:2438-39.

5. Reynolds LA, Closson RG, eds. Extemporaneous Ophthalmic Preparations. Vancouver: Applied Therapeutics, Inc. 1993.

6. McBride HA, Martinez DR, Trnag JM et al. Stability of gentamicin sulfate and tobramycin sulfate in extemporaneously prepared ophthalmic solutions at 8°C. *Am J Hosp Pharm* 1991;48:507-9.

7. Osborn E, Baum JL, et al. The stability of ten antibiotics in artificial tear solutions. *Am J Ophthalmol* 1976;82:775-80.

8. Oldham GB, Andrews V. The control of microbial contamination in unpreserved eye drops. (in press BJO 1996).

9. Fiscella RG, Proffitt DF, and Weisbecker CA. Stability of mitomycin for ophthalmic use. *Am J Hosp Pharm* 1992;49:2440.

10. Fiscella RG, Aramwit P. Ganciclovir for intravitreal injection. *Am J Health-Syst Pharm* 1995;52:422.

11. Trissel LA. Handbook on Injectable Drugs 8th ed. American Society of Hospital Pharmacists Incorporated 1994.

12. Ward C and Weck S. Dilution and storage of recombinant tissue plasminogen activator (Activase) in balanced salt solutions. *Am J Ophthalmol* 1990;109:98-99.

13. Parks DJ, Abrams DA, et al. Comparison of topical ciprofloxacin to conventional antibiotic therapy in the treatment of ulcerative keratitis. *Am J Ophthalmol* 1993;115:471-77.

14. O'Brien TP, Maguire MG, et al. Efficacy of ofloxacin vs cefazolin and tobramycin in the therapy for bacterial keratitis. *Arch Ophthalmol* 1995;113:1257-65.

15. Fiscella RG. Extemporaneously compounded ophthalmic antibiotic solutions: survey of usage and costs and pharmacotherapeutic considerations. (submitted to AJHP).

16. Yee E, Fiscella RG, and Winarko TK. Topical polyhexamethylene biguanide (pool cleaner) for treatment of *Ananthamoeba* keratitis. *Am J Hosp Pharm* 1993;50:2522-23.

OCULAR DOSAGE FORM *Drug Class*	**Commercial Strength**	**Ophthalmic Strength**	**Dilution Directions**	**Special Instructions**	**Comments**
TOPICAL					
Antibiotics					
Gentamicin (or Tobramycin)	40 mg/ml (injection) & 3 mg/ml (ophth soln)	9-14 mg/ml	Add 2 ml of injectable to 5 ml bottle (7 ml or 13.6 mg/ml)		Use same bottle eyedrops came in
Cefazolin	1 gram (vial-recon)	25-100 mg/ml	Recon vial with 3 ml water, qs to 10 ml with water - transfer to ophthalmic bottle	Artificial tear used to qs	Frozen stability appears to be good for at least 28 days - concerns are to ensure sterility when frozen
Vancomycin	0.5 gram (vial-recon)	25-50 mg/ml	Recon with 10 ml sterile water, transfer to ophthalmic bottle		Frozen stability good for 28 days Must ensure sterility when frozen Unbuffered pH is in 4 to 4.5 range
Other					
PHMB	20% solution	0.02%	Dilution with sterile water is best	First dilute an intermediate solution of *0.5% PHMB* then further dilute to 0.02% with sterile water	Stability is very good - 30 days Intermediate dilution is more accurate
PERIOCULAR					
Antibiotics					
Gentamicin	40 mg/ml vial	20 mg/0.5 ml	No dilution required		
Cefazolin	1 gram vial (recon)	100 mg/ 0.5 ml	Recon with sterile water		
Corticosteroids					
Dexamethasone	4 mg/ml or 10 mg/ml	2 mg/0.5 ml 5 mg/0.5 ml	No dilution required	Given sub-conjunctivally	Short half life 24 to 48 hours
Triamcinolone acetonide	40 mg/ml	20 mg/0.5 ml	No dilution required	Given sub-Tenon's	Long half life - may last weeks to months
Antimetabolites					
Mitomycin	5 mg vial (recon)	0.2-0.4 mg/ml	Dilute with sterile water	Solution soaked into sponge	Frozen stability in 0.2-0.4 mg range is good for 60 days[9]
INTRAOCULAR					
Antibiotics					
Vancomycin	500 mg (recon)	1 mg/0.05-0.1 ml	Recon with 10 ml normal saline	Take 2 ml of reconstituted solution add sterile vial; add 8 ml of sterile water (final conc. = 1 mg/0.1 ml)	Double check dilution; filter

OCULAR DOSAGE FORM *Drug Class*	Commercial Strength	Ophthalmic Strength	Dilution Directions	Special Instructions	Comments
Amikacin	100 mg/2 ml vial	400 mcg/0.05-0.1 ml	Dilute with sterile normal saline (NS)	Take 1 ml of amikacin, add 11.5 ml saline in vial (final conc. = 400 mcg/0.1 ml)	Double check dilution
Ceftazidime	1 g vial (recon)	2 mg/0.05-0.1 ml	Dilute with sterile water	Add 9.4 ml of water to 1 g ceftazidime vial. Transfer 2 ml of solution to vial, add 8 ml of NS (final conc. = 2 mg/0.1 ml)	Double check dilution
Antivirals					
Ganciclovir	500 mg vial (recon)	200-2000 mcg/0.05-0.1 ml	Dilute with sterile water	Recon with 2.5 ml NS; transfer 0.1 ml to sterile vial, add 9.9 ml NS *(final conc. = 200 mcg/0.1 ml)* or transfer 1 ml and add 9 ml NS *(final conc. = 2000 mcg/0.1 ml)*	Refrigerate for storage
Foscarnet	Solution 24 mg/ml	1200-2400 mcg/0.05-0.1 ml	Use directly from vial		
Others					
Tissue plasminogen activator (tPA) (alteplase)	20 mg vial	6.25-25 mcg/0.1 ml	Dilute 20 mg vial with 20 ml sterile water as per directions; further dilute 1 ml of above with 3 ml of NS (250 mcg/ml)		Frozen stability good for at least 1 year

ODF

15

Systemic Drugs Affecting the Eye

The eye, due to its rich blood supply, multiple tissue types and relatively small size, is highly susceptible to toxic substances. Many systemically administered drugs have the potential to cause adverse ocular effects, and nearly all ocular structures are vulnerable. This section considers the most common drugs that are documented to cause ocular toxicity, summarizing the salient features of the ocular effects.

DRUGS AFFECTING THE CORNEA AND LENS

Antimalarial Drugs

Quinacrine, chloroquine and hydroxychloroquine can cause changes in the cornea. In the early stages, diffuse punctate deposits appear in the corneal epithelium, and later the deposits aggregate into curved lines that converge and coalesce just below the central cornea. These opacities take on a whorl-like configuration. Less than half of patients affected by corneal changes have visual symptoms consisting of halos around lights, glare and photophobia. Visual acuity usually remains unchanged. Once drug therapy is discontinued, both subjective symptoms and objective corneal signs disappear.

Chlorpromazine

Chlorpromazine is the only phenothiazine to cause changes in the cornea and lens. Lenticular pigmentation can vary from fine, dot-like opacities on the anterior lens surface to a central, lightly pigmented, pearl-like, opaque mass surrounded by smaller clumps of pigment. Corneal pigmentary changes occur almost invariably only in patients who have concomitant lens opacities. Corneal pigmentation occurs at the level of the endothelium and Descemet's membrane primarily in the interpalpebral fissure area. These ocular changes rarely reduce visual acuity, but patients may occasionally report glare, halos around lights or hazy vision. The pigmentary deposits are generally irreversible even when drug therapy is reduced or discontinued.

Systemic Drugs Affecting The Eye		
Systemic Drug	**Examples**	**Structure/Function Affected**
Alcohol	alcohol	Extraocular muscles
Amiodarone	*Cordarone*	Cornea and lens
Antianxiety Agents	chlordiazepoxide (eg, *Librium*)	Extraocular muscles Causes cycloplegia
Anticholinergics	atropine scopolamine	Tear secretion Pupil (mydriasis) Causes cycloplegia
Antidepressants	amitriptyline (eg, *Elavil*)	Extraocular muscles Causes cycloplegia
Antihistamines	chlorpheniramine (eg, *Chlor-Trimeton*) diphenhydramine (eg, *Benadryl*)	Tear secretion Extraocular muscles Pupil (mydriasis) Causes cycloplegia
Antimalarials	chloroquine (eg, *Aralen Phosphate*) hydroxy-chloroquine (eg, *Plaquenil Sulfate*) quinacrine (eg, *Atabrine HCl*)	Cornea, lids, retina
Barbiturates	phenobarbital	Extraocular muscles
β-blockers	atenolol (eg, *Tenormin*)	Tear secretion Reduces intraocular pressure
Carbonic Anhydrase Inhibitors	acetazolamide (eg, *Diamox*)	Causes myopia
Central Nervous System Stimulants	amphetamines (eg, *Dexedrine*), cocaine, methylphenidate (eg, *Ritalin*)	Pupil (mydriasis) Lowers intraocular pressure
Chloramphenicol	*Chloromycetin*	Optic nerve
Chlorpromazine	*Thorazine*	Cornea and lens, lids Extraocular muscles
Cocaine	crack cocaine	Cornea and conjunctiva
Corticosteroids	prednisone cortisol	Lens Elevates intraocular pressure
Digitalis Glycosides	digoxin (eg, *Lanoxin*)	Retina
Diuretics	hydrochlorothiazide (eg, *HydroDIURIL*)	Causes myopia
Ethambutol	*Myambutol*	Optic nerve
Gold Salts	auranofin (*Ridaura*) gold sodium thiomalate (*Aurolate*)	Cornea and lens Conjunctiva and lids Extraocular muscles
Indomethacin	*Indocin*	Cornea, retina
Isotretinoin	*Accutane*	Conjunctiva and lids Tear secretion Retina
Opiates	morphine, codeine, heroin	Pupil (miosis)
Phenytoin	*Dilantin*	Extraocular muscles
Psoralens	methoxsalen (*Oxsoralen*)	Cornea and lens
Quinine	*Quinamm*	Retina
Salicylates	aspirin (eg, *Bayer*)	Extraocular muscles
Sulfonamides	sulfisoxazole (*Gantrisin*)	Causes myopia
Tamoxifen	*Nolvadex*	Retina
Tetracycline	*Sumycin*	Conjunctiva and lens
Thioridazine	*Mellaril*	Retina

Indomethacin

The incidence of corneal toxicity associated with indomethacin therapy is 11% to 16%. The corneal lesions appear either as fine stromal, speckled opacities or have a whorl-like distribution resembling that of chloroquine keratopathy. These changes diminish or disappear within 6 months after discontinuing indomethacin. No definite relationship has been established between dosage of drug and corneal changes.

Photosensitizing Drugs

Photosensitizing drugs are compounds that absorb optical radiation and undergo a photochemical reaction, resulting in chemical modifications of tissue. The psoralen compounds are classic examples of photosensitizing drugs and are widely used by dermatologists to treat psoriasis and vitiligo. This treatment, commonly referred to as PUVA therapy, involves administering methoxsalen (*Oxsoralen*) or related compounds, followed by exposure to UV radiation. Cataract formation is well documented in patients undergoing PUVA therapy.

Gold Salts

Following prolonged administration, gold salts can be deposited in various tissues of the body, a condition known as chrysiasis. Ocular chrysiasis can involve the conjunctiva, cornea and lens. Corneal chrysiasis consists of numerous gold deposits that appear as yellowish-brown, violet or red particles distributed irregularly in the stroma. The deposition of gold usually spares the peripheral 1 to 3 mm and superior ¼ to ½ of the cornea, and the deposits tend to localize to the posterior stroma. Lenticular chrysiasis appears as fine dust-like, yellowish, glistening deposits in the anterior capsule or anterior subcapsular region.

Corticosteroids

Systemic steroids can produce posterior subcapsular (PSC) cataracts that are clinically indistinguishable from complicated cataracts and cataracts caused by exposure to ionizing radiation. They often cannot be distinguished from age-related PSC cataracts. Even if the steroid dosage is reduced or discontinued, the cataract usually remains unchanged. Visual impairment is rare in patients with steroid-induced PSC cataracts. Most patients retain visual acuity of 20/40 or better, but patients may report light sensitivity, frank photophobia, reading difficulty or glare.

Amiodarone

Amiodarone causes a distinctive keratopathy early in the course of treatment. The onset may be as early as 6 days following initiation of treatment, but it more commonly appears after 1 to 3 months of therapy. Virtually all patients will demonstrate corneal changes after 3 months of treatment. The corneal deposits are bilateral and are initially similar to the horizontal configuration of a Hudson-Stahli line, but eventually assume the configuration of a whorl-like opacity in the corneal epithelium. Once amiodarone therapy is discontinued, the keratopathy gradually resolves within 6 to 18 months. Lenticular opacities generally cause no visual symptoms, but moderate to severe keratopathy can lead to complaints of blurred vision, glare and halos around lights or light sensitivity. Visual acuity is usually normal.

DRUGS AFFECTING THE CONJUNCTIVA AND LIDS

Isotretinoin

Ocular complications of isotretinoin (*Accutane*) include blepharoconjunctivitis, dry eye symptoms, contact lens intolerance and subepithelial corneal opacities. There appears to be a dose-dependent relationship between isotretinoin therapy and blepharoconjunctivitis.

Chlorpromazine

Discoloration of the conjunctiva, sclera and exposed skin has been reported with phenothiazine therapy. The discoloration is usually slate blue. Melanin-like granules have been observed in the superficial dermis.

Tetracyclines

Conjunctival deposits similar to those seen in epinephrine-treated glaucoma patients have been reported in patients treated with oral tetracycline. These deposits appear as dark-brown to black granules in the palpebral conjunctiva. When observed under ultraviolet light, the brown pigment concentrations give a yellow fluorescence characteristic of tetracycline.

DRUGS THAT DECREASE AQUEOUS TEAR SECRETION

Anticholinergics

Dryness of mucous membranes is a common side effect of anticholinergic drugs since atropine and related agents inhibit glandular secretion in a dose-dependent manner.

Antihistamines

H_1 antihistamines have varying degrees of atropine-like actions including the ability to alter tear film integrity. Both aqueous and mucin production may decrease with use of systemic antihistamines.

Isotretinoin

Dry eye symptoms are commonly reported with use of isotretinoin. The incidence has been estimated to be as high as 20%, and about 8% of patients experience contact lens intolerance.

Beta Blockers

Reduced tear secretion is a reported side effect of oral β-blockers. Most of the reported cases have occurred with practolol (not available in the US), but other β-blockers have also been implicated in patients with dry eye syndrome.

DRUGS CAUSING MYDRIASIS

The iris is an excellent indicator of autonomic activity because of the delicate balance between adrenergic and cholinergic innervation to the iris dilator and sphincter muscles, respectively. Adrenergic and cholinergic agents can thus easily influence pupil size and activity.

Anticholinergics

Drugs with pronounced anticholinergic action, such as *atropine* or related compounds, can cause significant mydriasis. Systemic administration of at least 2 mg of atropine can cause pupillary dilation and cycloplegia. Both mydriasis and reduced pupillary light response can occur when transdermal scopolamine (*Transderm Scop*) is used for 3 or more days. This usually occurs through direct contamination of the eye by rubbing with fingers following application of the patch.

Central Nervous System Stimulants

Central nervous system stimulants, such as *amphetamines, methylphenidate* and *cocaine*, can cause mydriasis. Likewise, central nervous system depressants, such as *phenobarbital* and antianxiety agents, can dilate the pupil through their action on the adrenergic division of the autonomic nervous system.

DRUGS CAUSING MIOSIS

Opiates (eg, heroin, morphine, codeine) characteristically constrict the pupil. Systemically administered *anticholinesterase agents* can also cause miosis.

DRUGS AFFECTING EXTRAOCULAR MUSCLES

Drugs affecting the autonomic nervous system, central vestibular system, or causing extrapyramidal effects may cause nystagmus, diplopia, extraocular muscle palsy or oculogyric crisis. Nystagmus can be caused by intoxication with *salicylates, phenytoin, antihistamines, gold salts* and *barbiturates*. Diplopia has been associated with the *phenothiazines, antianxiety agents* and *antidepressants*. *Alcohol* can impair both smooth pursuits and saccades.

DRUGS CAUSING MYOPIA

Systemically administered *sulfonamides* can induce transient myopia. The myopia is acute in onset and subsides within days or weeks following withdrawal of the medication. *Diuretics* and *carbonic anhydrase inhibitors* may also cause myopia.

DRUGS CAUSING CYCLOPLEGIA

Drugs with mild anticholinergic properties (eg, *antianxiety agents, antihistamines, tricyclic antidepressants)* and agents with strong anticholinergic effects (eg, *atropine, scopolamine*), can dilate the pupil and cause dry eye symptoms, but the cyloplegic effects are less commonly encountered in clinical practice. The most common drugs associated with clinical cycloplegia include *chloroquine* and *phenothiazines*.

DRUGS AFFECTING INTRAOCULAR PRESSURE

Drugs known to be capable of dilating the pupil can cause acute or subacute angle-closure glaucoma if the anterior chamber angle is narrow. *Steroids* are widely known to elevate intraocular pressure in the presence of open angles. Other drugs, such as β-*blockers*, can reduce intraocular pressure.

DRUGS AFFECTING THE RETINA

Chloroquine and Hydroxychloroquine

Chloroquine maculopathy consists of a granular hyperpigmentation surrounded by a zone of depigmentation, which is surrounded by another ring of pigment. This clinical picture can vary in intensity, but is characteristic of chloroquine retinopathy and is referred to as a "bull's eye" lesion. Variations of pigmentary disturbances can occur, and some patients may show retinal changes resembling retinitis pigmentosa.

Thioridazine

Thioridazine can cause significant retinal toxicity, leading to reduced visual acuity, color vision changes and disturbances of dark adaptation. These symptoms usually occur 30 to 90 days after treatment is begun. The fundus appearance is often normal during the early stages, but within several weeks or months a pigmentary retinopathy develops, characterized by clumps of pigment developing first in the periphery and then progressing toward the posterior pole.

Quinine

Acute vision loss is common in quinine toxicity (eg, overdose due to attempted suicide) and frequently consists of a clinical presentation of no light perception along with dilated and nonreactive pupils. In the early stages, visual fields usually demonstrate concentric contraction, and improvement of the visual fields may require days or months, but the field loss can sometimes become permanent.

Talc

Tablets of medication intended for oral use contain inert filler materials, such as talc (magnesium silicate), cornstarch, cotton fibers and other substances. Chronic drug abusers may prepare a suspension of medication for injection by dissolving the crushed tablet of *cocaine, methylphenidate, codeine* or other narcotic in water. The solution is then boiled and filtered through a crude cigarette or cotton filter prior to injection. The talc particles eventually embolize to the retinal circulation and produce a characteristic form of retinopathy. Multiple, tiny, yellow-white, glistening particles are scattered throughout the posterior pole and are more numerous in the capillary bed and small arterioles of the perimacular area. Retinal neovascularization can also occur.

Digitalis Glycosides

Digitoxin and *digoxin* can cause changes in color vision and impairment of vision. Various visual phenomena often precede cardiac abnormalities as the earliest symptoms of digitoxin intoxication. A common symptom is snowy vision, wherein objects appear to be covered with frost or snow.

Indomethacin

Indomethacin can induce pigmentary changes of the macula and other areas of the retina. The lesions usually consist of discrete pigment scattering and fine areas of depigmentation around the macula.

Tamoxifen

Tamoxifen can cause white or yellow refractile opacities in the macular and paramacular area, with or without macular edema. The patient can experience reduced visual acuity associated with the macular lesions, and the visual fields can demonstrate abnormalities.

Isotretinoin

Isotretinoin therapy in dosages of 1 mg/kg body weight daily can impair dark adaptation with or without excessive glare sensitivity. Once therapy is discontinued, both the abnormal dark adaptation and abnormal electroretinogram (ERG) usually resolve within several months.

DRUGS AFFECTING THE OPTIC NERVE

Ethambutol

Ethambutol can cause ocular symptoms of reduced visual acuity, color vision changes and visual field loss. Signs of ocular toxicity can appear several weeks following initial therapy, but the onset of ocular complications usually occurs several months after treatment is begun. The primary ocular manifestation of ethambutol toxicity is retrobulbar neuritis.

Chloramphenicol

Chloramphenicol causes both optic neuritis and retrobulbar neuritis. There is severe bilateral reduction of visual acuity accompanied by dense central scotomas. The optic discs are usually edematous and hyperemic, the retinal veins are engorged and tortuous and hemorrhages are often seen. Optic atrophy is a late complication.

Jimmy D. Bartlett OD, DOS
University of Alabama at Birmingham

For More Information

Bartlett JD, Jaanus SD, eds. Clinical Ocular Pharmacology, ed. 3. Boston: Butterworth-Heinemann, 1995.

Bartlett JD. Ophthalmic toxicity by systemic drugs. In: Chiou GCH, ed. Ophthalmic Toxicology. New York: Raven Press, 1992;167.

Fraunfelder FT. Drug Induced Ocular Side Effects and Drug Interactions, ed. 4. Philadelphia: Lea & Febiger, 1995.

Fraunfelder FT, Meyer SM. The national registry of drug-induced ocular side effects. *J Toxicol Cutaneous Ocul Toxicol* 1982;1:65.

Grant WM. Toxicology of the Eye, ed. 4. Springfield, IL: Charles C. Thomas, 1993.

Koneru PB, et al. Oculotoxicities of systemically administered drugs. *J Ocul Toxicol* 1986;2:385.

ODF

16

Systemic Medications Used for Ocular Conditions

Topical, peribulbar or intraocular drug administration may not be effective routes of administration for treatment of all eye diseases. Systemic medication is often required to achieve effective concentrations of drug in and around the ocular tissues. Included in this chapter are the more common indications and systemic medications employed for the treatment of these ocular conditions. Dosages may vary depending upon patient response, new recommendations and guidelines. Some conditions require concurrent treatment by other routes of administration (eg, topical drops, subconjunctival or intravitreal injections).

ANTIMICROBIAL AGENTS

Antimicrobial agents may be given by topical, intraocular, peribulbar and systemic routes of administration. Systemic antimicrobial agents are utilized for anterior segment, posterior segment or orbital infections, often in conjunction with topical treatment. Duration of treatment may vary, although generally 7 to 14 days is adequate in most cases. The etiology of the various conditions may vary, but the more prevalent causes are listed.

Antibacterials				
Condition	**Etiology**	**Antibiotic**	**Dose**	**Comment**
Blepharitis/ meibomian gland/acne rosacea	*Staphylococcal* species	Tetracycline	250-500 mg orally every 6 hours, may be reduced to 250 mg daily in some cases	Not for antibacterial effect Reduces free fatty acid byproducts Tetracycline contraindicated in pregnancy and in children < 10 years old Treat for ≥ 1 month for meibomian gland dysfunction
		Doxycycline	50-100 mg 1-2 times/day	
Internal hordeolum	*Staphylococcal* species	Dicloxacillin	250 mg orally every 6 hours	Use with caution in penicillin allergy
		Cephalexin	250-500 mg orally every 6 hours	Use with caution in penicillin allergy
Acute dacryocystitis	*Staphylococcal* sp., *pneumoniae* *H. influenzae*	Dicloxacillin	250 mg orally every 6 hours	Use with caution in penicillin allergy
		Cephalexin	250-500 mg orally every 6 hours	Use with caution in penicillin allergy
		Amoxicillin/ Clavulanate *(Augmentin)*	125-250 mg orally every 8 hours	Amoxicillin/clavulanate recommended in children *(H. influenzae)*

Antibacterials				
Condition	**Etiology**	**Antibiotic**	**Dose**	**Comment**
Conjunctivitis	*Gonococcal*[1] (ophthalmic)	Ceftriaxone		
		neonatal	25-50 mg/kg, up to 125 mg IV or IM	AAO practice standards require daily injections for 7 days
		adult	1 gram IV or IM daily	May treat up to 5 days
		Cefixime *(Suprax)*	400 mg orally for 1 dose	Ciprofloxacin 500 mg or ofloxacin 400 mg also indicated as a single dose treatment
	Chlamydial[1] (adult inclusion)	Doxycycline	100 mg orally twice daily	Treat for ≥ 3 weeks
		Tetracycline	500 mg orally three times daily	Treat for ≥ 3 weeks
		Erythro-mycin	500 mg orally four times daily	Treat for ≥ 3 weeks
		Ofloxacin *(Floxin)*	300 mg orally twice daily	Treat for 7 days
		Azithro-mycin *(Zithromax)*	1 gram orally once daily	Azithromycin may require only single dose
	(neonatal inclusion)	Erythro-mycin	50 mg/kg/day orally in 4 divided doses	Treat for 14 days
	H. influenza	Amoxicillin	125-250 mg orally every 8 hours	Often used in conjunction with topical therapy
Keratitis	*Pseudomonas* (various others possible)	Gentamicin	3 m/kg every 8 hours (request peak & trough serum levels)	Use if pending scleral involvement Antibiotic selection depends upon organism isolated
Lid trauma/ oculoplastics procedures	*Staphylococcus, Streptococcus, H. influenzae,* etc	Cephalexin	250-500 mg orally every 6 hours	Prophylaxis
		Dicloxacillin	250-500 mg orally every 6 hours	
		Amoxicillin/ Clavulanate (*Augmentin*)	125-500 mg orally every 8 hours	Suggest amoxicillin/clavulanate if *H. influenzae* suspected (more often in children)
Preseptal cellulitis	*Streptococcus, H. influenzae, Staphylococcus,* etc	Amoxicillin/ Clavulanate	250-875 mg orally 2-3 times daily	Oral antibiotics may be sufficient
Orbital Cellulitis	*Streptococcus, H. influenzae, Staphylococcus,* etc	Ceftriaxone	1 g IV every 12 hours	Intravenous therapy required
		and anti-staphylococcal penicillins (Nafcillin)	1-2 g IV every 4-6 hours	
Endophthalmitis/penetrating eye injury prophylaxis	*Staphylococcus, Streptococcus Bacillus,* etc	Aminoglycoside and Cefazolin	Gentamicin 3 mg/kg every 8 hours and Cefazolin 1 g every 8 hours	Not all clinicians use systemic therapy
Retinitis	*Toxoplasmosis*	Sulfadiazine and	1 g orally every 6 hours	Watch sulfa hypersensitivity Treat for 3-6 weeks
		Pyrimeth-amine *(Daraprim)* and	25 mg orally 1-2 times/day (loading dose 75 mg)	May need folinic acid to prevent bone marrow depression; treat for 3-6 weeks
		Clindamycin (optional)	300 mg orally every 6 hours	Treat for 3-6 weeks; pseudomembranous colitis is a risk

Antibacterials				
Condition	**Etiology**	**Antibiotic**	**Dose**	**Comment**
Neuro-syphilis	*Treponema pallidum*	Aqueous crystalline penicillin G	12 MU/day IV for 10 days	Caution if allergies; in HIV up to 24 MU/day for 14-21 days CNS toxicity in doses > 20 MU/day
		Ceftriaxone	1 g daily (IV or IM) for 14 days	

[1] Recommend concurrent treatment for gonorrhea and chlamydia.

Antivirals				
Condition	**Etiology**	**Antiviral**	**Dose**	**Comment**
Keratitis/ keratoconjunctivitis	Herpes zoster	Acyclovir *(Zovirax)*	600-800 orally 5 times/day for 7-10 days	Best if used within 72 hours of onset
		Valacyclovir *(Valtrex)*	1000 mg orally 3 times/day for 7 days	Best if used within 72 hours of onset
		Famciclovir *(Famivr)*	500 mg orally three times/day for 7 days	Best if used within 72 hours of onset
Cytomegalovirus (CMV) Retinitis		Ganciclovir	IV-induction - 5 mg/kg every 12 hours for 14-21 days; maintenance 5 mg/kg every day or 6 mg/kg 5 days per week	Bone marrow suppression; granulocytopenia, thrombocytopenia Dosing may vary with renal impairment
			Oral capsule - 1000 mg three times/day	Maintenance
		Foscarnet *(Foscavir)*	IV-induction - 60 mg/kg every day, Maintenance - 90-120 mg/kg every day	Renal toxicity, adjust for dose. Other side effects include headache, nausea, vomiting
		Cidofovir *(Vistide)*	IV-5 mg/kg once per week for 2 weeks then 5 mg/kg every 2 weeks	IV saline and oral probenecid given before and after each dose; dosage reduction required with increased serum creatinine.
Varicella or Herpes Simplex (ARN; PORN)		Acyclovir *(Zovirax)*	IV - 14 mg/kg every 8 hours (or 1500 mg/m^2)	Adequate hydration essential

Antifungals[2]				
Condition	**Etiology**	**Antifungals[2]**	**Dose**	**Comment**
Endophthalmitis	*Candida, Aspergillus, Fusarium,* etc	Itraconazole (*Sporanox*)	200-400 mg orally twice a day	Monitor liver function tests (LFTs)
		Ketoconazole (*Vizoral*)	200 mg orally every 6-8 hours	Monitor LFTs
		Amphotericin B	0.5-0.8 mg/kg/day IV	More effective in endogenous type Systemic toxicity (eg, hypokalemia, chills, nausea, vomiting, etc) Liposomal preparation less side effects
		Fluconazole (*Diflucan*)	100-200 mg orally 1-2 times/day (or IV)	Well tolerated, minimal side effects Antifungal spectrum limited
		Flucytosine (*Ancobon*)	50-150 mg/kg/day orally in 4 doses	Not used alone because of potential resistance

[2] Rifampin 600 mg/day has been added to regimen to supplement antifungal activity. Various protocols and combinations have been used. Most have not been studied adequately to recommend one regimen or antifungal agent. Some clinicians may add systemic antifungal agents to supplement treatment of *fungal keratitis*.

ANALGESICS

Various types of systemic analgesics may be used for pain. Nonnarcotic analgesics may be sufficient for minor eye pain. Acetaminophen and NSAIDs (eg, ibuprofen, aspirin or naproxen) are also commonly used. Narcotic-containing medication such as acetaminophen with codeine (*Tylenol #3*) or acetaminophen with hydrocodone (*Vicodin*) may be required for more severe pain. Pain will vary significantly among individuals. Therefore, careful assessment is required by the clinician to determine the appropriate amount of pain relief the patient may require.

Narcotic Analgesics				
Condition	**Etiology**	**Analgesic**	**Dose**	**Comment**
Keratitis	PRK/RK Corneal abrasions	Acetaminophen with codeine 30 mg (narcotic)	1-2 tabs every 4-6 hours	Short-term control of severe eye pain May cause drowsiness, nausea or constipation
		Acetaminophen with hydrocodone 5-7.5 mg	1-2 tabs every 4-6 hours	Short-term control of severe eye pain May cause drowsiness, nausea or constipation

Non-Narcotic Analgesics				
Condition	**Etiology**	**Analgesic**	**Dose**	**Comment**
Keratitis	Epithelial defect General eye pain	Acetaminophen 500 mg	1-2 tabs every 4-6 hours	For mild eye pain
		Ketorolac (*Toradol*) 10 mg	1 tab every 4-6 hours (40 mg per day maximum)	Not to exceed 5 days combined IM/IV and PO GI bleeding
		Ibuprofen 200 mg (OTC)	1-2 tabs every 4-6 hours	Take with food Some bleeding risk
		Tramadol (*Ultram*) 50 mg	1-2 tabs every 6 hours (400 mg per day maximum)	Drowsiness; potential for abuse

ANTIHISTAMINES

The systemic administration of antihistamines for signs or symptoms of seasonal allergies may benefit patients with ocular symptoms. Patients may not require topical medication for treatment of conjunctivitis if systemic antihistamines control or alleviate both systemic and ocular symptoms. Some patients do not wish to be on systemic antihistamines; therefore, local treatment with various topical agents may suffice. Other patients receiving systemic antihistamines may require supplemental therapy with topical medication to achieve adequate control of ocular symptoms.

Non-sedating antihistamines			
Condition	**Etiology**	**Antihistamine**	**Dose**
Conjunctivitis	Seasonal allergic	Loratadine (*Claritin*)	10 mg every day
		Astemizole (*Hismanal*)[1]	10 mg every day
		Cetirazine (*Zyrtec*)	10 mg every day
		Terfenadine[1]	60 mg twice daily

[1] Drug interactions of non-sedating antihistamines with erythromycin, antifungals, phenytoin or cyclosporine. May cause cardiac toxicity (torsades de pointes).

Sedating antihistamines				
Condition	**Etiology**	**Antihistamine**	**Dose**	**Comment**
Conjunctivitis	Seasonal allergic	Chlorpheniramine Diphenhydramine Many others	4-12 mg every 4-12 hours 25-50 mg every 4-6 hours	Sedation may be a problem Sedation

ANTI-INFLAMMATORY AGENTS

Systemic corticosteroids have been utilized in many ocular conditions, and their use is not limited to the conditions below. Systemic NSAIDs probably do not penetrate the eye in sufficient levels to provide for good intraocular anti-inflammatory effect and have somewhat limited application. Generally, immunosuppressive agents are reserved for more severe or unresponsive conditions.

Corticosteroids				
Condition	**Etiology**	**Corticosteroid**	**Dose**	**Comment**
Scleritis	Autoimmune vascular-collagen disease (eg, arthritis, SLE, Wegener's) Other etiologies include infectious, metabolic or granulomatous diseases	Prednisone	Variable - 20-100 mg/day	Watch for side effects including rebound inflammation, psychosis, electrolyte disturbance, peptic ulcer aggravation, hyperglycemia, asceptic necrosis, hypertension, pancreatitis Informed consent requires review with patient
Hyphema	Trauma Red blood cells	Prednisone	20 mg twice daily (adult)	Decreasing dose in children
Keratitis	Viral/bacterial	Prednisone	20-60 mg/day	If infection under control or if topical steroids cannot be used (ie, with an epithelial defect)
Vitritis	Post-op membrane	Prednisone	20-100 mg/day	Short course under 2 weeks; taper dose to prevent rebound inflammation
Retinitis	Toxoplasmosis	Prednisone	20-100 mg/day	Used if impending macular involvement or severe posterior segment inflammation
Optic neuropathy	Traumatic	Methylprednisolone	30 mg/kg loading dose then starting 2 hours later 15 mg/kg every 6 hours, usually for a maximum of 3-5 days	Megadose steroid Watch for side effects (hyperglycemia, steroid psychosis, aggravation of peptic ulcer, rebound inflammation, electrolyte imbalance)
Neuritis	Demyelinizing Optic	Methylprednisolone	250 mg every 6 hours for 3 days IV followed by oral prednisone 1 mg/kg/day for 11 days	Same as megadose

Nonsteroidal Anti-inflammatory Drugs (NSAIDs)				
Condition	**Etiology**	**NSAID**	**Dose**	**Comment**
Conjunctivitis	Vernal	Aspirin 325 mg	650 mg 3 times/day	May give additional relief with topical mast cell stabilizers or steroids
Scleritis	Diffuse or nodular; necrotizing	Indomethacin	75-150 mg/day	Take with food; combination with prednisone 60-80 mg/day is more effective than either alone
		Ibuprofen	400-800 mg/day 3-4 times per day (2400 mg max)	Take with food
		Naproxen	250-500 mg 2-3 times per day	Take with food
Myositis	Idiopathic orbital	Indomethacin	25-50 mg 3 times/ day	Not used often

IMMUNOSUPPRESSIVE AGENTS

Many of the immunosuppressive agents listed below have been utilized in other autoimmune-related diseases in addition to those listed. Most are reserved for cases unresponsive to initial therapy because of concerns for increased systemic toxicity and vigilant monitoring required. Doses may vary since extensive clinical studies are lacking.

Immunosuppressive Agents				
Condition	**Etiology**	**Agent**	**Dose**	**Comment**
Uveitis	Unknown Autoimmune	Azothioprine[1]	1-2.5 mg/kg/day orally (50 mg 3 times/day)	Bone marrow depression, nausea, vomiting
		Bromocriptine	Variable	Headache, nausea, vomiting, fatigue, dizzy
		Cyclosporine A[1] *(Sandimmune)*	4-5 mg/kg/day orally (variable)	Nephrotoxicity, hypertension, gingival hyperplasia, hypertrichosis, etc
		Methotrexate	12.5-15 mg/week	Watch bone marrow depression, nausea, vomiting, pneumonitis
Cicatricial pemphigoid	Unknown	Dapsone	25 mg/day orally for week 1, increase to 50 mg/day variable dosing	Hemolytic anemia, nausea, vomiting, anorexia, methemoglobInemia
		Azathioprine *(Imuran)*	1-2 mg/kg/day orally	Bone marrow depression, nausea, vomiting Often combined with corticosteroids
		Cyclophosphamide[1] *(Cytoxan Lyophilized, Neosar)*	2-3 mg/kg/day orally	Hemorrhagic cystitis, nausea, vomiting, alopecia, thrombocytopenia
Behçet's syndrome	Unknown	Chlorambucil (*Leukeran*)	Up to 2.5 mg orally 4 times/day	Bone marrow depression, mutagenicity; start with low dose, increase slowly
		Colchicine	1-1.5 mg/day orally	Nausea, vomiting, diarrhea

[1] Also used in Behçet's syndrome.

AMINOCAPROIC ACID

Aminocaproic acid (*Amicar*) is an antifibrinolytic agent used orally for the prevention of secondary rebleeds in traumatic hyphemas. Corticosteroids may also be effective, cost less and exhibit fewer side effects than aminocaproic acid.

Aminocaproic Acid

Condition	Etiology	Drug	Dose	Comment
Hyphema	Traumatic	Aminocaproic acid (*Amicar*)	50 mg/kg orally every 4 hours for 5 days; not to exceed 5 g every 4 hours (max 30 g/day)	Treat for 5 days Nausea, vomiting, hypotension

OCULAR HYPOTENSIVE AGENTS

Systemic ocular hypotensive agents are some of the most effective agents for decreasing intraocular pressure (IOP). Carbonic anhydrase inhibitors effectively decrease IOP, but are associated with various systemic side effects. Hyperosmotic agents are especially effective in reducing very elevated IOPs, although the underlying cause must be corrected to prevent rebound increase in IOP. Hyperosmotic agents are generally indicated for short-term control of IOP with effects lasting for 6 to 8 hours.

Carbonic Anhydrase Inhibitors

Condition	Etiology	CAI	Dose	Comment
Glaucoma	Open-angle	Acetazolamide	125-500 mg orally every 6-12 hours	Systemic side effects include GI intolerance, parasthesias, hypokalemia, CNS (drowsiness, lethargy, depression), renal stones, sulfa hypersensitivity, etc)
		Methazolamide	25-50 mg orally 2-3 times/day	Same as acetazolamide, more CNS, less GI
	Acute	Acetazolamide	500 mg injectable IV	Systemic side effects include GI intolerance, parasthesias, hypokalemia, CNS (drowsiness, lethargy, depression), renal stones, sulfa hypersensitivity, etc)

Hyperosmotic Agents

Condition	Etiology	Osmotic Agent	Dose	Comment
Glaucoma	Acute Pre-operative (to lower IOP)	Glycerin 50-75% (*Osmoglyn*)	1-1.5 g/kg orally	May cause hyperglycemia in diabetics Sweet taste may cause nausea and vomiting
		Isosorbide 45% (*Ismotic*)	1.5-2 g/kg orally	Less nausea and vomiting than glycerin
		Mannitol IV 15-25% (*Osmitrol*)	1.5-2 g/kg IV	Watch crystal formation; use with in-line IV filter, keep warm Infuse over 30 minutes Watch for electrolyte disturbances, thirst, diuresis, potential cardiovascular overload

VITAMINS/MINERALS

Various vitamins and minerals have established roles in the treatment of ophthalmic conditions. Others are not well documented.

Vitamin/ Minerals				
Condition	**Etiology**	**Vitamin/Mineral**	**Dose**	**Comment**
Dry eye/keratitis	Vitamin A deficiency	Vitamin A	50,000 U every day	Fat soluble vitamin, toxicity includes dry mucous membranes, increased eye irritation
Optic Neuritis	Nutritional or toxic	Vitamin B_{12} hydroxyco-balamin	1000 U IM daily, reduce dose to weekly then monthly	Cyanocobalamin may not be as effective
	Drug toxicity (INH)	Pyridoxine (B_6)	50 mg daily	Often given concurrently with INH
Macular degeneration	Deficiency of antioxidant vitamins (eg, E, C and A) Zinc Selenium Copper	*Ocuvite,* *Icaps Plus* Various Mfr.	1 tablet 1-2 times daily	Causative agent not well established; recent evidence has suggested beta-carotene may not be beneficial

For More Information

Olin BR, Hebel SK, eds. Drug Facts & Comparisons. Facts & Comparisons. St. Louis: 1997.

Tabbara KF, Hyyndiuk RA, eds. Infections of the Eye, ed 2. Boston: Little, Brown and Company, 1996.

Bartlett JD, Jaanus SD, eds. Clinical Ocular Pharmacology, ed 3. Boston: Butterworth-Heinemann, 1995.

Sanford JP, Gilbert DN, Sande MA, eds. Guide to Antimicrobial Therapy. Dallas: Antimicrobial Therapy Inc., 1995.

Preferred Practice Pattern Series, American Academy of Ophthalmology, San Francisco CA.

Optometric Clinical Practice Guidelines, American Optometric Association, St. Louis MO.

ODF

17

Drugs With Off-Labeled Ophthalmic Uses

For many years, the drug package insert was interpreted as a legal standard for drug use. However, the legal implications of the package insert have been challenged, and in some cases, various courts have recognized that drugs may be used for clinical indications other than those specified in the package insert. It is possible for prescribed dosage schedules to differ from those specified in the package insert if such a schedule is consistent with sound scientific rationale and medical practice.

Since it has been recognized that the package insert may not contain the most recent information about a drug, it is now generally agreed that the clinician should be free to use a drug for an indication not in the package insert if two conditions have been met:

1. When such use is part of the rational practice of medicine intended for the benefit of the patient;

2. Documented evidence exists for use of a drug in the manner prescribed.

When using an approved drug for an unlabeled purpose, the patient should be informed regarding the nature of the intended therapy, and the practitioner is advised to obtain the patient's written permission (informed consent) before beginning treatment. Since drug-related side effects are a significant cause of malpractice litigations, it is essential that patients understand the risks of potential side effects. In determining what constitutes sound medical practice in malpractice litigations, the package insert is admissible into evidence, but it does not establish conclusively the standards of acceptable practice or that departure from the directions contained in the package insert constitutes negligence. One of the best protections against unfavorable malpractice verdicts is to prescribe medications in the best interests of the patient according to rational standards of practice.

The drugs listed in the following table have been approved by the Food and Drug Administration (FDA), but not for the ophthalmic purposes listed. Each agent, however, has been documented to be useful for the diagnosis or therapy of certain ocular conditions.

Drugs With Off-labeled Ophthalmic Uses		
Generic *(Trade)*	Labeled Indication	Unlabeled Ophthalmic Use
Acetylcysteine (*Mucomyst*)	Mucolytic agent in broncho-pulmonary conditions	Topical mucolytic treatment of vernal, giant papillary conjunctivitis, filamentary keratitis
Acyclovir (*Zovirax*)	Treatment of varicella-zoster and genital herpes simplex	Treatment of epithelial HSV keratitis
Aminocaproic acid (*Amicar*)	Antifibrinolytic agent for the treatment of excessive bleeding	Oral treatment of traumatic hyphema
Aspirin (eg, *Bayer*)	Anti-inflammatory, analgesic, antipyretic agent	Oral treatment of vernal conjunctivitis
Diclofenac sodium (*Voltaren*)	Treatment of postoperative cataract inflammation	Anti-inflammatory treatment following argon laser trabeculoplasty, treatment of seasonal allergic conjunctivitis, pain associated with radial keratotomy and photorefractive keratectomy
Fluorescein sodium (eg, *Fluorescite*)	Topical or IV diagnostic ophthalmic dye	Oral fluorography for diagnosis of retinal vascular diseases
Ketorolac tromethamine (*Acular*)	Treatment of seasonal allergic conjunctivitis	Treatment of pain associated with corneal trauma
Lodoxamide (*Alomide*)	Treatment of vernal keratoconjunctivitis	Treatment of seasonal allergic conjunctivitis
Polyhexamethylene biguanide	Swimming pool and contact lens disinfectant	Treatment of *Acanthamoeba* keratitis
Sodium hyaluronate (*Amvisc*) Chondroitin sulfate (*Viscoat*)	Viscoelastic agents in intraocular surgery	Topical treatment of severe dry eye disorders
Suprofen (*Profenal*)	Prevention of intraoperative miosis during cataract extraction	Topical treatment of contact lens-associated GPC

ACETYLCYSTEINE

Acetylcysteine (*Mucomyst*) has been approved for use as a mucolytic agent in acute and chronic bronchopulmonary conditions. The agent is administered by nebulization for its local effect on the bronchopulmonary tree. The product contains disodium edetate and sodium hydroxide and, thus, has a significant odor accompanying its clinical use. When used on the eye, acetylcysteine dissolves mucous threads and decreases tear viscosity. The drug is commonly prepared for topical ocular use by diluting the commercial preparation to 2% to 5% in artificial tears or physiologic saline.

ACYCLOVIR

Acyclovir *(Zovirax)* has been approved for treatment of genital herpes simplex (HSV). During initial episodes of the disease, oral acyclovir can decrease the duration of viral shedding and healing time of the genital lesions, decrease the severity of symptoms and reduce the development of new lesions. Acyclovir ointment is also approved for treatment of initial genital herpes, and IV acyclovir seems to be effective for severe initial episodes of the disease. Acyclovir is also the treatment of choice for biopsy-proven herpes simplex encephalitis. In the treatment of HSV keratitis, 3% acyclovir ointment may be useful to treat epithelial involvement. Although acyclovir is effective for treating HSV epithelial keratitis, there is no clear superiority of the drug when compared with other commercially available antiviral agents.

AMINOCAPROIC ACID

Aminocaproic acid *(Amicar)* is an antifibrinolytic agent approved for treatment of excessive bleeding from systemic hyperfibrinolysis and urinary fibrinolysis. The drug may also be useful for the treatment of some patients with traumatic hyphema. Some studies have shown the drug to be effective in reducing the rate of rebleeding from about 30% to 3% or 4%. Dosage is 100 mg/kg body weight every 4 hours to a maximum dose of 30 g daily. It may be possible to administer one-half of this dosage to reduce side effects while maintaining efficacy. It has been established that the drug is ineffective in children.

ASPIRIN

The efficacy of salicylates in the treatment of ocular inflammation has been infrequently studied in human models, but several reports have suggested that aspirin may be valuable for intractable cases of vernal conjunctivitis. Patients who remain symptomatic following treatment with cromolyn sodium, steroids, or a combination of agents may demonstrate improvement in both symptoms and signs when aspirin is added to the therapeutic regimen.

DICLOFENAC SODIUM

Diclofenac sodium (*Voltaren*) is a topically applied nonsteroidal anti-inflammatory agent currently approved for treatment of inflammation following cataract surgery. The drug is effective possibly through its antiprostaglandin mechanism. In a recent study, the anti-inflammatory effect of diclofenac was evaluated following argon laser trabeculoplasty (ALT). Diclofenac or placebo drops were given once before and after trabeculoplasty and then 4 times daily for 4 days. The increase of anterior chamber flare was completely inhibited by topical diclofenac. Thus, 0.1% diclofenac may represent an effective anti-inflammatory therapy following ALT. Studies have also demonstrated the safety and efficacy of topical diclofenac for treatment of seasonal allergic conjunctivitis and pain associated with corneal refractive surgery.

FLUORESCEIN SODIUM

Fluorescein sodium (eg, *Fluorescite*) is approved for topical and IV use (Ophthalmic Dyes chapter). Oral fluorography was reintroduced in 1979, allowing fluorescein studies without the potential systemic effects attributable to IV fluorescein. Various studies using oral fluorography have established this technique as a viable alternative for the diagnosis of certain retinal vascular diseases. The procedure is especially useful for conditions in which late dye leakage is expected. Oral fluorography is performed using either bulk powder fluorescein sodium USP or the commercially available vials of 10% injectable fluorescein sodium. The dosage typically used is 1000 mg to 1500 mg of fluorescein sodium mixed with a citrus drink and allowed to cool in crushed ice.

LIQUID PERFLUOROCARBONS

Liquid perfluorocarbons are heavier than water liquids that are used to push the retina against the back of the eye with the patient in the supine position. They are clear, have low viscosity and low surface tension, and are immiscible with water. Their refractive indices vary with some being so close to aqueous that it is hard to see the interface between the perfluorocarbon and the aqueous. With others, the refractive index is significantly different from that of aqueous, and a clear meniscus is visible between the perfluorocarbon and the physiologic intraocular fluids or BSS. Some are intended for intraoperative use only but others have been left in eyes for prolonged periods of time.

They are ideally suited for unrolling the flap of a giant retinal tear. After vitrectomy, the perfluorocarbon can be injected by hand through a cannula whose tip is positioned posterior to, or under, the flap of the giant tear. As the perfluorocarbon flows into the eye, it will settle on the back of the retina pushing it against the posterior choroid. Subretinal fluid will be displaced anteriorly and flow into the central vitreous cavity through the giant retinal tear as the perfluorocarbon is injected. Because of the low viscosity, the perfluorocarbon liquid may flow into the subretinal space if it is brought anterior to the edge of the tear. Commonly, a partial fill is used to partially unroll the tear, further vitrectomy is done to relieve traction on the anterior edge of the tear, and then more perfluorocarbon is added to further flatten the retina. Endolaser can be given through the perfluorocarbon. Gas is then infused into the eye through the pars plana infusion port as the perfluorocarbon is aspirated. Perfluorocarbons have vapor pressures that vary from less than 1 to greater than with 57. The residue of those with high vapor pressures do not need to be rinsed out because they quickly vaporize into the intraocular gas. If the vapor pressure is low, however, the inside of the retina should be rinsed with about 0.5 ml of BSS to remove residual perfluorocarbons. This rinse is then aspirated off the posterior retina.

Perfluorocarbons are also heavier than intraocular lenses. Hence, they can be used to float a displaced intraocular lens off the posterior retina probably making it safer and easier to reposition or remove. The injection of a perfluorocarbon may be especially helpful when there is a concomitant retinal detachment as it will simultaneously push the retina against the back of the eye holding it away from the intraocular instruments and lift the intraocular lens anteriorly.

Perfluorocarbons can be used to push the retina posteriorly in detachments complicated by fibrovascular tissue proliferation as in proliferative diabetic retinopathy or by preretinal fibrous membranes as in eyes with massive periretinal proliferation. This can make the membranes easier to visualize and dissect in some cases. However, because of their low surface tension, the perfluorocarbon liquids will quickly flow through any posterior retinal breaks into the subretinal space if there is residual traction present around the breaks. An additional posterior retinotomy can then be made to remove the perfluorocarbon.

Some perfluorocarbons have been left in eyes to provide prolonged tamponade of the inferior retina. Eventually the perfluorocarbon liquid must be removed in a second operation.

POLYHEXAMETHYLENE BIGUANIDE

Chlorhexidine, a biguanide compound (Zeneca Pharmaceuticals), is an antiseptic that is used to treat open wounds, gingivitis and skin infections. It has been used by some clinicians for *Acanthamoeba* keratitis, usually in combination treatment with propamidine isethionate drops 0.1%. Chlorhexidine 0.02% eyedrops are not commercially available and have to be extemporaneously compounded from a stock solution. Chlorhexidine 0.02% has been effective for treatment of *Acanthamoeba* ketatitis that did not respond to polyhexamethylene biguanide (PHMB) 0.02%. Debate exists as to which compound, chlorhexidine or PHMB, is more effective for the treatment of *Acanthamoeba* keratitis.

Polyhexamethylene biguanide (PHMB) is a polymeric environmental disinfectant commonly used for disinfecting swimming pools and, more recently, as a contact lens disinfectant. This agent has a broad spectrum of activity, effective against both gram-positive and gram-negative bacteria. There have been recent reports of PHMB effectiveness in treatment of *Acanthamoeba* keratitis when conventional therapy has failed. When topical therapy employing propamidine and neomycin is ineffective, treatment with topical PHMB may be successful. The formulation can be prepared, under sterile conditions, from the stock 20% solution and diluted 1:1000 for administration as a 0.02% solution.

VISCOELASTIC AGENTS

Sodium hyaluronate (*Amvisc*) and chondroitin sulfate (*Viscoat*), are approved as vitreous replacement substances and for use during intraocular surgery to protect the corneal endothelium. When prepared as a 0.1% topical solution in saline, sodium hyaluronate may be beneficial for patients with severe dry eye syndromes. The beneficial effects of sodium hyaluronate have been attributed to its viscoelastic properties, which lubricate and protect the ocular surface. Most patients achieve control of symptoms with topical instillation up to 4 times daily.

SUPROFEN

When used as a 1% solution, topically applied suprofen (*Profenal*), a propionic acid derivative, has been shown to be superior to placebo in the treatment of contact lens-associated giant papillary conjunctivitis (GPC). In a randomized, double-masked comparison, suprofen provided a greater reduction of both signs and symptoms such as papillae and mucous strands.

Jimmy D. Bartlett OD, DOS
University of Alabama at Birmingham

For More Information

Absolon MJ, Brown S. Acetylcysteine in keratoconjunctivitis sicca. *Br J Ophthalmol* 1968;52:310.

Camacho H, Bajaire B, Mejia LF. Silicone oil in the management of giant retinal tears. *Ann Ophthalmol* 1992;24:45.

Cerqueti PM, et al. Lodoxamide treatment of allergic conjunctivitis. *Int Arch Allergy Appl Immunol* 1994;105:185.

Collum LMT, et al. Randomized double-blind trial of acyclovir and idoxuridine in dendritic corneal ulceration. *Br J Ophthalmol* 1980;64:766.

DeLuise VP, Peterson WS. The use of topical Healon tears in the management of refractory dry-eye syndrome. *Ann Ophthalmol* 1984;1:823.

Donnenfeld ED, et al. Controlled evaluation of a bandage contact lens and a topical nonsteroidal anti-inflammatory drug in treating traumatic corneal abrasions. *Ophthalmology* 1995;102:979.

Eller AW, et al. A survey of intraocular silicone oil use in the United States. *Ophthalmology* 1992;99:1174.

Herbort CP, et al. Anti-inflammatory effect of diclofenac drops after argon laser trabeculoplasty. *Arch Ophthalmol* 1993;111:481.

Hung SO, et al. Oral acyclovir in the management of dendritic herpetic corneal ulceration. *Br J Ophthalmol* 1984;68:398.

Irwin R. Practical aspects of oral fluorography. *J Ophthal Photog* 1981;4:16.

Jackson WB, et al. Treatment of herpes simplex keratitis: Comparison of acyclovir and vidarabine. *Can J Ophthalmol* 1984;19:107.

Kelley JS, Kincaid M. Retinal fluorography using oral fluorescein. *Arch Ophthalmol* 1979;97:2331.

Kraft SP, et al. Traumatic hyphema in children. Treatment with epsilon-aminocaproic acid. *Ophthalmology* 1987;94:1232.

Kutner B, et al. Aminocaproic acid reduces the risk of secondary hemorrhage in patients with traumatic hyphema. *Arch Ophthalmol* 1987;105:206.

Larkin DFP, et al. Treatment of *Acanthamoeba* keratitis with polyhexamethylene biguanide. *Ophthalmology* 1992;99:185.

Limberg MB, et al. Topical application of hyaluronic acid and chondroitin sulfate in treatment of dry eyes. *Am J Ophthalmol* 1987;103:194.

McGetrick JJ, et al. Aminocaproic acid decreases secondary hemorrhage after traumatic hyphema. *Arch Ophthalmol* 1983;101:1031.

Mengher LS, et al. Effect of sodium hyaluronate (0.1%) on break-up time (NIBUT) in patients with dry eyes. *Br J Ophthalmol* 1986;70:442.

Meyer E, et al. Efficacy of antiprostaglandin therapy in vernal conjunctivitis. *Br J Ophthalmol* 1987;71:497.

Mindel JS, Goldstein JI. Non-approved use of Food and Drug Administration approved drugs. *Am J Ophthalmol* 1979;88:626.

Noble MJ, Cheng H. Oral fluorescein and cystoid macular edema: Detection in aphakic and pseudophakic eyes. *Br J Ophthalmol* 1984;68:221.

Palmer DJ, et al. A comparison of two dose regimens of epsilon aminocaproic acid in the prevention and management of secondary traumatic hyphemas. *Ophthalmology* 1986;93:102.

Potter JW, et al. Oral fluorography. *J Am Optom Assoc* 1985;56:784.

Roth SH. Drug use, the package insert, and the practice of medicine. *Arch Intern Med* 1982;142:871.

Stuart JC, Linn JG. Dilute sodium hyaluronate (Healon) in the treatment of ocular surface disorders. *Ann Ophthalmol* 1985;17:190.

Wood TS, et al. Suprofen treatment of contact lens associated GPC. *Ophthalmology* 1988;96:822.

ODF

18

Orphan And Investigational Drugs

In addition to the Food and Drug Administration (FDA) approved drugs and the drugs with unlabeled ophthalmic uses (see the Drugs with Off-labeled Ophthalmic Uses chapter), two other groups of drugs are of interest to eye-care practitioners: Investigational New Drugs (INDs) and Orphan Drugs. INDs are drugs not yet approved by the FDA, but are being investigated by a pharmaceutical company or sponsor. Orphan drugs are drugs made available by manufacturers for the treatment of rare diseases.

ORPHAN DRUGS

The term "orphan drug" first appeared in the medical literature in a 1968 editorial. It was used to disclaim nonapproved substances as drugs and included compounds such as lithium carbonate, d-xylose and sodium fluoride. These products were frequently labeled "for chemical purposes, not for drug use," "for research use only, not for clinical use," and "for manufacturing use only." Orphan drug has since been applied to drugs and devices used in the treatment or diagnosis of rare diseases.

The FDA established the Office of Orphan Products Development in 1982. These products consist of drugs, biologicals (eg, vaccines), medical devices and foods for the diagnosis, treatment or prevention of rare diseases.

Government Incentives To Assist In Orphan Drug Development
♦ Developers of orphan drugs have 7 years of exclusive licensing, during which time the product may not be marketed by another company in the US without the sponsor's permission.
♦ Developers may claim up to 63% of the cost of clinical investigations as a tax credit.
♦ The FDA can grant up to $70,000 in support of a sponsor's orphan drug clinical research. The Orphan Drug Act authorizes $4,000,000 per year for these research grants.
♦ The FDA can assist sponsors of orphan drugs in the development of investigational guidelines and protocols.
♦ When appropriate, the FDA can modify approval requirements for specific orphan drugs (eg, modify the size of study populations).
♦ The FDA can assign to orphan drugs a high review priority. The review phase (time from a new drug application submission to approval) for nine orphan drugs receiving approval in 1985 and 1986 was 2.7 years.

Tatro, DS. Orphan drugs. *Drug Newsletter* 1988 Apr;7(4):26.

Ophthalmic drugs established by the FDA as Orphan Drugs are listed in the following table.

Orphan Drugs		
Drug Generic *(Trade)*	**Indication**	**Manufacturer/Sponsor**
Acid implant (Intravitreal, Ganciclovir-free)	Cytomegalovirus retinitis.	Chiron Vision 4560 Horton Street Emeryville, CA 94608
Aminocaproic acid	Topical treatment of traumatic hyphema of the eye.	Orphan Medical 13911 Ridgedale Drive Minnetonka, MN 55305
Botulinum toxin type A (*Botox*) (*Dysport*)	To treat essential blepharospasm and synkinetic closure of the eyelid associated with VIII cranial nerve aberrant regeneration.	Allergan/Porton P.O. Box 19534 Irvine, CA 94501
Bromhexine (*Bisolvon*)	Treatment of mild to moderate keratoconjunctivitis sicca in patients with Sjogren's Syndrome.	Boehringer Ingelheim 90 East Ridge P.O. Box 368 Ridgefield, CT 06877
Chondroitinase	To treat patients undergoing virectomy.	Storz Ophthalmics American Cyanamid Co. Pearl River, NY 10965
Cyclosporine (*Optimmune*)	Treatment of severe keratoconjunctivitis sicca associated with Sjogren's Syndrome.	Allergan, Inc. P.O. Box 19534 Irvine, CA 94501
Cyclosporine 2% Ophthalmic Ointment (*Sandimmune*)	Treatment of high-risk corneal transplant and use in corneal melting syndromes of known or presumed immunologic etiopathogenesis, including Mooren's ulcer.	Allergan, Inc. P.O. Box 19534 Irvine, CA 94501
Dehydrex	Treatment of recurrent corneal erosion unresponsive to conventional therapy.	Holles Labs 30 Forest Notch Cohasset, MA 02025
Epidermal Growth Factor, Human	Acceleration of corneal epithelial regeneration and healing of stromal tissue in non-healing corneal defects.	Chiron Corporation 4560 Horton Street Emeryville, CA 94608
Fibronectin	Treatment of non-healing corneal ulcers or epithelial defects that have been unresponsive to conventional therapy and whose underlying cause has been eliminated.	Chiron Ophthalmics with New York Blood Center 310 E. 67th Street New York, NY 10021
Filgrastim (*Neupogen*)	Treatment of AIDS patients with CMV treated with ganciclovir.	Amgen Inc. 1900 Oak Terrace Lane Thousand Oaks, CA 91320-1789
Lodoxamide tromethamlne (*Alomide*)	Treatment of vernal conjunctivitis.	Alcon Labs 6201 South Freeway Ft. Worth, TX 76134
Matrix Metalloproteinase Inhibitor (*Galardin*)	Treatment of corneal ulcers.	Glycomed Inc. 860 Atlantic Ave. Alameda, CA 94501
Mytomycin-C	To treat refractory glaucoma as an adjunct to AB externo glaucoma surgery.	IOP Inc.
Ofloxacin	Treatment of bacterial corneal ulcers.	Allergan Inc. P.O. Box 19534 Irvine, CA 92713-9534
Pilocarpine HCl (*Salagen*)	Treatment of xerostomia induced by radiation therapy for head and neck cancer; xerostomia and keratoconjunctivitis sicca in Sjogren's syndrome.	MGI Pharma, Inc.
Propamidine Isethionate 0.1% (*Brolen*)	Treatment of *Acanthamoeba keratitis.*	Bausch and Lomb, Inc. 1400 N. Goodman Street Rochester, NY 14692
Retinoin	To treat squamous metaplasia of the ocular surface epithelia (conjunctiva or cornea) with mucus deficiency and keratinization.	Hannan Ophthalmic Marketing

Orphan Drugs		
Drug Generic *(Trade)*	**Indication**	**Manufacturer/Sponsor**
Urogastrone	Acceleration of corneal epithelial regeneration and healing of stromal incisions from transplant surgery.	Chiron Vision 4560 Horton St. Emeryville, CA 94608

The Orphan Drug Act has provided an environment for the development of products for rare diseases and should continue to facilitate this process. In 1984, the Orphan Drug Act was amended to define a rare disease or condition as that which (a) affects fewer than 200,000 persons or (b) affects more than 200,000 persons and for which the manufacturing company has no reasonable prospect of recovering research and development costs from sales within the US. Occasionally, a drug which is already commercially available may achieve orphan status for an indication that does not involve a large patient population. The incentives provided by both the Orphan Drug Act and other federal initiatives make it possible for commercial manufacturers to produce drugs for FDA approval at minimal costs. Individuals with rare diseases can be assured that efforts will continue to be made to find a treatment.

Published information about orphan drugs is made available by various agencies. These sources can be contacted to obtain information about the acquisition or availability of an orphan drug product.

Information Sources For Rare Diseases And Orphan Drug Treatment		
Organization	**Information**	**Telephone**
National Organization for Rare Disorders (NORD) P.O. Box 8923 New Fairfield, CT 06812-8923	Information on rare diseases and their treatment.	(203) 746-6518
Federal Register. Dockets Management Branch (HFA-305) Food and Drug Administration Room 4-62 5600 Fishers Lane Rockville, MD 20857	List of orphan drugs and biologicals, designated uses, sponsor's name and address. Available under Docket #84N-0102.	not available
Office of Orphan Products Development (HF-35) Food and Drug Administration 5600 Fishers Lane Rockville, MD 20857	Technical information on orphan drug product development, product availability, research grants, drug sponsorship.	(301) 443-2043

Tatro, DS. Orphan Drugs. *Drug Newsletter* 1988 Apr;7(4):26.

INVESTIGATIONAL NEW DRUGS

The FDA is responsible for determining if a new drug is safe and effective before it is approved for marketing. During the IND process, scientific and statistical information about the drug is gathered. The FDA cannot release information pertaining to formulas, manufacturing processes or identification of patients involved in clinical trials. However, the Freedom of Information Act does allow release of specially prepared information which does not contain trade or confidential information.

New Drug Development		
Stage	**Description**	**Duration**
Preclinical Trials	Research and development, initial drug synthesis and animal testing.	1 to 3 years (average 18 months)
IND filing	Allows interstate transport and human testing.	30 days
Clinical Trials		2 to 10 years (average 5 years)
Phase I:	Determine drug safety, tolerance, pharmacokinetics in 20 to 100 normal adult males.	Several months

New Drug Development		
Stage	**Description**	**Duration**
Phase II:	Given to 100 to 200 people with the disease to determine effectiveness and dose response.	Up to 2 years
Phase III:	Assessment of safety and efficacy in 800 to 1000 patients. Studies include drug interactions, use in the elderly and in liver and kidney disease.	1 to 4 years
NDA Review	NDA submitted to FDA for approval to market.	2 months to 7 years (average 24 months)
Post-market surveillance	Adverse reaction reporting, survey/samples and inspections.	Ongoing

A practitioner may obtain a Treatment IND allowing the use of IND drugs in a controlled situation. There are two ways to obtain a Treatment IND: 1) Contact the drug sponsor or 2) contact the FDA directly.

The sponsor usually provides a practitioner with technical information about the drug and a description of the approved treatment protocol. When the sponsor is unwilling to provide the treatment protocol, an individual may contact the FDA. The practitioner must meet all of the FDA's requirements for a Treatment IND. The FDA must respond to the request for a Treatment IND within 30 days of the application.

Investigational Drugs			
Drug Name Generic *(Trade)*	**Developmental Stage**	**Class/Use**	**Manufacturer/ Sponsor**
4197X-RA	Phase II	Monoclonal antibody based immunotoxin for use following primary extracapsular cataract surgery to prevent secondary cataract.	Houston Biotechnology Inc.
Adaprolol Maleate	Phase II	For treatment of glaucoma using Site-Active targeted delivery system.	Pharmos Corp.
Adenosine Regulating Agents	Research	ARAs for ophthalmic indications.	Allergan
AF2975	Phase I	Tear stimulation.	Angelini
AGN-191045	Phase II	Prostaglandin prodrug/treatment of ocular hypertension and chronic open-angle glaucoma.	Allergan
Alpha-1 antichymotrypsin (*LEX001*)	Research	Treatment of inflammatory diseases of the eye.	Lexin Pharmaceutical Corp.
Alpha-2 Agonist	Research	Treatment for glaucoma.	Synaptic Pharmaceutical Corp.
Aminocaproic acid (*ACA*)	Clinicals	Treatment of hyphema.	Chronimed, Inc.
Aminocaproic acid (*ACA*)	Pre-IND Filing	Treatment of traumatic hyphema.	Orphan Medical
Analgesic, ophthalmic	Phase I	Topical analgesic for ocular pain associated with chronic conditions such as dry eye, and for pain following ophthalmic surgery.	Telor Ophthalmic Pharmaceuticals
APC-366-2	Research	Tryptase inhibitor/nonsteroidal anti-inflammatory for treatment of conjunctivitis.	Bayer
APC-366-C	Research	Tryptase inhibitor/nonsteroidal anti-inflammatory for treatment of conjunctivitis.	Arris Pharmaceutical Corp.
Batimastat (*BB-94*)	Phase I Completed	Prevention of postsurgical recurrence of pyterygium using DuraSite delivery.	InSite Vision/ British Biotech
Benzoporphyrin derivative (*BPD*)	Phase I	Photodynamic therapy for treatment of age-related macular degeneration.	Quadra Logic Technologies Inc.

Investigational Drugs			
Drug Name Generic *(Trade)*	**Developmental Stage**	**Class/Use**	**Manufacturer/ Sponsor**
Beta-glucan receptor antagonists	Research	Prevention and treatment of inflammatory diseases and disorders such as allergic conjunctivitis.	Alpha-Beta Technology, Inc.
BL-016/FL-1003	Preclinicals	Monokine and leukotriene antagonist for control of the migration of neutrophils and lymphocytes, reduction of acute and chronic (immune) inflammation.	Forest Pharm
Botulinum toxin type A	Phase II	Treatment of synkinetic closure of the eyelid associated with VII cranial nerve aberrant regeneration.	Biopure Corporation
Bromhexine HCl (*Bisolvon*)	Phase II/III	Treatment for mild-to-moderate keratoconjunctivitis sicca associated with Sjogren syndrome.	Boehringer Ingelheim/Pharmaceutical Discovery Group
CBT-101	Phase I/II	Pentapeptide/treatment of glaucoma.	Carlbiotech Ltd. A/S
Cell adhesion molecule (CAM) inhibitors	Research	Treatment of ophthamologic infectious diseases.	Chiron Corp.
Cell transplant product, universal retinal epithelial	Research	Treatment of eye diseases, including age-related macular degeration.	Cell Genesys, Inc.
CI-922	Phase I	Treatment for inflammatory conditions, including conjunctivitis.	Parke-Davis Division (Warner-Lambert)
CI-949	Phase I/II	Treatment for allergic and inflammatory conditions, including conjunctivitis.	Parke-Davis Division (Warner-Lambert)
Cidofovir (*GS-504*)	Preclinicals	Treatment of a variety of ophthalmic viruses including adenovirus.	Gilead Sciences, Inc.
Clostridium botulinum toxin type A (*Dysport*)	Phase III	Treatment of ocular muscle disorders including blepharospasm.	Speywood Pharmaceuticals, Inc.
Clostridium botulinum toxin type A (*Dysport*)	Undisclosed	Treatment of ocular muscle disorders including torticollis.	Speywood Pharmaceuticals, Inc.
Clostridium botulinum toxin type F	Undisclosed	Treatment of essential blepharospasm, spasmodic torticollis.	Speywood Pharmaceuticals, Inc.
Corneal collagen shield	Preclinicals	Drug delivery to the eye.	Chiron Corp.
Corneal mortar	Preclinicals	Wound healing agent for use in radial keratomy.	Chiron Corp.
Cyclocreatine (*AM-285*)	Preclinicals	Treatment for cyclomegalovirus retinitis.	Repligen Corp.
Cyclosporine	Phase III	Immunosuppressive agent.	Sandoz Pharmaceuticals, Inc.
Cyclosporine (*Sandimmune*)	Approved	Immunosuppresive agent for the treatment of keratoconjunctivitis sicca.	Allergan
Dehydrex	Phase III	Treatment of recurrent corneal erosion.	Holles Labs
Dexanabinol (*HU-211*)	Phase I	Treatment of glaucoma and optic neuropathies.	Pharmos Corp.
Dronabinol (*Marinol*)	Clinicals	Treatment of glaucoma.	Unimed Pharmaceuticals, Inc.
Ethacrynate sodium (*Xarano*)	Phase III	Prevention/reduction of transient postoperative increases in IOP following cataract eye surgery.	Telor Ophthalmic Pharmaceuticals
Ethacrynic acid analogues	Preclinicals	Antiglaucoma products for control of IOP by increasing outflow from eye.	Telor Ophthalmic Pharmaceuticals

Investigational Drugs			
Drug Name Generic *(Trade)*	**Developmental Stage**	**Class/Use**	**Manufacturer/ Sponsor**
EY-128	Phase I	To control pupil constriction during cataract surgery (surgical miosis).	Telor Ophthalmic Pharmaceuticals
Fibronectin	Phase III	Treatment of non-healing corneal ulcers or epithelial defects unres- ponsive to conventional therapy.	New York Blood Center, Inc.
Fluorometholone (*MethaSite*)	Amended NDA filed	Treatment of allergic conjunctivitis, reduction in postoperative eye inflammation, using DuraSite sustained release twice-daily delivery system.	Ciba Vision/InSite Vision
Foscarnet sodium/ddl *trisodium phosphono-formate/dideoxyinosine*	Undisclosed	Treatment of cytomegalovirus (CMV) retinitis.	Astra USA, Inc.
Glycosaminoglycans	Research	Treatment of conditions affecting eye.	CytRx Corp.
Growth factors	Research	Protection of the cornea and retina.	Houston Biotechnology, Inc.
Heparanase	Research	Treatment for a variety of burns, surgical/incisional wounds, including ophthalmic injuries.	ImClone Systems, Inc./Lederle Labs
Hyaluronic acid (HA) (hyalectin; (*Hyalf*)	PMA Submitted	Surgical aid in ophthalmic surgery.	Fidia Pharmaceutical Corp.
Hypericin (aromatic polycyclic dione) (APD-1) (*VIMRxyn*)	Preclinicals	Treatment of cytomegalovirus (CMV) retinitis.	VIMRx Pharmaceuticals
Imaging agents	Research	Detection and localization of cancer cells.	Mallinckrodt Medical/OP-TIMEDx
Immunotoxin, monoclonal antibody (MAb)-based	Research	Treatment for proliferative vitreoretinopathy and eye muscle spasms.	Houston Biotechnology Inc.
Implant delivery technology	Phase III	Antiviral implant for treatment of cytomegalovirus (CMV) retinitis in AIDS patients.	Chiron Corp.
Insulin-like growth factor (IGF)/BP3 complex (*SomatoKine*)	Phase III	Treatment of surgical/traumatic wounds and ophthalmic diseases.	Celtrix Pharmaceuticals, Inc.
ISIS-2922	Phase III	Treatment of cytomegalovirus (CMV) retinitis in AIDS patients.	Eisai America/ ISIS Pharmaceuticals
ISV-205	Preclinicals	Antiglaucoma agent for protection of the trabecular meshwork and prevention of disease progression.	InSite Vision
Levobunolol HCl (*BetaSite*)	Phase III	Treatment of glaucoma, using DuraSite sustained release eye drop delivery.	Insite Vision
Levobunolol HCl/ dipivefrin HCl	NDA filed	Chronic treatment of glaucoma and ocular hypertension.	Allergan
Lexipafant (BB-882)	Preclinicals	Treatment for ocular inflammation.	British Biotech/ InSite Vision
LGD-1057	Phase I	9-CIS retinoic acid/treatment for non-cancer indications, eye disease.	Ligant Pharmaceuticals, Inc.
LGD-1057 analogues	Research	9-CIS retinoic acid analogues/treatment for oncologic eye disease.	Ligant Pharmaceuticals/Allergan
LGD-1069	Phase I/IIa	Reinoid X receptors/selective retinoid-retinoic acid receptor, treatment of eye disease.	Ligant Pharmaceuticals, Inc.
LGD-1069 analogues	Research	Reinoid X receptors/retinoid-retinoic acid analogues/ treatment of cancer, premalignancy, eye disease.	Ligant Pharmaceuticals, Inc.

Investigational Drugs			
Drug Name Generic *(Trade)*	**Developmental Stage**	**Class/Use**	**Manufacturer/ Sponsor**
Loteprednol etabonate (*Lotemax*)	NDA filed	Treatment of contact lens associated giant papillary conjunctivitis, seasonal allergic conjunctivitis and uveitis using Site-Active targeted delivery technology.	Pharmos Corp.
Loteprednol etabonate *Lotemax*	Clinicals	Treatment of ophthalmic inflammations and allergies, using Site-Active targeted delivery technology.	Pharmos Corp.
Loteprednol etabonate/ tobramycin	Preclinicals	Combination anti-inflammatory/anti-infective.	Pharmos Corp.
Mitotoxin conjugate	Research	Proprietary mitotoxin conjugate of fibroblast growth factor linked to saporin/topical glaucoma therapies.	Prizm Pharmaceuticals, Inc.
Molgramostim/ganciclovir *Leucomax*	Phase III	Biosynthetic GM-CSF in combination with ganciclovir treatment for cytomegalovirus (CMV) retinitis.	Sandoz Pharmaceuticals Corp.
Monoclonal antibodies	Research	Antiangiogenesis agent for treatment of ophthalmic eye disorders.	Ixsys, Inc.
MSI-239/erythroycin	Preclinicals	Treatment of keratitis.	Magainin Pharmaceuticals
MSI-420	Preclinicals	Antimicrobial wound healing agent for eye infection and promotion of corneal epithelialization.	Magainin Pharmaceuticals
N-acetylcysteine (NAC) (*Fluimucil*)	Phase III	Treatment of severe dry eye syndrome.	Zambon Corp.
Nedocromil sodium (*Tilade*)	Phase III Completed	Ophthalmic solution.	Medeva/Allergan
Neurotrophic factor, lung derived (LDNF)	Research	Treatment of glaucoma.	Houston Biotechnology, Inc.
Neutrophic factors (NTFs)	Research	Treatment of neurodegenerative and other diseases, including ocular diseases.	Glaxo Wellcome/ Regeron Pharmaceuticals, Inc.
OcuNex	Phase II	Treatment of dry eye syndrome and promotion of healing after eye injuries, infections or eye surgery.	Telios Pharmaceuticals, Inc.
Oligonucleotide-based therapeutics	Research	Treatment of inflammatory and viral diseases of the eye, using InSite delivery system.	Genta, Inc./InSite Vision
Pantetheine (*OC-2*)	Phase II/III	Prevention of cataracts.	Oculon Corp.
Pilocarpine	Phase II Completed	Treatment of glaucoma, using Submicron Emulsion (SME) delivery system.	Pharmos Corp.
Pilocarpine (*PilaSite*)	Phase III	Treatment of chronic glaucoma, using DuraSite sustained release eye drop delivery system.	Ciba Vision/InSite Vision
Pilocarpine HCl (*MGI-647; Salagen*)	Phase III	Treatment of xerostomia and keratoconjunctivitis sicca in Sjogren syndrome.	MGI PHARMA, Inc.
Pilolactam (AGN-191053)	Phase I/II	Treatment for chronic glaucoma.	Allergan
Pimagedine HCl	Preclinicals	Prevention of certain complications of aging, including cataracts.	Alteon, Inc./ Hoechst Marion Roussel
Pimagedine HCl	Phase II	Treatment of retinopathy.	Alteon Inc./ Hoechst Marion Roussel
Procaterol	Phase II	Treatment of allergic conjunctivitis.	Otskua American Pharmaceutical

Investigational Drugs			
Drug Name Generic *(Trade)*	**Developmental Stage**	**Class/Use**	**Manufacturer/ Sponsor**
Proparacaine (*ISV-701*)	Phase I/II Completed	Topical anesthetic/adjunct in ophthalmic surgery, using DuraSite sustained release delivery system.	InSite Vision
Prostaglandin Compound	Preclinicals	Treatment of chronic glaucoma and ocular hypertension.	Allergan
Protein kinase C (PKC)	Research	Treatment for ocular inflammation.	Sphinx Pharmaceuticals Corp.
RMP-7	Research	Bradykinin analogue for drug delivery to the eye/receptor mediated permeabilizer (RMP) delivery technology for ocular indications.	Alkermes, Inc.
RMP-7/adjunct	Preclinicals	Bradykinin analogue/adjunct, treatment of cytomegalovirus (CMV) retinitis, using receptor mediated permeabilizer (RMP) delivery technology.	Alkermes, Inc.
Servirumab (MSL-109; monoclonal antibody (MAb)	Phase I Completed	Treatment for cytomegalovirus (CMV) infection in AIDS patients (retinitis).	Protein Design Labs/Sandoz Pharm.
Smooth muscle agent, presbyopia	Phase I/II Completed	Treatment of presbyopia.	Telor Ophthalmic Pharmaceuticals
Sodium hyaluronate (*BioLon*)	Clinicals	Surgical aid for protection of the corneal endothelium during intraocular surgery.	Bio-Technology General Corp.
Tirilazad mesylate (*ISV-600, U-74006*)	Preclinicals	Antioxidant with non-systemic ophthalmic applications, using DuraSite delivery system.	InSite Vision/ Pharmacia & Upjohn
Tobramycin/prednisolone (*ToPreSite*)	Phase III	Combination anti-inflammation agents in DuraSite formulation and after cataract surgery.	InSite Vision
Transforming growth factor (TGF)-beta receptors	Research	Types II and III receptors/treatment for ophthalmic and fibrotic diseases.	Celtrix Pharmaceuticals
Transforming growth factor beta-1 (TGF-b1)	Preclinicals	Healing agent for ophthalmic use.	Escalon Ophthalmics, Inc./ Genentech, Inc.
Transforming growth factor beta-2 (TGF-b2) (*BetaKine*)	Phase II	Treatment of age-related macular degeneration of the retina.	Celtrix Pharmaceuticals
Transforming growth factor beta-2 (TGF-b2) (*BetaKine*)	Phase III	Treatment of macular holes.	Celtrix Pharmaceuticals
Transforming growth factor beta-2 (TGF-b2) (*BetaKine*)	Preclinicals	Treatment of post-surgical corneal wounds.	Celtrix Pharmaceuticals
Transforming growth factor beta-2 (TGF-b2) (*BetaKine*)	Phase II	Treatment of retinal (macular) edema.	Celtrix Pharmaceuticals
Verapamil (*Caloptic*)	Phase III	Treatment for ocular hypertension and other symptoms of glaucoma.	Cooper Vision Pharmaceuticals
Viscoelastic substance	Preclinicals	Substance for use in ophthalmic surgery.	Chiron Corp.
(*Vision AID*)	Clinicals	Treatment of *Retinitis pigmentosa*.	Platon J. Collipp, MD
Zenarestat (*FK-366*)	Phase II	Treatment of diabetic cataract.	Fujisawa USA
Zopolrestat (*CP-73,850*)	Phase III	Treatment of retinopathy.	Pfizer, Inc.

ODF 1998

American Optometric Association Guidelines

The following sections are excerpted from the American Optometric Association *Clinical Practice Guidelines* for management of conjunctivitis, open-angle glaucoma and acute anterior uveitis. Clinicians should not rely on these guidelines alone for patient care and management but, instead, should refer also to other sources for more detailed discussion of patient care information. These guidelines are copyrighted by the American Optometric Association and reprinted courtesy of that organization.

Frequency and Composition of Evaluation and Management Visits for Conjunctivitis

Type of Patient	Frequency of Followup	History	Visual Acuity	Slit Lamp Biomicroscopy	Ophthalmoscopy	Management Plan
Allergic Conjunctivitis	Mild—every 5-7 days Moderate—every 3-5 days Severe—every 1-3 days	Yes	Yes	Yes	As indicated	Identify/remove allergen Use of nonpreserved lubricants, cold compresses, topical pharmaceuticals, systemic antihistamines Educate patient
Bacterial Conjunctivitis	Mild—every 5-7 days Moderate—every 3-5 days Severe—every 1-3 days	Yes	Yes	Yes	As indicated	Identify organism and specific antimicrobial agent Hyperacute form: obtain smears and cultures, do saline lavage Use of topical and/or systemic antibiotics Refer for evaluation and treatment of underlying systemic condition Educate patient
Viral Conjunctivitis	Mild—every 5-7 days Moderate—every 3-5 days Severe—every 1-3 days	Yes	Yes	Yes	As indicated	Use of cold compresses, lubricants, ocular decongestants Herpes simplex: use of antiviral agent Herpes zoster: use of topical antibiotic/steroid combinations Educate patient

Frequency and Composition of Evaluation and Management Visits for Conjunctivitis						
Type of Patient	Frequency of Followup	History	Visual Acuity	Slit Lamp Biomicroscopy	Ophthalmoscopy	Management Plan
Chlamydial Conjunctivitis	Mild—every 5-7 days Moderate—every 3-5 days Severe—every 1-3 days	Yes	Yes	Yes	As indicated	Use of systemic antibiotics Refer for evaluation and treatment of underlying systemic condition Educate patient

Frequency and Composition of Evaluation and Management Visits for Open Angle Glaucoma							
Type of Patient	Frequency of Examination	Tonometry	Gonioscopy	ON/NFL Assessment	Stereoscopic ON and FNL Photography	Perimetry*	Management Plan
New glaucoma patient or new glaucoma suspect	Weekly or biweekly to achieve target pressure	Multiple readings may be necessary to establish baseline	Standard classification and drawing at initial visit	Dilate; optic nerve drawing at initial visit	As part of initial glaucoma evaluation	Repeat to establish baseline	Prepare problem list with treatment plan
Glaucoma suspect	6-12 months, depending on level of risk	Multiple readings may be necessary to establish baseline	Annual	Dilate every other visit	Every 2 years	Annual	Review
Stable – mild stage	4-6 months	Every visit	Annual	Dilate every other visit	Annual	Annual	Review
Stable – moderate stage	2-4 months	Every visit	Annual	Dilate every other visit	Annual	6 months	Review
Stable – severe state	1-3 months	Every visit	6 months	Dilate every other visit	Annual	3-4 months	Review
Unstable – IOP poorly controlled; ON or VF progressing	Weekly or biweekly until stability is established	Every visit	Initial visit and each time other clinical findings warrant a reassessment	Dilate at initial visit and each time other clinical findings warrant reassessment	Annual or each time ON or NFL changes	4-6 weeks or as needed to establish new baseline	Formulate new plan until stable
Recently established stability	1-3 months	Every visit; re-establish baseline	Depends on severity of the glaucoma	Dilate every interim visit	Annual or each time ON or NFL changes	Depends on severity of the disease	Review

* Threshold automated perimetry is recommended.

Acute Anterior Uveitis: Treatment and Followup*

1. Mild uveitis (Optional depending on symptoms)
   a. Cyclopentolate, 1% (tid) or homatropine, 5% (bid-tid)
   b. Prednisolone, 1% (bid-qid)[a]
   c. Oral aspirin or ibuprofen, 2 tablets (q 4 h)[b]
   d. Consider beta blockers if IOP is elevated
   e. Re-evaluate 4–7 days (or prn if worsening)

2. Refer to primary care physician for systemic evaluation (when indicated)

3. Moderate uveitis
   a. Homatropine, 5% (qid) or scopolamine, 0.25% (bid)
   b. Prednisolone, 1% (qid)[a]
   c. Oral aspirin or ibuprofen, 2 tablets (q 4 h)[b]
   d. Consider beta blockers if IOP is elevated
   e. Dark glasses
   f. Advise patient carefully (eg, pain, course, compliance)
   g. Re-evaluate in 2 to 4 days (or prn)

4. Severe uveitis
   a. Atropine, 1% (bid-tid) or homatropine, 5% (q 4 h)
   b. Prednisolone, 1% (q 2 to 4 h)[a]
   c. Oral aspirin or ibuprofen, 2 tablets (q 3 to 4 h)[b]
   d. Consider beta blockers if IOP is elevated
   e. Dark glasses
   f. Advise patient carefully
   g. Re-evaluate in 1 to 2 days

[a] Shake steroid suspensions well before using. May use dexamethasone or fluorometholone steroid ointments at bedtime.
[b] Contraindicated in the presence of concurrent hyphema.

---

* Adapted from Catania LJ. Primary care of the anterior segment, 2nd ed. Norwalk, CT: Appleton & Lange, 1995;372.

ODF 1998

Excipient Glossary

Acetic acid: Buffering (acidifying), tonicity agent.

Acetone sodium bisulfite: Antioxidant (0.01% to 1%).

Acetoxyphenylmercury, see Phenylmercuric acetate.

Acetylcysteine: Mucolytic, corneal vulnerary; antioxidant.

Alcohol (ethanol, ethyl alcohol): Solvent, preservative.

Alkyl ether sulfate, see Sodium lauryl sulfate.

Aluminum tristearate: Astringent.

Amphoteric 10: Wetting, solubilizing, emulsifying agent.

Anhydrous lanolin, see Lanolin anhydrous.

Anhydrous liquid lanolin: Absorbent ointment base.

Anhydrous sodium carbonate, see Sodium carbonate.

Antibacterial: Kill, suppress bacteria growth.

Antifungal: Kill, suppress fungus growth.

Antimicrobial: Kill, suppress microorganism growth.

Antioxidants: Prevent, delay deterioration of products by oxygen.

Ascorbic acid (vitamin C): Antioxidant (0.01% to 0.1%.)

Astringent: Topical agent causing contraction of tissues or arresting of secretions.

Bacqucil, see Polyhexamethylene biguanide.

Bacteriostatic: Agent that inhibits bacteria growth or reproduction.

Baking soda, see Sodium bicarbonate.

Benzalkonium chloride: Antimicrobial preservative (0.05% to 0.02%) (0.01% most common). Most effective at pH 8.

Benzene ethanol, see Phenylethyl alcohol.

Benzethonium chloride: Antimicrobial preservative. Maximum concentration for direct instillation into eye is 1:10,000 (0.01%).

Benzoate of soda, see Sodium benzoate.

Benzyl alcohol: Antimicrobial preservative at concentrations less than 2%. Solvent at concentrations of greater than 5%. Also used as local anesthetic, antiseptic.

Benzyl carbinol, see Phenylethyl alcohol.

Boric acid: Tonicity, antiseptic, buffering agent at 2%.

Bovine catalase, see Catalase.

Buffering agents: Substances which stabilize pH of solutions against changes produced by introduction of acids or bases.

Camphor: Counterirritant, local anesthetic; topical cream; not for use in eye.

Carbamide: Antibacterial.

Carbomer 934P: Suspending, emulsifying agent in suspensions and gels.

Carbopol 940, see Carbomer 934P.

Carboxymethylcellulose sodium: Viscosity-increasing, suspending agent.

Catalase (bovine catalase): Enzymes which promote reactions involving decomposition of hydrogen peroxide to water and oxygen.

Cationic cellulose derivative polymer: Wetting agent.

Cellulose methyl ether, see Methylcellulose.

Cetanol, see Cetyl alcohol.

Cetyl alcohol (cetanol, palmityl alcohol): Used in ointment as a stiffening, emulsifying agent.

Cetylpyridinium chloride: Antimicrobial preservative and disinfectant.

Chlorhexidine: Antibacterial and antiseptic.

Chlorhexidine gluconate: Preservative in concentrations of 0.01% and disinfection of contact lenses in concentrations of 0.002% to 0.006%.

Chlorobutanol: Antimicrobial preservative (0.15% to 0.5%). Should be used in solutions pH 5 to 5.5.

Chlorobutanol anhydrase, see Chlorobutanol.

Cholesterol: Emulsifying, solubilizing agent in ointments.

Citnatin, see Sodium citrate.

Citric acid (2-hydroxy-1,2,3-propane-tricarboxylic acid): Sequestering, buffering (acidifying) and antioxidant agent.

Citrosodine, see Sodium citrate.

CMC, see Carboxymethylcellulose sodium.

Demulcent: Soothes and relieves irritated, inflamed or abraded areas.

Dextran 40: Tonicity, demulcent, wetting agent.

Dextran 70: Viscosity-increasing, tonicity, demulcent, wetting agent.

Dextrose: Tonicity agent.

Dibasic sodium phosphate, see Disodium hydrogen phosphate.

Disinfectant: Destroys or inhibits growth or activity of pathogenic microorganisms.

Disodium hydrogen phosphate, see Sodium phosphate.

Disodium hydrogen phosphate dihydrate: Buffering agent.

Disodium laureth sulfosuccinate: Wetting agent.

Edetates, see EDTA.

Edetate disodium, see EDTA.

Edetic acid, see EDTA.

EDTA (edetates, edetate disodium, edetic acid, ethylenediamine-tetraacetic acid): Enhances activity of preservatives (0.1%); antioxidant synergist, antibacterial. Chelating agent which sequesters trace metal ions necessary for autooxidation reactions and microbial growth (0.005% to 0.1%).

Emulsifying agent: Agent used to stabilize an emulsion.

Emulsion: Preparation of one liquid distributed in small globules throughout the body of a second immiscible liquid.

Ethanol, see Alcohol.

Ethoxylated polyoxypropylene glycol: Surfactant.

Ethyl alcohol, see Alcohol.

Ethylenediaminetetraacetic acid, see EDTA.

Eucalyptol: Antiseptic.

Fatty acid amide: Surfactant.

Fungicide: Agent that destroys fungus.

Gelatin: Viscosity-increasing, emulsifying, suspending agent.

Gelatin A, see Gelatin.

Germicide: Agent that kills microorganisms.

Glycerin: Viscosity-increasing, tonicity, agent; lubricant; preservative; solvent.

Glycerol monostearate: Emulsifying, solubilizing agent.

Glycerol stearate, see Glyceryl monostearate.

Glyceryl monostearate (glycerol monostearate, glycerol stearate): Emulsifying, solubilizing, thickening agent.

Glycols, see Propylene glycol.

Hamamelis water: Astringent.

Humectant: Moistening agent.

Hydrochloric acid: Acidifying agent.

Hydrogen peroxide: Disinfectant.

Hydroxyethyl cellulose: Viscosity-increasing, suspending agent.

Hydroxypropyl methylcellulose (methyl hydroxypropylcellulose, methylcellulose propylene glycol ether): Viscosity-increasing, demulcent, suspending agent.

Hydroxypropyl methylcellulose 2906, see Hydroxypropyl methylcellulose.

Hydroxypropyl methylcellulose 2910, see Hydroxypropyl methylcellulose.

Hypertonicity agent, see Tonicity agent.

Isopropanol, see Isopropyl alcohol.

Isopropyl alcohol (isopropanol): Solvent, disinfectant.

Lactose: Diluent.

Lanolin: Ointment base, emulsion.

Lanolin alcohol: Paraffin-base substance containing 6% alcohol used in preparation of water-in-oil creams and ointments; emulsifying, solubilizing agent.

Lanolin anhydrous: Used in preparation of absorbent ointment base.

Lanolin oil: Emulsifying, suspending agent.

Laureth-23: Surfactant, emulsifying, solubilizing, wetting agent.

Lauryl sulfate salt of imidazoline, see Sodium lauryl sulfate.

Light mineral oil, see Mineral oil.

Liquid paraffin, see Mineral oil.

Liquid petrolatum, see Mineral oil.

Magnesium chloride: Electrolyte.

Magnesium chloride hexahydrate, see Magnesium chloride.

Manita, see Mannitol.

Manna sugar, see Mannitol.

Mannite, see Mannitol.

Mannitol (manita, manna sugar, mannite): Tonicity agent.

Menthol: Counterirritant, local analgesic; not for use in the eye.

Mercurial preservatives, see Thimerosal.

Mercurothiolate, see Thimerosal.

Merphenyl nitrate, see Phenylmercuric nitrate.

Methylcellulose (cellulose methyl ether): Viscosity-increasing, wetting, soaking, suspending agent.

Methylcellulose propylene glycol ether, see Hydroxypropyl methylcellulose.

Methyl glycol, see Propylene glycol.

Methyl hydroxypropylcellulose, see Hydroxypropyl methylcellulose.

Methylparaben, see Parabens.

Methyl/propylparaben, see Parabens.

Microclens polymeric: Cleaner.

Mineral oil (liquid paraffin, liquid petrolatum): Vehicle, emollient, solvent.

Monosodium phosphate, see Sodium phosphate.

Mucolytic agent: To destroy, liquify or dissolve mucus.

Octoxynol 40: Detergent, emulsifying, dispersing agent.

Octylphenoxypolyethoxyethanol: Surfactant.

Palmityl alcohol, see Cetyl alcohol.

Parabens: Parahydroxybenzoic acid esters mixtures sometimes used as antimicrobial preservative. FDA found them unacceptable as ophthalmic solution preservatives.

PEG, see Polyethylene glycol.

PEG-15 tallow polyamine, see Polyethylene glycol.

PEG-78 glyceryl monococoate, see Polyethylene glycol.

PEG-80 glyceryl cocoate, see Polyethylene glycol.

PEG-80 sorbitan laurate, see Polyethylene glycol.

PEG-90M, see Polyethylene glycol.

PEG-150 distearate, see Polyethylene glycol.

PEG-200 glyceryl monotallowate, see Polyethylene glycol.

PEG 300, see Polyethylene glycol.

PEG 400, see Polyethylene glycol.

PEG 8000, see Polyethylene glycol.

Petrolatum: Emollient, ointment base.

Petroleum jelly, see Petrolatum.

Phenethyl alcohol, see Phenylethyl alcohol.

Phenol: Germicide, preservative.

Phenylethanol, see Phenylethyl alcohol.

Phenylethyl alcohol (benzene ethanol, benzyl carbinol, phenethyl alcohol, phenylethanol): Antimicrobial preservative (0.25% to 0.5%).

Phenylmercuric acetate (acetoxyphenylmercury): Mercurial antimicrobial preservative (0.002% to 0.004%).

Phenylmercuric borate (phenylmercuriborate, phenomerborum): Antimicrobial preservative, antiseptic agent (0.002% to 0.004%).

Phenylmercuric nitrate (merphenyl nitrate): Mercurial antiseptic, antimicrobial preservative (0.002% to 0.004%).

Phosphonic acid, see Phosphoric acid.

Phosphoric acid: Buffering (acidifying), tonicity agent; solvent.

Poloxamer: Solubilizing, wetting, gelling, emulsifying, viscosity-increasing agent; ointment base.

Poloxamer 185, see Poloxamer.

Poloxamer 188, see Poloxamer.

Poloxamer 282, see Poloxamer.

Poloxamer 407, see Poloxamer.

Poloxalene: Surfactant.

Polycarbophil: Vehicle which increases bioavailability by prolonging medication release.

Polyethylene base, see Polyethylene glycol.

Polyethylene glycol (PEG, polyoxyethylene glycol): Viscosity-increasing, gelling, solubilizing, suspending agent; water-soluble ointment base; solvent.

Polyethylene glycol 400, see Polyethylene glycol.

Polyhema (polyhydroxyethylmethacrylate): Ingredient used in drug matrices.

Polyhexamethylene biguanide (bacqucil): Disinfectant.

Polyhydroxyethylmethacrylate, see Polyhema.

Polyoxyethylene glycol, see Polyethylene glycol.

Polyoxyethylene polyoxpropylene: Emulsifying, wetting, solubilizing agent; defoamer; detergent, lubricant.

Polyoxyl 35 castor oil: Emulsifying, solubilizing, wetting agent; surfactant.

Polyoxyl 40 stearate: Surfactant, emulsifier.

Polyquaternium-1: Disinfection agent used in contact lens care systems.

Polysorbate 20: Wetting, solubilizing agent; emulsifying surfactant.

Polysorbate 60: Wetting, solubilizing agent; emulsifying surfactant.

Polysorbate 80: Viscosity-increasing, wetting, solubilizing agent; emulsifying surfactant.

Polyvidone, see Povidone.

Polyvinyl alcohol (PVA): Suspending, viscosity-increasing agent; emulsifier; lubricant; protectant.

Polyvinylpyrrolidone, see Povidone.

Potassium bicarbonate: Buffering, tonicity agent.

Potassium borate: Buffering, tonicity agent.

Potassium carbonate: Buffering (alkalinizing), tonicity agent.

Potassium chloride: Tonicity agent.

Potassium citrate: Buffering, tonicity agent.

Potassium phosphate: Buffering, tonicity agent.

Potassium sorbate: Antimicrobial preservative.

Potassium tetraborate: Buffering, tonicity agent.

Povidone (polyvidone, polyvinylpyrrolidone, PVP): Suspending, dispersing, viscosity-increasing agent.

Preservatives: Prevent or inhibit microorganism growth.

Propylene glycol (1,2-propanediol, propane-1,2-diol, methyl glycol): Viscosity-increasing, tonicity, suspending agent; humectant; solvent; preservative.

Propylene oxide: Lubricant, surfactant, oil demulsifier, solvent.

Propylparaben, see Parabens.

PVA, see Polyvinyl alcohol.

PVP, see Povidone.

Quaternium-15: Emulsifying agent, detergent-germicide, surfactant.

Retinol palmitate: Antioxidant.

Silica gel: Stabilizing, suspending agent.

Sodium acetate: Tonicity, buffering agent.

Sodium acetate trihydrate, see Sodium acetate.

Sodium acid carbonate, see Sodium bicarbonate.

Sodium benzoate (benzoate of soda): Antifungal and bacteriostatic preservative (0.1%).

Sodium bicarbonate (baking soda, sodium acid carbonate, sodium hydrogen carbonate): Buffering, tonicity, alkalinizing agent.

Sodium biphosphate: Buffering, tonicity agent.

Sodium bisulfite: Antioxidant (0.01% to 0.3%), stabilizing agent.

Sodium borate: Buffering, alkalinizing agent.

Sodium carbonate: Buffering, tonicity, alkalinizing agent.

Sodium cellulose glycolate, see Carboxymethylcellulose sodium.

Sodium chloride: Tonicity agent.

Sodium citrate (citnatin, citrosodine, trisodium citrate): Buffering, tonicity, alkalinizing agent. Buffer (0.3% to 2%).

Sodium citrate dihydrate, see Sodium citrate.

Sodium CMC, see Carboxymethylcellulose sodium.

Sodium dihydrogen phosphate hydrate, see Sodium phosphate.

Sodium ethylmercurothiosalicylate, see Thimerosal.

Sodium hydrogen carbonate, see Sodium bicarbonate.

Sodium hydroxide: Buffering, tonicity, alkalinizing agent.

Sodium lactate: Emulsifying agent.

Sodium lauryl sulfate: Emulsifying, solubilizing, wetting agent; detergent, surfactant.

Sodium metabisulfite: Antioxidant (0.01% to 0.3%).

Sodium perborate: Antiseptic.

Sodium phosphate: Buffering, tonicity agent.

Sodium phosphate, dibasic, see Disodium hydrogen phosphate.

Sodium phosphate, monobasic, see Disodium hydrogen phosphate.

Sodium propionate: Preservative, antifungal.

Sodium thiosulfate: Antioxidant, antifungal.

Solvent: Vehicle or substance that dissolves another substance.

Sorbic acid (2,4-hexadienoic acid, 2-propenylacrylic acid): Antimicrobial and preservative (0.05% to 0.2%); frequently used in combination with other antimicrobials.

Sorbitol: Vehicle, humectant, viscosity-increasing agent.

Stearic acid (octadecanoic acid, cetylacetic acid, stearophanic acid): Solidifying, emulsifying, solubilizing agent.

Sulfasuccinate: Emulsifying, wetting, dispersing agent.

Tartaric acid: Buffering and acidifying agent.

Thimerosal (mercurial preservatives, mercurothiolate, sodium ethylmercurothiosalicylate, thiomersalate): Mercurial antiseptic, antimicrobial preservative (0.005% to 0.02%).

Thiomersalate, see Thimerosal.

Thiourea: Antioxidant.

Titanium dioxide: UV absorbent; scatters UV light at 290 to 700nm.

Tonicity agent: Enables ophthalmic solutions to be isotonic with natural tears.

Tri-quaternary cocoa-based phospholipid: Buffering agent.

Tris (hydroxymethyl) amino methane, see Tromethamine.

Trisodium citrate, see Sodium citrate.

Tromethamine (tris [hydroxymethyl] aminomethane): Emulsifying, buffering agent.

Tween 21, see Polysorbate 80.

Tyloxapol: Wetting, solubilizing, emulsifying agent.

Viscosity-increasing agent: Prolongs contact time of product with eye, increasing drug absorption and activity.

Vitamin C, see Ascorbic acid.

Wetting agent: Reduces surface tension of eye.

White petrolatum, see Petrolatum.

Zinc sulfate: Weak antiseptic; recommended concentrations of 0.05% to 0.25%.

ODF 1998

Manufacturers and Distributors Index

00074
Abbott Laboratories
1 Abbott Park Road
Abbott Park, IL 60064-3500
847-937-6100

Advanced Vision Research
7 Alfred St., Suite 330
Woburn, MA 01801
617-932-8327

17478
Akorn, Inc.
100 Akorn Drive
Abita Springs, LA 70420
504-893-9300

00065, 00998
Alcon Laboratories, Inc.
6201 South Freeway
Ft. Worth, TX 76134
817-293-0450

00023
Allergan, Inc.
2525 DuPont Drive
Irvine, CA 92715-9534
800-433-8871

17314
Alza Corp.
950 Page Mill Road
Palo Alto, CA 94303-0802
415-494-5000

89709, 90605
Amcon Laboratories
40 N. Rock Hill Road
St. Louis, MO 63119
314-961-5758

00517
American Regent
1 Luitpold Drive
Shirley, NY 11967
516-924-4000

00003, 00015
Apothecon
P.O. Box 4500
Princeton, NJ 08543-4500
800-321-1335

Astra Pharmaceuticals Products
See Astra USA, Inc

00186
Astra USA, Inc.
50 Otis Street
Westborough, MA 01581
508-366-1100

Barnes-Hind
See PBH Wesley Jessen

10119
Bausch & Lomb Personal Products Division
1400 N. Goodman Street
P.O. Box 450
Rochester, NY 14692-0450
716-338-6000

24208, 57782
Bausch & Lomb Pharmaceuticals
8500 Hidden River Pkwy.
Tampa, FL 33637
813-975-7700

00338, 47679
Baxter Healthcare Corp.
Route 120 and Wilson Road
Round Lake, IL 60073
800-933-0303

12843, 16500
Bayer Corp. (Consumer Division)
P.O. Box 5967
Parsippany, NJ 07054
800-331-4536

31280
Becton Dickinson & Co.
One Becton Drive
Franklin Lakes, NJ 07417-1881
201-847-6800

55390
Bedford Laboratories
300 Northfield Road
Bedford, OH 44146
216-232-3320

50486
Blairex Labs, Inc.
P.O. Box 2127
Columbus, IN 47202-2127
812-378-1864

00081
Burroughs Wellcome Co.
See Glaxo Wellcome

00436
Century Pharmaceuticals, Inc.
10377 Hague Rd.
Indianapolis, IN 46256-3399
317-849-4210

Chiron Vision
555 W. Arrow Highway
Claremont, CA 91711
909-624-2020

Ciba Self-Medication, Inc.
See Novartis

00346
Ciba Vision Ophthalmics
11460 Johns Creek Pkwy.
Duluth, GA 30136
404-418-4101

Clintec Nutrition
Three Pkwy. North,
Suite 500
Deerfield, IL 60015
708-317-2800

00961
Cook-Waite Laboratories, Inc.
90 Park Ave.
New York, NY 10016
212-907-2000

59426
CooperVision
10 Faraday
Irvine, CA 92618
714-597-8130

54799
Cynacon/OCuSOFT
P.O. Box 429
Richmond, TX 77406-0429
800-233-5469

55994
Dakryon Pharmaceuticals
2579 S. Loop
Suite 8
Lubbock, TX 79423-1400
806-745-2872

10310
Del Pharmaceuticals, Inc.
163 East Bethpage
Plainview, NY 11803
516-293-7070

00777
Dista Products Co.
Lilly Corp. Center
Indianapolis, IN 46285
317-276-4000

Eagle Vision, Inc.
6263 Poplar Ave.
Suite 650
Memphis, TN 38119
901-767-3937

00641
Elkins-Sinn, Inc.
See Wyeth Ayerst

Escalon Ophthalmics, Inc.
Montgomery Knoll
182 Tamarack Circle
Skillman, NJ 08558
800-486-4848

Falcon Ophthalmics, Inc.
6201 S. Freeway
Fort Worth, TX 76134
800-343-2133

Fisons Consumer Health
See Novartis

00585
Fisons Corp.
See Medeva

00258, 00456, 00535
Forest Pharmaceutical, Inc.
13622 Lakefront Drive
St. Louis, MO 63045
314-344-8870

00168
E. Fougera and Co.
60 Baylis Road
Melville, NY 11747
516-454-6996

10432
Freeda Vitamins, Inc.
36 E. 41st Street
New York, NY 10017-6203
212-685-4980

00469, 57317
Fujisawa USA, Inc.
3 Parkway North Center
Deerfield, IL 60015-2548
708-317-0600

00781
Geneva Pharmaceuticals
2599 W. Midway Blvd.
P.O. Box 469
Broomfield, CO 80038-0469
800-525-8747

00081, 00173
Glaxo Wellcome
Five Moore Drive
Research Triangle Pk, NC 27709
919-248-2100

00182
Goldline Laboratories, Inc.
See Zenith Goldline

Hauck
See Roberts Pharmaceuticals

47992
Holles Laboratories, Inc.
30 Forest Notch
Cohasset, MA 02025-1198
617-383-0741

00548
I.M.S., Ltd.
1886 Santa Anita Ave.
South El Monte, CA 91733
818-913-4660

00814
Interstate Drug Exchange (IDE)
1500 New Horizons Blvd.
Amityville, NY 11701-1130
516-957-8300

Iolab Pharmaceuticals
See Ciba Vision Ophthalmics

00137
Johnson & Johnson
Grandview Road
Skillman, NJ 08558-9418
908-524-0400

KabiVitrum, Inc.
See Pharmacia & Upjohn

00588
Keene Pharmaceuticals, Inc.
P.O. Box 7
Keene, TX 76059-0007
817-645-8083

La Haye Laboratories, Inc.
2205 152nd Ave. N.E.
Redmond, WA 98052
206-644-2020

Lacrimedics, Inc.
9008 Newby St.
Rosemead, CA 91770

10651
Lavoptik, Inc.
661 Western Ave.
St. Paul, MN 55103
612-489-1351

00005
Lederle Laboratories
North Middletown Road
Pearl River, NY 10965-1299
914-732-5000

23558
Lee Pharmaceuticals
1444 Santa Anita Blvd.
South Elmonte, CA 91733
800-950-5337

00002, 59075
Eli Lilly and Co.
Lilly Corp. Center
Indianapolis, IN 46285
317-276-2000

Lyphomed
See Fujisawa USA, Inc.

00904
Major Pharmaceuticals
1640 W. Fulton
Chicago, IL 60612
312-666-9600

Marlin Industries
P.O. Box 560
Grover City, CA 93483-0560
805-473-2743

00259
Mayrand, Inc.
915 Bridge Street
Winston Salem, NC 27101
910-765-4252

00264
McGaw, Inc.
P.O. Box 19791
Irvine, CA 92713-9791
714-660-2000

00348, 75137
Medeva Pharmaceuticals
755 Jefferson Road
Rochester, NY 14623-0000
888-963-3382

Medtech Laboratories, Inc.
3510 N. Lake Creek
P.O. Box 1108
Jackson, WY 83011-1108
307-733-1680

Menicon USA, Inc.
333 West Pontiac Way
Clovis, CA 93612
800-636-4266

00006
Merck & Co.
P.O. Box 4
West Point, PA 19486
215-652-5000

00682, 46672
Mikart, Inc.
2090 Marietta Blvd. N.W.
Atlanta, GA 30318
404-351-1125

00839
H.L. Moore Drug Exchange, Inc.
389 John Downey Drive
New Britain, CT 06050
203-826-3600

53489
Mutual Pharmaceutical, Inc.
1100 Orthodox Street
Philadelphia, PA 19124
215-288-6500

Novartis Pharmaceuticals
556 Morris Avenue
Summit, NJ 07901
908-277-5000

Novartis Self-Medication
581 Main Street
Woodbridge, NJ 07095
908-602-6600

00362
Novocol Chemical Mfr. Co.
P.O. Box 11926
Wilmington, DE 19850
302-328-1102

Novocol Pharmaceutical
25 Wolseley Court
Cambridge, Ontario N1R 6X3

51944
Ocumed, Inc.
119 Harrison Ave.
Roseland, NJ 07068
201-226-2330

OCuSOFT
See Cynacon/OCuSOFT

Optikem International, Inc.
2172 S. Jason Street
Denver, CO 80223
303-936-1137

52238
Optopics Laboratories, Corp.
32 Main Street
P.O. Box 210
Fairton, NJ 08320-0210
609-451-9350

59148
Otsuka America Pharmaceutical
2440 Research Blvd.
Rockville, MD 98101
206-682-5300

00071
Parke-Davis
201 Tabor Road
Morris Plains, NJ 07950
800-223-0432

00349
Parmed Pharmaceuticals, Inc.
4220 Hyde Park Blvd.
Niagara Falls, NY 14305
716-284-5666

00418
Pasadena Research Labs
See Taylor Pharmaceuticals

00927
Pfeiffer Co.
43-45 N. Washington
P.O. Box 100
Wilkes-Barre, PA 18701
717-826-9000

00069, 00663, 74300
Pfizer US Pharmaceutical Group
235 E. 42nd Street
New York, NY 10017-5755
800-438-1985

Pharmacia
See Pharmacia & Upjohn

00013, 00016
Pharmacia & Upjohn
P.O. Box 16529
Columbus, OH 43216-6529
614-764-8100

Pharmafair
See Bausch & Lomb Pharmaceuticals

00813
Pharmics, Inc.
P.O. Box 27554
Salt Lake City, UT 84127
801-972-4138

00077
Pilkington Barnes Hind
See PBH Wesley Jessen

PBH Wesley Jessen
7976 Engineer Road
San Diego, CA 92111
619-614-7600

47144
Polymer Technology Corp.
100 Research Drive
Wilmington, MA 01887
800-343-1445

00034
Purdue Frederick Co.
100 Connecticut Ave.
Norwalk, CT 06850-3590
203-853-0123

00603, 52446
Qualitest Products, Inc.
1236 Jordan Road
Huntsville, AL 35811
205-859-4011

00686
Raway Pharmacal, Inc.
15 Granit Road
Accord, NY 12404-0047
914-626-8133

Roberts Hauck
See Roberts Pharmaceuticals 54092

54092
Roberts Pharmaceuticals
4 Industrial Way West
Eatontown, NJ 07724
908-389-1182

00004, 00033, 00140, 18393, 42987
Roche Laboratories
340 Kingsland Street
Nutley, NJ 07110-1199
800-526-6367

00049
Roerig
See Pfizer

00074
Ross Laboratories
6480 Busch Blvd.
Columbus, OH 43229
614-624-3333

00536
Rugby Labs, Inc.
898 Orlando Ave.
West Hempstead, NY 11552
516-536-8565

00024
Sanofi Winthrop Pharmaceuticals
90 Park Ave.
New York, NY 10016
800-446-6267

00364
Schein Pharmaceutical, Inc.
100 Campus Drive
Florham Park, NJ 07932
914-278-3724

00274
Scherer Laboratories, Inc.
16200 N. Dallas Pkwy.
Suite 165
Dallas, TX 75248
800-858-9888

00085
Schering-Plough Corp.
2000 Galloping Hill Road
Kenilworth, NJ 07033
908-298-4000

00085
Schering-Plough Healthcare Products
110 Allen Road
Liberty Corner, NJ 07938
908-298-4000

49731
Sherman Pharmaceuticals, Inc.
P.O. Box 1377
Mandeville, LA 70470-1377
504-893-0007

00766
SmithKline Beecham Consumer Healthcare
1500 Littleton
Parsippany, NJ 07054
201-631-8700

00007, 00029, 00108, 00128
SmithKline Beecham Pharmaceuticals
One Franklin Plaza
P.O. Box 7929
Philadelphia, PA 19103
215-751-4000

Sola/Barnes-Hind
See PBH Wesley Jessen

51318
Stellar Pharmacal Corp.
1990 N.W. 44th Street
Pompano Beach, FL 33064
800-845-7827

00402
Steris Laboratories, Inc.
620 N. 51st Ave.
Phoenix, AZ 85043
602-278-1400

57706
Storz Ophthalmics
3365 Tree Court Industrial
St. Louis, MO 63122-6694
314-225-5051

Syntex Laboratories
See Roche Laboratories

00677
United Research Laboratories
3600 Marshall Lane
P.O. Box 8546
Bensalem, PA 19020-8546
215-638-2626

00009
Upjohn Co.
See Pharmacia & Upjohn

54891
Vision Pharmaceuticals, Inc.
P.O. Box 400
Mitchell, SD 57301-0400
605-996-3356

00619
Walker Pharmacal Co.
4200 Laclede Ave.
St. Louis, MO 63108
314-533-9600

00008
Wyeth-Ayerst Laboratories
P.O. Box 8299
Philadelphia, PA 19101
610-688-4400

Zenith
See Zenith-Goldline

Zenith-Goldline
1900 W. Commercial Blvd.
Ft. Lauderdale, FL 33309
305-491-4002

CHAPTER SUMMARIES

The following tables are provided as a quick-look product guide. The tables cover Chapter 2 (Ophthalmic Dyes) through Chapter 12 (Nonsurgical Adjuncts) and contain a summary of product information including: generic name, trade name, manufacturer(s), ingredient(s), strength(s), doseform(s) and how supplied. For complete information about a particular product, please consult the index for the appropriate page number.

Ophthalmic Dyes		
Generic Name Trade Name	**Dose Form/ Strength**	**How Supplied**
Fluorescein Sodium		
AK-Fluor (*Akorn*)	Injection: 10%	In 5 ml amps and vials.
Fluorescite (*Alcon*)	Injection: 10%	In 5 ml amps with syringes.
Funduscein-10 (*Ciba Vision*)	Injection: 10%	In 5 ml amps.
Ophthifluor (*Deklerht*)	Injection: 10%	In 5 ml amps.
AK-Fluor (*Akorn*)	Injection: 25%	In 2 ml amps and vials.
Fluorescite (*Alcon*)	Injection: 25%	In 2 ml amps.
Funduscein-25 (*Ciba Vision*)	Injection: 25%	In 3 ml amps.
Fluorescein Sodium (*Various, eg, Alcon*)	Solution: 2%	In 1, 2 and 15 ml.
Ful-Glo (*PBH Wesley Jessen*)	Strips: 0.6 mg	In 300s.
Fluorets (*Akorn*)	Strips: 1 mg	In 100s.
Fluor-I-Strip-A.T. (*Wyeth-Ayerst*)	Strips: 1 mg	In 300s.[1]
Fluor-I-Strip (*Wyeth-Ayerst*)	Strips: 9 mg	In 300s.[1]
Fluorexon		
Fluoresoft (*Various, eg, Akorn, Holles*)	Solution: 0.35%	In 0.5 ml pipettes (12s).
Indocyanine Green		
Cardio-Green (CG) (*Becton-Dickinson*)	Powder for Injection: 25 mg, 50 mg	In 10 ml amps of aqueous solvent (2s).
Lissamine Green		
Lissamine Green (*Dakryon*)	Solution: 0.1%, 0.5%, 1%	Bot. 5 ml. In 3s.
Rose Bengal		
Rose Bengal (*PBH Wesley Jessen*)	Strips: 1.3 mg/strip	In 100s.
Rosets (*Akorn*)	Strips: 1.3 mg/strip	In 100s.

[1] With boric acid, polysorbate 80, 0.5% chlorobutanol.

Local Anesthetics, Injectable		
Generic Name Trade Name	**Dose form/ Strength**	**How Supplied**
Lidocaine HCl and Lidocaine Combinations		
Xylocaine MPF (*Astra*)	Injection: 4%	In 5 ml amps and 5 ml disp. Syringe with laryngotracheal cannula.
Duo-Trach Kit (*Astra*)	Injection: 4%	In 5 ml pre-filled syringe with cannula.
Mepivacaine HCl		
Carbocaine (*Sanofi Winthrop*)	Injection: 1%	In 30 ml vials and 50 ml vials.[1]
Mepivacaine HCl (*Various, eg, Zenith-Goldline, Schein*)	Injection: 1%	In 50 ml vials.
Polocaine (*Astra*)	Injection: 1%	In 50 ml vials.
Polocaine MPF (*Astra*)	Injection: 1%	In 30 ml vials.
Carbocaine (*Sanofi Winthrop*)	Injection: 1.5%	In 30 ml vials.
Polocaine MPF (*Astra*)	Injection: 1.5%	In 30 ml vials.
Carbocaine (*Sanofi Winthrop*)	Injection: 2%	In 20 ml vials and 50 ml vials.[1]
Polocaine (*Astra*)	Injection: 2%	In 50 ml vials.
Polocaine MPF (*Astra*)	Injection: 2%	In 20 ml vials.
Mepivacaine (*Various, eg, Zenith-Goldline, IDE, Moore, Schein*)	Injection: 2%	In 50 ml vials.
Bupivacaine HCl and Bupivacaine Combinations		
Bupivacaine HCl (*Abbott*)	Injection: 0.75%	In 20 ml amps and 20 ml *Abboject*.
Marcaine HCl (*Sanofi Winthrop*)	Injection: 0.75%	In 30 ml amps and 10 and 30 ml vials.
Marcaine Spinal (*Sanofi Winthrop*)	Injection: 0.75%	In 2 ml single dose amps.[2]
Sensorcaine (*Astra*)	Injection: 0.75%	In 30 ml amps.
Sensorcaine MPF (*Astra*)	Injection: 0.75%	In 30 ml amps and 10 and 30 ml vials.
Sensorcaine MPF Spinal (*Astra*)	Injection: 0.75%	In 2 ml amps.[2]
Marcaine HCl (*Sanofi Winthrop*)	Injection: 0.75% with 1:200,000 epinephrine	In 30 ml amps.[3]

Sensorcaine MPF (*Astra*)	Injection: 0.75% with 1:200,000 epinephrine	In 30 ml amps and 10 and 30 ml vials.[4]
Etidocaine HCl		
Duranest MPF (*Astra*)	Injection:1%	In 30 ml single dose vials.
Duranest MPF (*Astra*)	Injection: 1% with 1:200,000 epinephrine	In 30 ml single dose vials.[4]
Duranest MPF (*Astra*)	Injection: 1.5% with 1:200,000 epinephrine	In 20 ml amps.[4]

[1] With methylparaben.
[2] With 8.25% dextrose.
[3] With sodium metabisulfite and EDTA.
[4] With sodium metabisulfite.

Local Anesthetics, Topical

Generic Name Trade Name	**Dose form/ Strength**	**How Supplied**
Tetracaine HCl		
Tetracaine HCl (*Various, eg, Alcon, Ciba Vision, Optopics, Schein*)	Solution: 0.5%	In 1, 2 and 15 ml.
AK-T-Caine PF (*Akorn*)	Solution: 0.5%	In 15 ml.
Pontocaine HCl (*Sanofi Winthrop*)	Solution: 0.5%	In 15 ml Mono-drop and 59 ml.[1]
Proparacaine HCl		
Proparacaine HCl (*Various, eg, Moore, Raway, Rugby*)	Solution: 0.5%	In 2, 15 ml and UD 1 ml.
Alcaine (*Alcon*)	Solution: 0.5%	In 15 ml Drop-Tainers.[2,3]
Ophthaine (*Apothecon*)	Solution: 0.5%	In 15 ml.[4,5]
Ophthetic (*Allergan*)	Solution: 0.5%	In 15 ml.[5,6]
Miscellaneous Local Anesthetic Combinations		
Fluoracaine (*Akorn*)	Solution: 0.5% proparacaine HCl and 0.25% fluorescein sodium	In 5 ml.[5,7]
Fluorescein Sodium with Proparacaine HCl (*Taylor Pharmaceuticals*)	Solution: 0.5% proparacaine HCl and 0.25% fluorescein sodium	In 5 ml.[8]
Fluress (*PBH Wesley Jessen*)	Solution: 0.4% benoxinate HCl and 0.25% fluorescein sodium	In 5 ml with dropper.[9]
Flurate (*Bausch & Lomb*)	Solution: 0.4% benoxinate HCl and 0.25% fluorescein sodium	In 5 ml.
Flu-Oxinate (*Taylor Pharmaceuticals*)	Solution: 0.4% benoxinate HCl and 0.25% fluorescein sodium	In 5 ml.[10]

[1] With 0.4% chlorobutanol and 0.75% sodium chloride.
[2] With glycerin and 0.01% benzalkonium Cl.
[3] Refrigerate after opening.
[4] With glycerin, 0.2% chlorobutanol and benzalkonium Cl.
[5] Refrigerate.
[6] With 0.01% benzalkonium Cl, glycerin and sodium Cl.
[7] With glycerin, povidone, polysorbate 80 and 0.01% thimerosal.
[8] With povidone, glycerin, EDTA and 0.01% thimerosal.
[9] With povidone, boric acid and 1% chlorobutanol.
[10] Povidone, glycerin, EDTA and 1% chlorobutanol.

Mydriatics		
Generic Name Trade Name	**Dose form/ Strength**	**How Supplied**
Phenylephrine HCl		
Phenylephrine HCl (*Various, eg, Steris*)	Solution: 2.5%	In 15 ml.
AK-Dilate (*Akorn*)	Solution: 2.5%	In 2 and 15 ml.[1]
Mydfrin 2.5% (*Alcon*)	Solution: 2.5%	In 3 and 5 ml Drop-Tainers.[2]
Neo-Synephrine (*Sanofi Winthrop*)	Solution: 2.5%	In 15 ml.[3]
Phenoptic (*Optopics*)	Solution: 2.5%	In 2, 5 and 15 ml.
Phenylephrine HCl (*Various, eg, Ciba Vision, Steris*)	Solution: 10%	In 2 and 5 ml.
AK-Dilate (*Akorn*)	Solution: 10%	In 2 and 5 ml.[1]
Neo-Synephrine (*Sanofi Winthrop*)	Solution: 10%	In 5 ml.[4]
Neo-Synephrine Viscous (*Sanofi Winthrop*)	Solution: 10%	In 5 ml.[5]

[1] With benzalkonium chloride.
[2] With 0.01% benzalkonium chloride, EDTA and sodium bisulfite.
[3] With 1:7500 benzalkonium chloride.
[4] With 1:10,000 benzalkonium chloride and methylcellulose.
[5] With 1:10,000 benzalkonium chloride.

Cycloplegic Mydriatics

Generic Name Trade Name	Dose form/ Strength	How Supplied
Atropine Sulfate		
Atropine Sulfate Ophthalmic *(Various, eg, Bausch & Lomb, Fougera, Zenith-Goldline, Pharmafair)*	Ointment: 1%	In 3.5 and UD 1 g.
Isopto Atropine (*Alcon*)	Solution: 0.5%	In 5 ml Drop-Tainers.[1]
Atropine Sulfate (*Various, eg, Alcon, Allergan, Bausch & Lomb, Zenith-Goldline*)	Solution: 1%	In 2, 5 and 15 ml and UD 1 ml.
Atropine Care (*Akorn*)	Solution: 1%	In 2, 5 and 15 ml.[2]
Atropine-1 (*Optopics*)	Solution: 1%	In 2, 5 and 15 ml.
Atropisol (*Ciba Vision*)	Solution: 1%	In 1 ml Dropperettes.[3]
Isopto Atropine (*Alcon*)	Solution: 1%	In 5 and 15 ml Drop-Tainers.[1]
Atropine Sulfate (*Alcon*)	Solution: 2%	In 2 ml.
Homatropine HBr		
Isopto Homatropine (*Alcon*)	Solution: 2%	In 5 and 15 ml Drop-Tainers.[4]
Homatropine HBr (*Various, eg, Alcon, Ciba Vision*)	Solution: 5%	In 1, 2 and 5 ml.
AK-Homatropine (*Akorn*)	Solution: 5%	In 5 ml.
Isopto Homatropine (*Alcon*)	Solution: 5%	In 5 and 15 ml Drop-Tainers.[5]
Scopolamine HBr (Hyoscine HBr)		
Isopto Hyoscine (*Alcon*)	Solution: 0.25%	In 5 and 15 ml Drop-Tainers.[6]
Cyclopentolate HCl		
Cyclogyl (*Alcon*)	Solution: 0.5%	In 2, 5 and 15 ml Drop-Tainers.[3]
Cyclopentolate HCl (*Various, eg, Bausch & Lomb, Schein, Steris*)	Solution: 1%	In 2, 5 and 15 ml.
AK-Pentolate (*Akorn*)	Solution: 1%	In 2 and 15 ml.[3]
Cyclogyl (*Alcon*)	Solution: 2%	In 2, 5 and 15 ml Drop-Tainers.[3]
Pentolair (*Bausch & Lomb*)	Solution: 1%	In 2 and 15 ml squeeze bottles.[7]
Tropicamide		
Tropicamide (*Various, eg, Bausch & Lomb*)	Solution: 0.5%	In 2 and 15 ml.
Mydriacyl (*Alcon*)	Solution: 0.5%	In 15 ml Drop-Tainers.[7]
Opticyl (*Optopics*)	Solution: 0.5%	In 2 and 15 ml.
Tropicacyl (*Akorn*)	Solution: 0.5%	In 2 and 15 ml.

Tropicamide (*Various, eg, Bausch & Lomb*)	Solution: 1%	In 15 ml.
Mydriacyl (*Alcon*)	Solution: 1%	In 3 and 15 ml Drop-Tainers.[7]
Opticyl (*Optopics*)	Solution: 1%	In 2 and 15 ml.
Tropicacyl (*Akorn*)	Solution: 1%	In 2 and 15 ml.[8]

[1] With 0.01% benzalkonium chloride, 0.5% hydroxypropyl methylcellulose and boric acid.
[2] With 0.01% benzalkonium chloride, hydroxypropyl methylcellulose and boric acid.
[3] With benzalkonium chloride, EDTA and boric acid.
[4] With 0.01% benzalkonium chloride, 0.5% hydroxypropyl methylcellulose and polysorbate 80.
[5] With 0.005% benzethonium chloride and 0.5% hydroxypropyl methylcellulose.
[6] With 0.01% benzalkonium chloride and 0.5% hydroxypropyl methylcellulose.
[7] With 0.01% benzalkonium chloride and EDTA.
[8] With 0.1% benzalkonium chloride and EDTA.

Mydriatic Combinations

Trade Name	**Dose form/ Strength**	**How Supplied**
Cyclomydril (*Alcon*)	Solution: 0.2% cyclopentolate HCl and 1% phenylephrine HCl	In 2 and 5 ml Drop-Tainers.[1]
Murocoll-2 (*Bausch & Lomb*)	Drops: 0.3% scopolamine HBr and 10% phenylephrine HCl	In 5 ml.[2]

[1] With 0.01% benzalkonium chloride, EDTA and boric acid.
[2] With 0.01% benzalkonium chloride, sodium metabisulfite and EDTA.

Decongestants

Generic Name Trade Name	Dose Form/ Strength	How Supplied
Naphazoline HCl		
Allerest Eye Drops (*Ciba Vision*)	Solution: 0.012%	In 15 ml.[1]
Clear Eyes (*Ross*)	Solution: 0.012%	In 15 and 30 ml.[2]
Clear Eyes ACR (*Ross*)	Solution: 0.012%	In 15 and 30 ml.[3]
Degest 2 (*Akorn*)	Solution: 0.012%	In 15 ml.[4]
Naphcon (*Alcon*)	Solution: 0.012%	In 15 ml.[5]
Allergy Drops (*Bausch & Lomb*)	Solution: 0.012%	In 15 ml.[6]
Vaso Clear (*Ciba Vision*)	Solution: 0.02%	In 15 ml.[7]
Vaso Clear A (*Ciba Vision*)	Solution: 0.02%	In 15 ml.[8]
Comfort Eye Drops (*PBH Wesley Jessen*)	Solution: 0.03%	In 15 ml.[9]
Maximum Strength Allergy Drops (*Bausch & Lomb*)	Solution: 0.03%	In 15 ml.[10]
Naphazoline HCl (*Various, eg, Zenith-Goldline, Rugby*)	Solution: 0.1%	In 15 ml.
AK-Con (*Akorn*)	Solution: 0.1%	In 15 ml.[5]
Albalon (*Allergan*)	Solution: 0.1%	In 15 ml.[11]
Nafazair (*Bausch & Lomb*)	Solution: 0.1%	In 15 ml.[5]
Naphcon Forte (*Alcon*)	Solution: 0.1%	In 15 ml Drop-Trainers.[5]
Vasocon Regular (*Ciba Vision*)	Solution: 0.1%	In 15 ml.[12]
Oxymetazoline		
OcuClear (*Schering-Plough*)	Solution: 0.025%	In 30 ml.[13]
Visine L.R. (*Pfizer*)	Solution: 0.025%	In 15 and 30 ml.[13]
Phenylephrine HCl		
AK-Nefrin (*Akorn*)	Solution: 0.12%	In 15 ml.[14]
Prefrin Liquifilm (*Allergan*)	Solution: 0.12%	In 20 ml.[15]
Relief (*Allergan*)	Solution: 0.12%	Preservative free. In UD 0.3 ml.[16]
Zincfrin Solution (*Alcon*)	Solution: 0.12%	In 15 and 30 ml Drop-Tainers.[16]

Tetrahydrozoline HCl		
Tetrahydrozoline HCl (*Various, eg, Moore, Rugby*)	Solution: 0.05%	In 15 and 30 ml.
AR Eye Drops-Astringent Redness Reliever (*Bausch & Lomb*)	Solution: 0.05%	In 15 ml.[17]
Collyrium Fresh (*Wyeth-Ayerst*)	Solution: 0.05%	In 15 ml.[18]
Eye Drops (Bausch & Lomb)	Solution: 0.05%	In 15 ml.[5]
Eye Drops Extra (*Bausch & Lomb*)	Solution: 0.05%	In 15 ml.[19]
Eyesine (*Akorn*)	Solution: 0.05%	In 15 ml.[5]
Geneye (*Zenith-Goldline*)	Solution: 0.05%	In 15 ml.[5]
Geneye Extra (*Zenith-Goldline*)	Solution: 0.05%	In 15 ml.[20]
Mallazine Eye Drops (*Roberts Hauck*)	Solution: 0.05%	In 15 ml.[5]
Murine Plus (*Ross*)	Solution: 0.05%	In 15 ml and 30 ml.[21]
Optigene 3 (*Pfeiffer*)	Solution: 0.05%	In 15 ml.[5]
Tetrasine (*Optopics*)	Solution: 0.05%	In 15 and 22.5 ml.[1]
Tetrasine Extra (*Optopics*)	Solution: 0.05%	In 15 ml.[20]
Visine (*Pfizer*)	Solution: 0.05%	In 15, 22.5 and 30 ml.[5]
Visine Allergy Relief (*Pfizer*)	Solution: 0.05%	In 15 and 30 ml.[22]
Visine Moisturizing (*Pfizer*)	Solution: 0.05%	In 15 and 30 ml.[23]

[1] With benzalkonium chloride, EDTA.
[2] With benzalkonium chloride, EDTA, 0.2% glycerin, boric acid.
[3] With benzalkonium chloride, EDTA, 0.25% zinc sulfate, 0.2% glycerin.
[4] With 0.0067% benzalkonium chloride, 0.02% EDTA, hydroxyethylcellulose, povidone.
[5] With 0.01% benzalkonium chloride, EDTA.
[6] With 0.2% PEG-300, 0.01% benzalkonium chloride.
[7] With 0.01% benzalkonium chloride, 0.25% polyvinyl alcohol, 1% PEG-400, EDTA.
[8] With 0.005% benzalkonium chloride, EDTA, 0.25% zinc sulfate, 0.25% polyvinyl alcohol, 1% PEG-400.
[9] With 0.005% benzalkonium chloride and 0.02% EDTA.
[10] With 0.01% benzalkonium chloride, 0.5% hydroxypropyl methylcellulose and EDTA.
[11] With 0.004% benzalkonium chloride, EDTA, 1.4% polyvinyl alcohol.
[12] With benzalkonium chloride, polyvinyl alcohol, EDTA, PEG-800.
[13] With 0.01% benzalkonium chloride and 0.1% EDTA.
[14] With 0.005% benzalkonium chloride, 1.4% polyvinyl alcohol and EDTA.
[15] With 1.4% polyvinyl alcohol, 0.004% benzalkonium chloride and EDTA.
[16] With 0.01% benzalkonium chloride, polysorbate 80, 0.25% zinc sulfate.
[17] With 0.25% zinc sulfate.
[18] With 0.01% benzalkonium chloride, 0.1% EDTA and 1% glycerin.
[19] With 1% polyethylene gylcol 400.
[20] With 1% polyethylene glycol 400, benzalkonium chloride and EDTA.
[21] With benzalkonium chloride, EDTA, 1.4% polyvinyl alcohol and 0.6% povidone.
[22] With 0.01% benzalkonium chloride, EDTA, 0.25% zinc sulfate.
[23] With 0.013% benzalkonium chloride, 0.1% EDTA and 1% PEG-400.

Antihistamines

Generic Name Trade Name	Dose Form/ Strength	How Supplied
Cromolyn Sodium Crolom (*Bausch & Lomb*)	Solution: 4%	In 2.5 and 10 ml bottles with controlled drop tip.
Levocabastine HCl Livostin (Ciba Vision)	Suspension: 0.05%	In 2.5, 5 and 10 ml dropper bottles. With 0.15 mg benzalkonium chloride, propylene glycol, EDTA.
Lodoxamide Tromethamine Alomide (*Alcon*)	Solution: 0.1%	10 ml Drop-Tainers.
Olopatadine HCl Patanol (*Alcon*)	Solution: 0.1%[1]	5 ml Drop-Tainers.

[1]With 0.01% benzalkonium chloride.

Decongestants and Antihistamines

Trade Name	Decongestant	Antihistamine	How Supplied
Naphazoline HCl & Antazoline Phosphate Solution (*Various, eg, Moore, Schein, Steris*)	naphazoline HCl 0.05%	antazoline phosphate 0.5%	In 5 and 15 ml.
Naphazoline HCl & Pheniramine Maleate Solution (*Various, eg, Moore*)	naphazoline HCl 0.025%	pheniramine maleate 0.3%	In 15 ml.
Naphazoline Plus Solution (*Parmed*)	naphazoline HCl 0.025%	pheniramine maleate 0.3%	In 15 ml.[1]
Naphcon-A Solution (*Alcon*)	naphazoline HCl 0.025%	pheniramine maleate 0.3%	In 15 ml Drop-Tainers.[1]
Opcon-A Solution (*Bausch & Lomb*)	naphazoline HCl 0.027%	pheniramine maleate 0.315%	In 15 ml.[2]
Vasocon-A Solution (*Ciba Vision*)	naphazoline HCl 0.05%	antazoline phosphate 0.5%	In 15 ml.[3]

[1]With 0.01% benzalkonium chloride, EDTA.
[2]With 0.5% hydroxypropyl methylcellulose, 0.01% benzalkonium chloride, 0.1% EDTA, boric acid.
[3]With 0.01% benzalkonium chloride, PEG-8000, polyvinyl alcohol, EDTA.

Corticosteroids

Generic Name Trade Name	Dose Form/ Strength	How Supplied
Dexamethasone		
Dexamethasone Sodium Phosphate (*Various, eg, Rugby, Ciba Vision, Steris*)	Solution: 0.1% dexamethasone phosphate (as sodium phosphate)	In 5 ml.
AK-Dex (*Akorn*)	Solution: 0.1% dexamethasone phosphate (as sodium phosphate)	In 5 ml.[1]
Decadron Phosphate (*Merck*)	Solution: 0.1% dexamethasone phosphate (as sodium phosphate)	In 5 ml Ocumeters.[2]
Dexamethasone (*Steris*)	Suspension: 0.1% dexamethasone	In 5 ml.
Maxidex (*Alcon*)	Suspension: 0.1% dexamethasone	In 5 ml and 15 ml Drop-Tainers.[3]
Dexamethasone Sodium Phosphate (*Various, eg, Zenith-Goldline, Major*)	Ointment: 0.05% dexamethasone phosphate (as sodium phosphate)	In 3.5 g.
AK-Dex (*Akorn*)	Ointment: 0.05% dexamethasone phosphate (as sodium phosphate)	In 3.5 g.[4]
Decadron Phosphate (*Merck*)	Ointment: 0.05% dexamethasone phosphate (as sodium phosphate)	In 3.5 g.[5]
Maxidex (*Alcon*)	Ointment: 0.05% dexamethasone phosphate (as sodium phosphate)	In 3.5 g.[5]
Fluorometholone		
Fluor-Op (*Ciba Vision*)	Suspension: 0.1%	In 5, 10 and 15 ml.[6]
FML (*Allergan*)	Suspension: 0.1%	In 1, 5, 10 and 15 ml.[6]
Flarex (*Alcon*)	Suspension: 0.1% fluorometholone acetate	In 2.5, 5 and 10 ml Drop-Tainers.[7]
eFLone (*Ciba Vision*)	Suspension: 0.1% fluorometholone acetate	In 5 and 10 ml.[7]
FML Forte (*Allergan*)	Suspension: 0.25% fluorometholone acetate	In 2, 5, 10 and 15 ml.[8]
FML S.O.P. (*Allergan*)	Ointment: 0.1%	In 3.5 g.[9]
Medrysone		
HMS (*Allergan*)	Suspension: 1%	In 5 and 10 ml.[10]
Prednisolone		
Pred Mild (*Allergan*)	Suspension: 0.12% prednisolone acetate	In 5 and 10 ml.[11]
Econopred (*Alcon*)	Suspension: 0.125% prednisolone acetate	In 5 and 10 ml Drop-Tainers.[12]

Prednisolone Sodium Phosphate (*Various, eg, Steris*)	Solution: 0.125% prednisolone sodium phosphate	In 5 and 15 ml.
AK-Pred (*Akorn*)	Solution: 0.125% prednisolone sodium phosphate	In 5 ml.[13]
Inflamase Mild (*Ciba Vision*)	Solution: 0.125% prednisolone sodium phosphate	In 3, 5 and 10 ml.[14]
Econopred Plus (*Alcon*)	Suspension: 1% prednisolone acetate	In 5 and 10 ml Drop-Tainers.[12]
Pred Forte (*Allergan*)	Suspension: 1% prednisolone acetate	In 1, 5, 10 and 15 ml.[11]
Prednisolone Acetate Ophthalmic (*Falcon*)	Suspension: 1% prednisolone acetate	In 5 and 10 ml.[12]
Prednisolone Sodium Phosphate (*Various, eg, Bausch & Lomb, Rugby*)	Solution: 1% prednisolone sodium phosphate	In 5, 10 and 15 ml.
AK-Pred (*Akorn*)	Solution: 1% prednisolone sodium phosphate	In 5 and 15 ml.[13]
Inflamase Forte (*Ciba Vision*)	Solution: 1% prednisolone sodium phosphate	In 3, 5, 10 and 15 ml.[14]
Rimexolone		
Vexol (*Alcon*)	Suspension: 1%	In 5 and 10 ml Drop-Tainers.[15]

[1] With 0.01% benzalkonium chloride, EDTA and hydroxyethylcellulose.
[2] With polysorbate 80, EDTA, 0.1% sodium bisulfite, 0.25% phenylethanol, 0.02% benzalkonium chloride.
[3] With 0.01% benzalkonium chloride, EDTA, 0.5% hydroxypropyl methylcellulose, polysorbate 80.
[4] With lanolin anhydrous, parabens, PEG-400, white petrolatum and mineral oil.
[5] With white petrolatum and mineral oil.
[6] With 0.004% benzalkonium chloride, EDTA, polysorbate 80 and 1.4% polyvinyl alcohol.
[7] With 0.01% benzalkonium chloride, EDTA, hydroxyethylcellulose and tyloxapol.
[8] With 0.005% benzalkonium chloride, EDTA, polysorbate 80 and 1.4% polyvinyl alcohol.
[9] With 0.0008% phenylmercuric acetate, white pertrolatum, mineral oil, petrolatum and lanolin alcohol.
[10] With 0.004% benzalkonium chloride, EDTA, 1.4% polyvinyl alcohol and hydroxypropyl methylcellulose.
[11] With benzalkonium chloride, EDTA, polysorbate 80, hydroxypropyl methylcellulose and sodium bisulfite.
[12] With 0.01% benzalkonium chloride, EDTA, polysorbate 80, hydroxypropyl methylcellulose and glycerin.
[13] With 0.01% benzalkonium chloride, EDTA, hydroxypropyl methylcellulose and sodium bisulfite.
[14] With 0.01% benzalkonium chloride and EDTA.
[15] With 0.01% benzalkonium chloride, polysorbate 80 and EDTA in carbapol gel.

Nonsteroidal Anti-Inflammatory Agents (NSAIDS)

Generic Name Trade Name	Dose Form/ Strength	How Supplied
Diclofenac Sodium Voltaren (*Ciba Vision*)	Solution: 0.1%	In 2.5 and 5 ml dropper bottles.[1]
Flurbiprofen Sodium Ocufen (*Allergan*)	Solution: 0.03%	In 2.5, 5 and 10 ml dropper bottles.[2]
Flurbiprofen Sodium Ophthalmic (*Various, eg, Bausch & Lomb*)	Solution: 0.03%	In 2.5 ml.[2]
Ketorolac Tromethamine Acular (*Allergan*)	Solution: 0.5%	In 5 ml dropper bottles.[3]
Suprofen Profenal (*Alcon*)	Solution: 1%	In 2.5 ml Drop-Tainers.[4]

[1]With 1 mg/ml EDTA, boric acid, polyoxyl 35 castor oil, 2 mg/ml sorbic acid and tromethamine.
[2]With 1.4% polyvinyl alcohol, 0.005% thimerosal and EDTA.
[3]With 0.01% benzalkonium Cl, 0.1% EDTA and octoxynol 40.
[4]With 0.005% thimerosal, 2% caffeine and EDTA.

Artificial Tear Solutions

Trade Name	Dose form/Strength	How Supplied
Absorbotear (*Alcon*)	Solution: 0.4% hydroxyethylcellulose, 1.67% povidone, water soluble polymers, 0.004% thimerosal, 0.1% EDTA	In 15 ml.
Akwa Tears (*Akorn*)	Solution: 0.01% benzalkonium Cl, 1.4% polyvinyl alcohol, sodium phosphate, EDTA, NaCl	In 15 ml.
AquaSite (*Ciba Vision*)	Solution: 0.2% PEG-400, 0.1% dextran 70, polycarbophil, NaCl, EDTA, sodium hydroxide	Preservative free. In 0.6 ml (single-use 24s) and 15 ml.
Artificial Tears (*Various, eg, Parmed, Rugby, Schein*)	Solution: 0.01% benzalkonium chloride. May also contain EDTA, NaCl, polyvinyl alcohol, hydroxypropyl methylcellulose	In 15 and 30 ml.
Artificial Tears Plus (*Various, eg, Rugby, Steris*)	Solution: 1.4% polyvinyl alcohol, 0.6% povidone, 0.5% chlorobutanol, NaCl	In 15 ml.
Bion Tears (*Alcon*)	Solution: 0.1% dextran 70, 0.3% hydroxypropyl methylcellulose 2910, NaCl, KCl, sodium bicarbonate	Preservative free. In single-use 0.45 ml containers (28s).
Celluvisc (*Allergan*)	Solution: 1% carboxymethylcellulose, NaCl, KCl, sodium lactate	Preservative free. In 0.3 ml (UD 30s).
Comfort Tears (*PBH Wesley Jessen*)	Solution: Hydroxyethylcellulose, 0.005% benzalkonium chloride, 0.02% EDTA	In 15 ml.
Dakrina (*Dakryon*)	Solution: Povidone, polyvinyl alcohol, antioxidant retinyl palmitate, boric acid, 0.09% EDTA, 0.001% WSCP, NaCl, KCl	In 15 ml.
Dry Eyes (*Bausch & Lomb*)	Solution: 1.4% polyvinyl alcohol, 0.01% benzalkonium chloride, sodium phosphate, EDTA, NaCl	In 15 ml.
Dry Eye Therapy (*Bausch & Lomb*)	Solution: 0.3% glycerin, NaCl, KCl, sodium citrate, sodium phosphate	Preservative free. In 0.3 ml (UD 32s).
Dwelle (*Dakryon*)	Solution: 0.09% EDTA, NaCl, KCl, boric acid, povidone, 0.001% NPX	In 15 ml.
Eye-Lube-A (*Optopics*)	Solution: 0.25% glycerin, EDTA, sodium chloride, benzalkonium Cl	In 15 ml.
Gen Teal (*Ciba Vision*)	Solution: Hydroxypropyl methylcellulose, boric acid, NaCl, KCl, phosphoric acid, sodium perborate	In 15 ml.

HypoTears (*Ciba Vision*)	Solution: 1% polyvinyl alcohol, PEG-400, 1% dextrose, 0.01% benzalkonium Cl, EDTA	In 15 and 30 ml.
HypoTears PF (*Ciba Vision*)	Solution: 1% polyvinyl alcohol, PEG-400, 1% dextrose, EDTA	Preservative free. In 0.6 ml (30s).
Isopto Plain (*Alcon*)	Solution: 0.5% hydroxypropyl methylcellulose 2910, 0.01% benzalkonium chloride, NaCl, sodium phosphate, sodium citrate	In 15 ml Drop-Tainers
Isopto Tears (*Alcon*)	Solution: 0.5% hydroxypropyl methylcellulose 2910, 0.01% benzalkonium chloride, NaCl, sodium phosphate, sodium citrate	In 15 and 30 ml.
Just Tears (*Blairex*)	Solution: Benzalkonium chloride, EDTA, 1.4% polyvinyl alcohol, NaCl, KCl	In 15 ml.
Liquifilm Tears (*Allergan*)	Solution: 1.4% polyvinyl alcohol, 0.5% chlorobutanol, NaCl	In 15 and 30 ml.
LubriTears (*Bausch & Lomb*)	Solution: 0.3% hydroxypropyl methylcellulose 2906, 0.1% dextran 70, EDTA, KCl, NaCl, 0.01% benzalkonium chloride	In 15 ml.
Moisture Drops (*Bausch & Lomb*)	Solution: 0.5% hydroxypropyl methylcellulose, 0.1% povidone, 0.2% glycerin, 0.01% benzalkonium chloride, EDTA, NaCl, boric acid, KCl, sodium borate	In 15 and 30 ml.
Murine (*Ross*)	Solution: 0.5% polyvinyl alcohol, 0.6% povidone, benzalkonium chloride, dextrose, EDTA, NaCl, sodium bicarbonate, sodium phosphate	In 15 and 30 ml.
Murocel (*Bausch & Lomb*)	Solution: 1% methylcellulose, propylene glycol, NaCl, 0.046% methylparaben, 0.02% propylparaben, boric acid, sodium borate	In 15 ml.
Nature's Tears (*Rugby*)	Solution: 0.4% hydroxypropyl methylcellulose 2910, KCl, NaCl, sodium phosphate, 0.01% benzalkonium chloride	In 15 ml.
Nu-Tears (*Optopics*)	Solution: 1.4% polyvinyl alcohol, EDTA, sodium chloride, benzalkonium chloride, KCl	In 15 ml.
Nu-Tears II (*Optopics*)	Solution: 1% polyvinyl alcohol, 1% PEG-400, EDTA, benzalkonium chloride	In 15 ml.

OcuCoat (*Storz Ophthalmics*)	Solution: 0.1% dextran 70, 0.8% hydroxypropyl methylcellulose, sodium phosphate, KCl, NaCl, 0.01% benzalkonium chloride, dextrose	In 15 ml.
OcuCoat PF (*Storz Ophthalmics*)	Solution: 0.1% dextran 70, 0.8% hydroxypropyl methylcellulose, sodium phosphate, KCl, NaCl, dextrose	Preservative free. In 0.5 ml single-dose containers (28s).
Puralube Tears (*Fougera*)	Solution: 1% polyvinyl alcohol, 1% PEG 400, EDTA, benzalkonium chloride	In 15 ml.
Refresh (*Allergan*)	Solution: 1.4% polyvinyl alcohol, 0.6% povidone, NaCl	Preservative free. In 0.3 ml (UD 30s, 50s).
Refresh Plus (*Allergan*)	Solution: 0.5% carboxymethyl-cellulose sodium, KCl, NaCl	Preservative free. In 0.3 ml single-use containers (30s and 50s).
Tear Drop (*Parmed*)	Solution: Polyvinyl alcohol, NaCl, EDTA, 0.01% benzalkonium Cl	In 15 ml.
TearGard (*Lee*)	Solution: 0.25% sorbic acid, 0.1% EDTA, hydroxyethylcellulose	Thimerosal free. In 15 ml.
Teargen (*Zenith-Goldline*)	Solution: 0.01% benzalkonium Cl, EDTA, NaCl, polyvinyl alcohol	In 15 ml.
Tearisol (*Ciba Vision*)	Solution: 0.5% hydroxypropyl methylcellulose, 0.01% benzalkonium chloride, EDTA, boric acid, KCl	In 15 ml.
Tears Naturale (*Alcon*)	Solution: 0.1% dextran 70, 0.01% benzalkonium chloride, 0.3% hydroxypropyl methylcellulose, NaCl, EDTA, hydrochloric acid, sodium hydroxide, KCl	In 15 and 30 ml.
Tears Naturale II (*Alcon*)	Solution: 0.1% dextran 70, 0.3% hydroxypropyl methylcellulose 2910, 0.001% polyquarternium-1, NaCl, KCl, sodium borate	In 15 and 30 ml Drop-Tainers.
Tears Naturale Free (*Alcon*)	Solution: 0.3% hydroxypropyl methylcellulose 2910, 0.1% dextran 70, NaCl, KCl, sodium borate	Preservative free. In 0.6 ml single-use containers.
Tears Plus (*Allergan*)	Solution: 1.4% polyvinyl alcohol, NaCl, 0.6% povidone, 0.5% chlorobutanol	In 15 and 30 ml.
Tears Renewed (*Akorn*)	Solution: 0.01% benzalkonium chloride, EDTA, 0.1% dextran 70, NaCl, 0.3% hydroxypropyl methylcellulose 2906	In 2, 15 and 30 ml.

Thera Tears[1] (*Advanced Vision*)	Solution: 0.25% sodium carboxymethylcellulose, NaCl, KCl, sodium phosphate	Preservative free. In 0.6 ml single-use containers.
Ultra Tears (*Alcon*)	Solution: 15 hydroxypropyl methylcellulose 2910, 0.01% benzalkonium chloride, NaCl	In 15 ml.
Viva-Drops (*Vision Pharm*)	Solution: Polysorbate 80, sodium chloride, EDTA, retinyl palmitate, mannitol, sodium citrate, pyruvate	Preservative free. In 10 and 15 ml.

[1] Advanced Vision Research, 7 Alfred St., Suite 330, Woburn, MA 01801 (617) 932-8327.

Ocular Lubricants

Trade Name	Dose form/Strength	How Supplied
Akwa Tears (*Akorn*)	Ointment: White petrolatum, mineral oil, lanolin	Preservative free. In 3.5 g.
Dry Eyes (*Bausch & Lomb*)	Ointment: White petrolatum, mineral oil, lanolin	Preservative free. In 3.5 g.
Artificial Tears (*Rugby*)	Ointment: White petrolatum, anhydrous liquid lanolin, mineral oil	In 3.5 g.
Duratears Naturale (*Alcon*)	Ointment: White petrolatum, anhydrous liquid lanolin, mineral oil	Preservative free. In 3.5 g.
LubriTears (*Bausch & Lomb*)	Ointment: White petrolatum, mineral oil, lanolin, 0.5% chlorobutanol	In 3.5 g.
HypoTears (*Ciba Vision*)	Ointment: White petrolatum, light mineral oil	Preservative and lanolin free. In 3.5 g.
Puralube (*Fougera*)	Ointment: White petrolatum, light mineral oil	In 3.5 g.
Tears Renewed (*Akorn*)	Ointment: White petrolatum, light mineral oil	Preservative and lanolin free. In 3.5 g.
Stye (*Del Pharm*)	Ointment: 55% white petrolatum, 32% mineral oil, boric acid, stearic acid, wheat germ oil	In 3.5 g.
Lacri-Lube NP (*Allergan*)	Ointment: 55.5% white petrolatum, 42.5% mineral oil, 2% petrolatum/lanolin alcohol	Preservative free. In 0.7 g (UD 24s).
Lacri-Lube S.O.P. (*Allergan*)	Ointment: 56.8% white petrolatum, 42.5% mineral oil, chlorobutanol, lanolin alcohols	In 3.5 and 7 g.
Refresh PM (*Allergan*)	Ointment: 56.8% white petrolatum, 41.5% mineral oil, lanolin alcohols, sodium chloride	Preservative free. In 3.5 g.

Artificial Tear Insert		
Trade Name	**Dose form/Strength**	**How Supplied**
Lacrisert (*Merck*)	Insert: 5 mg hydroxpropyl cellulose	Preservative free. In 60s with applicator.

Punctal Plugs		
Trade Name	**Dose form/Strength**	**How Supplied**
Herrick Lacrimal Plug (*Lacrimedics*)	Plug: Silicone plug	In 0.3 and 0.5 mm sizes (packs of 2 plugs).
Punctum Plug (*Eagle Vision, Ciba Vision*)	Plug: Silicone plug	In 0.5, 0.6, 0.7 and 0.8 mm sizes (packs of 2 plugs). Contains one inserter tool.
Punctum Plug (*FCI Ophthalmics*)	Plug: Silicone plug	In 0.4, 0.7, 0.8 and 1.0 mm sizes (packs of 2 plugs).

Collagen Implants		
Trade Name	**Dose form/Strength**	**How Supplied**
Collagen Implant (*Lacrimedics*)	Implant: Collagen implant	In 0.2, 0.3, 0.4, 0.5 and 0.6 mm sizes (72s).
Temporary Punctal/ Canalicular Collagen Implant (*Eagle Vision, Ciba Vision*)	Implant: Collagen implant	In 0.2, 0.3, 0.4, 0.5 and 0.6 mm sizes (72s).

Cleaning/Lubricant for Artificial Eyes		
Generic Name Trade Name	**Dose form/ Strength**	**How Supplied**
Tyloxapol Enuclene (*Alcon*)	Solution: 0.25%	0.02% benzalkonium Cl. In 15 ml Drop-Tainers.

Antibiotics

Generic Name Trade Name	Dose form/ Strength	How Supplied
Bacitracin		
Bacitracin (*Various*)	Ointment: 500 units/g	In 3.5 and 3.75 g.
AK-Tracin (*Akorn*)	500 units/g	Preservative free. In 3.5 g.[1]
Polymyxin B Sulfate		
Polymyxin B Sulfate Sterile (*Roerig*)	Powder for Solution: 500,000 units	In 20 ml vials.
Chloramphenicol		
Chloramphenicol (*Various*)	Solution[2]: 5 mg/ml	In 7.5 and 15 ml.
AK-Chlor (*Akorn*)	5 mg/ml	In 7.5 and 15 ml.[3]
Chloroptic (*Allergan*)	5 mg/ml	In 2.5 and 7.5 ml.[4]
Chloramphenicol (*Various*)	Ointment: 10 mg/g	In 3.5 g.
AK-Chlor (*Akorn*)	10 mg/g	In 3.5 g.[5]
Chloromycetin (*Parke-Davis*)	10 mg/g	Preservative free. In 3.5 g.[6]
Chloroptic S.O.P. (*Allergan*)	10 mg/g	In 3.5 g.[7]
Chloromycetin (*Parke-Davis*)	Powder for Solution: 25 mg/vial	Preservative free. In 15 ml with diluent.
Erythromycin		
Erythromycin (*Various*)	Ointment: 5 mg/g	In 3.5 g.
Ilotycin (*Dista*)	5 mg/g	In 3.5 g.[8]
Gentamicin Sulfate		
Gentamicin Ophthalmic (*Various*)	Solution: 3 mg/ml	In 5 and 15 ml.
Garamycin (*Schering*)	3 mg/ml	In 5 ml dropper bottles.[9]
Genoptic (*Allergan*)	3 mg/ml	In 1 and 5 ml dropper bottles.[10]
Gentacidin (*Ciba Vision*)	3 mg/ml	In 5 ml dropper bottles.[9]
Gentak (*Akorn*)	3 mg/ml	In 5 and 15 ml dropper bottles.[9]
Gentamicin Ophthalmic (*Various*)	Ointment: 3 mg/g	In 3.5 g.
Garamycin (*Schering*)	3 mg/g	In 3.5 g.[11]
Genoptic S.O.P. (*Allergan*)	3 mg/g	In 3.5 g.[11]
Gentacidin (*Ciba Vision*)	3 mg/g	In 3.5 g.[1]
Gentak (*Akorn*)	3 mg/g	In 3.5 g.[11]

Tobramycin		
Tobramycin (*Various*)	Solution: 0.3%	In 5 ml bottle.
AKTob (*Akorn*)	0.3%	In 5 ml.[12]
Defy (*Akorn*)	0.3%	In 5 ml.
Tobrex (*Alcon*)	0.3%	In 5 ml Drop-Tainers.[13]
Tobrex (*Alcon*)	Ointment: 3 mg/g	In 3.5 g.[14]
Ciprofloxacin		
Ciloxan (*Alcon*)	Solution: 0.3% (equivalent to 3 mg base)	In 2.5 and 5 ml Drop-Tainers.[15]
Norfloxacin		
Chibroxin (*Merck*)	Solution: 3 mg/ml	In 5 ml Ocumeters.[16]
Ofloxacin		
Ocuflox (*Allergan*)	Solution: 0.3%	In 1, 5 and 10 ml.[17]

[1] With white petrolatum and mineral oil.
[2] Refrigerate until dispensed.
[3] With 0.5% chlorobutanol, boric acid, sodium borate, hydroxypropryl methylcellulose, sodium hydroxide and hydrochloric acid.
[4] With 0.5% chlorobutanol, PEG-300, polyoxyl 40 stearate and sodium hydroxide or hydrochloric acid.
[5] With white petrolatum, mineral oil and polysorbate 60.
[6] With liquid petrolatum and polyethylene base.
[7] With 0.5% chlorobutanol, white petrolatum, mineral oil, polyoxyl 40 stearate, petrolatum (and) lanolin alcohol and PEG-300.
[8] With white petrolatum, mineral oil and parabens.
[9] With 0.1 mg/ml benzalkonium chloride, sodium phosphate and NaCl.
[10] With benzalkonium chloride, 1.4% polyvinyl alcohol, EDTA, sodium phosphate dibasic, NaCl and hydrochloric acid or sodium hydroxide.
[11] With white petrolatum and parabens.
[12] With 0.01% benzalkonium chloride, boric acid and soidum sulfate.
[13] With 0.01% benzalkonium chloride, tyloxapol and boric acid.
[14] With white petrolatum, mineral oil and 0.5% chlorobutanol.
[15] With 0.006% benzalkonium chloride, 4.6% mannitol and 0.05% EDTA.
[16] With 0.0025% banzalkonium chloride and EDTA.
[17] With 0.005% benzalkonium chloride.

Combination Antibiotics		
Trade Name	**Antibiotics**	**How Supplied**
Triple Antibiotic Ophthalmic Ointment (*Various, eg, Fougera*)	Polymyxin B Sulfate (units/g or ml): 10,000 Neomycin Sulfate (mg/g or ml): 3.5 Bacitracin Zinc (units/g): 400	In 3.5 g.
Bacitracin Neomycin Polymyxin B Ointment (*Various, eg, Fougera*)		In 3.5 g.
AK-Spore Ointment (*Akorn*)		Preservative free. White petrolatum, mineral oil. In 3.5 g.
Neosporin Ophthalmic Ointment (*Glaxo Wellcome*)		White petrolatum. In 3.5 g.
Ocutricin Ointment (*Bausch & Lomb*)		White petrolatum, mineral oil. In 3.5 g.
Neomycin Sulfate-Polymyxin B Sulfate-Gramicidin Solution (*Various, eg, Rugby, Steris*)	Polymyxin B Sulfate (units/g or ml): 10,000 Neomycin Sulfate (mg/g or ml): 1.75 Gramicidin: 0.025 mg/ml	In 2 and 10 ml.
AK-Spore Solution (*Akorn*)		In 2 and 10 ml.[1]
Neosporin Ophthalmic Solution (*Glaxo Wellcome*)		In 10 ml Drop Dose.[1]
Bacitracin Zinc and Polymyxin B Ointment (*Bausch & Lomb*)	Polymyxin B Sulfate (units/g or ml): 10,000 Bacitracin Zinc (units/g): 500	White petrolatum and mineral oil. In 3.5 g.
AK-Poly-Bac Ointment (*Akorn*)		Preservative free. White petrolatum, mineral oil. In 3.5 g.
Polysporin Ophthalmic Ointment (*Glaxo Wellcome*)		White petrolatum. In 3.5 g.
Terramycin w/Polymyxin B Ointment (*Roerig*)	Polymyxin B Sulfate (units/g or ml): 10,000 Oxytetracycline HCl: 5 mg/g	White and liquid petrolatum. In 3.5 g.
Terak Ointment		White and liquid petrolatum. In 3.5 g.
Trimethoprim Sulfate and Polymyxin B Sulfate Ophthalmic Solution (*Bausch & Lomb*)	Polymyxin B Sulfate (units/g or ml): 10,000 Trimethoprim: 1 mg/ml	In 10 ml.[2]
Polytrim Ophthalmic Solution (*Allergan*)		In 10 ml.[2]

[1] With 0.001% thimerosal, 0.5% alcohol, propylene glycol, polyoxyethylene polyoxypropylene.
[2] With 0.004% benzalkonium chloride and NaCl.

Sulfonamides		
Generic Name Trade Name	**Dose form/ Strength**	**How Supplied**
Sulfisoxazole Diolamine	Solution:	
Gantrisin (*Roche*)	4%	With 1:100,000 phenylmercuric nitrate. In 15 ml with dropper.
Sulfacetamide Sodium		
Sulfacetamide Sodium (*Various, eg, Bausch & Lomb, Fougera, Geneva, Moore, Optopics, Rugby, Schein, Steris, URL, Zenith-Goldline*)	Solution: 10%	In 15 ml.
AK-Sulf (*Akorn*)	10%	In 2, 5 and 15 ml.[1]
Bleph-10 (*Allergan*)	10%	In 2.5, 5 and 15 ml.[2]
Ocusulf-10 (*Optopics*)	10%	In 2, 5 and 15 ml.[3]
Sodium Sulamyd (*Schering*)	10%	In 5 and 15 ml.[1]
Sulf-10 (*Ciba Vision*)	10%	In 1 ml Dropperettes[4] and 15 ml dropper bottles.[5]
Isopto Cetamide (*Alcon*)	15%	In 5 and 15 ml Drop-Tainers.[6]
Sulfacetamide Sodium (*Various, eg, Schein, Steris*)	30%	In 15 ml.
Sodium Sulamyd (*Schering*)	30%	In 15 ml.[7]
Sodium Sulfacetamide (*Various, eg, Fougera, Moore, URL*)	Ointment: 10%	In 3.5 g.
AK-Sulf (*Akorn*)	10%	In 3.5 g.[8]
Bleph-10 (*Allergan*)	10%	In 3.5 g.[9]
Cetamide (*Alcon*)	10%	In 3.5 g.[10]
Sodium Sulamyc (*Schering*)	10%	In 3.5 g.[11]
Sulfonamide/Deconges-tant Combination		
Vasosulf (*Ciba Vision*)	Solution: 15% sodium sulfacet-amide and 0.125% phenylephrine HCl	With sodium thiosulfate, poloxamer 188 and parabens. In 5 and 15 ml.

[1] 3.1 mg sodium thiosulfate pentahydrate, 5 mg methylcellulose, 0.5 mg methylparaben and 0.1 mg propylparaben per ml.
[2] With 1.4% polyvinyl alcohol, 0.005% benzalkonium chloride, polysorbate 80, sodium thiosulfate and EDTA.
[3] With parabens, 1.4% polyvinyl alcohol and sodium thiosulfate.
[4] With sodium thiosulfate and 0.005% thimerosal.
[5] With 0.1% hydroxypropyl methylcellulose 2208, sodium thiosulfate and 0.01% thimerosal.
[6] With 0.05% methylparaben, 0.01% propylparaben, 0.5% hydroxypropyl methylcellulose 2910 and 0.3% sodium thiosulfate.
[7] With 1.5 mg sodium thiosulfate pentahydrate, 0.5 mg methylparaben and 0.1 mg propylparaben per ml.
[8] With 0.5 mg methylparaben, 0.1 mg propylparaben, 0.25 mg benzalkonium chloride and petrolatum base per g.
[9] With 0.0008% phenylmercuric acetate, white petrolatum, mineral oil, petrolatum and lanolin alcohol.

[10] With 0.05% methylparaben, 0.01% propylparaben, white petrolatum, anhydrous liquid lanolin and mineral oil.
[11] With 0.5 mg methylparaben, 0.1 mg propylparaben, 0.25 mg benzalkonium chloride and petrolatum base per g.

Steroid and Sulfonamide Combinations, Suspensions and Solutions

Trade Name	Steroid	Sulfonamide	How Supplied
FML-S Suspension (*Allergan*)	0.1% fluorometholone	1% sodium sulfacetamide	In 5 and 10 ml.[1]
Blephamide Suspension (*Allergan*)	0.2% prednisolone acetate	10% sodium sulfacetamide	In 2.5, 5 and 10 ml.[2]
Isopto Cetapred Suspension (*Alcon*)	0.25% prednisolone acetate	10% sodium sulfacetamide	In 5 and 15 ml Drop-Tainers.[3]
AK-Cide Suspension (*Akorn*) Metimyd Suspension (*Schering*)	0.5% prednisolone acetate	10% sodium sulfacetamide	In 5 ml dropper bottle.[4] In 5 ml.[5]
Sulfacetamide Sodium and Prednisolone Sodium Phosphate (*Schein*) Sulster Solution (*Akorn*) Vasocidin Solution (*Ciba Vision*)	0.25% prednisolone acetate	10% sodium sulfacetamide	In 5 and 10 ml.[6] In 5 and 10 ml.[7] In 5 and 10 ml.[8]

[1] EDTA, 1.4% polyvinyl alcohol, 0.006% benzalkonium chloride, polysorbate 80, povidone, sodium thiosulfate and sodium chloride.
[2] EDTA, 1.4% polyvinyl alcohol, polysorbate 80, sodium thiosulfate, benzalkonium chloride.
[3] 0.5% hydroxypropyl methylcellulose 2910, EDTA, polysorbate 80, sodium thiosulfate, 0.025% benzalkonium chloride, 0.05% methylparaben, 0.01% propylparaben.
[4] 5 mg phenethyl alcohol, tyloxapol, sodium thiosulfate, 0.25 mg benzalkonium chloride and EDTA per ml.
[5] 0.5 % phenylethyl alcohol, 0.025% benzalkonium chloride, sodium thiosulfate, EDTA, tyloxapol.
[6] 0.01% mg thimerosal, EDTA, boric acid.
[7] 0.01% mg thimerosal, EDTA.
[8] EDTA, 0.01% thimerosal, poloxamer 407.

Steroid and Sulfonamide Combinations, Ointments

Trade Name	Steroid	Sulfonamide	How Supplied
Blephamide (*Allergan*)	0.2% prednisolone acetate	10% sodium sulfacetamide	In 3.5 g.[1]
Cetapred (*Alcon*)	0.25% prednisolone acetate	10% sodium sulfacetamide	In 3.5 g.[2]
AK-Cide (*Akorn*)	0.5% prednisolone acetate	10% sodium sulfacetamide	In 3.5 applicator tube.[3]
Metimyd (*Schering*)			In 3.5 g.[4]
Vasocidin (*Ciba Vision*)			In 3.5 g.[5]

[1] 0.0008% phenylmercuric acetate, mineral oil, white petrolatum, lanolin alcohol.
[2] Mineral oil, white petrolatum, lanolin oil, 0.05% methylparaben 0.01% propylparaben.
[3] 0.5 mg methylparaben, 0.1 mg propylparaben per g, mineral oil, white petrolatum.
[4] Mineral oil, white petrolatum, 0.05% methylparaben, 0.01% propylparaben.
[5] Mineral oil, white petrolatum.

Steroid and Antibiotic Ointments

Trade Name	Steroid (per g)	Antibiotic (per g)	How Supplied
Bacitracin Zinc/ Neomycin Sulfate/ Polymyxin B Sulfate/ Hydrocortisone (*Various, eg, Fougera*)	1% hydrocortisone	Neomycin sulfate equivalent to 0.35% neomycin base, 400 units bacitracin zinc, 10,000 units polymyxin B sulfate	In 3.5 g.
AK-Spore H.C. (*Akorn*)			Preservative free. In 3.5 g.[1]
Cortisporin (*Glaxo Wellcome*)			In 3.5 g.[2]
Neotricin HC (*Bausch & Lomb*)	1% hydrocortisone acetate	Neomycin sulfate equivalent to 0.35% neomycin base, 400 units bacitracin zinc, 10,000 units polymyxin B sulfate	In 3.5 g.[1]
Pred-G S.O.P. (*Allergan*)	0.6% prednisolone acetate	Gentamicin sulfate equivalent to 0.3% gentamicin base	In 3.5 g.[3]
NeoDecadron (*Merck*)	0.05% dexamethasone phosphate (as sodium phosphate)	Neomycin sulfate equivalent to 0.35% neomycin base	In 3.5 g.[1]
TobraDex (*Alcon*)	0.1% dexamethasone	0.3% tobramycin	In 3.5 g.[4]
Neomycin/Polymyxin B Sulfate/Dexamethasone (*Various, eg, Fougera, Rugby*)	0.1% dexamethasone	Neomycin sulfate equivalent to 0.35% neomycin base, 10,000 units polymyxin B sulfate	In 3.5 g.
AK-Trol (*Akorn*)			In 3.5 g.[5]
Dexacidin (*Ciba Vision*)			In 3.5 g.[1]
Dexasporin (*Bausch & Lomb*)			In 3.5 g.[1]
Maxitrol (*Alcon*)			In 3.5 g.[6]

[1] White petrolatum, mineral oil.
[2] White petrolatum.
[3] 0.5 % chlorobutanol, white petrolatum, mineral oil, petrolatum, lanolin alcohol.
[4] 0.5 % chlorobutanol, white petrolatum, mineral oil.
[5] White petrolatum, lanolin oil, mineral oil, parabens.
[6] White petrolatum, anhydrous liquid lanolin, parabens.

Steroid and Antibiotic Solutions and Suspensions

Trade Name	Steroid (per ml)	Antibiotic (per ml)	How Supplied
Chloromycetin/Hydrocortisone for Suspension (*Parke-Davis*)	0.5% hydrocortisone acetate[1] (2.5% as powder)	0.25% chloramphenicol[1] (1.25% as powder)	In 5 ml w/diluent and dropper.[2]
Neomycin/Polymyxin B Sulfate/Hydrocortisone (*Various, eg, Rugby, Schein*)	1% hydrocortisone	Neomycin sulfate equivalent to 0.35% neomycin base and 10,000 units polymyxin B sulfate	In 7.5 and 10 ml.[3]
AK-Spore H.C. Ophthalmic Suspension (*Akorn*)			In 7.5 ml.[3]
Cortisporin Suspension (*Glaxo Wellcome*)			In 7.5 ml Drop Dose.[3]
Terra-Cortril Suspension (*Roerig*)	1.5% hydrocortisone acetate	0.5% oxytetracycline (as HCl)	In 5 ml.[4]
Poly-Pred Suspension (*Allergan*)	0.5% prednisolone acetate	Neomycin sulfate equivalent to 0.35% neomycin base, 10,000 units polymyxin B sulfate	In 5 and 10 ml.[5]
Pred-G Suspension (*Allergan*)	1% prednisolone acetate	Gentamicin sulfate equivalent to 0.3% gentamicin base	In 2, 5 and 10 ml.[6]
Neomycin Sulfate/Dexamethasone Sodium Phosphate Solution (*Various, eg, Rugby, Schein, Zenith-Goldline*)	0.1% dexamethasone phosphate (as sodium phosphate)	Neomycin sulfate equivalent to 0.35% neomycin base	In 5 ml.
NeoDecadron Solution (*Merck*)			In 5 ml Ocumeters.[7]
Neo-Dexameth (*Major*)			In 5 ml.[8]
AK-Neo-Dex Solution (*Akorn*)			In 5 ml.[9]
TobraDex Suspension (*Alcon*)	0.1% dexamethasone	0.3% tobramycin	In 2.5 and 5 ml Drop-Tainers.[10]
Neomycin/Polymyxin B Sulfate/Dexamethasone Suspension (*Various, eg, Rugby, Schein*)	0.1% dexamethasone	Neomycin sulfate equivalent to 0.35% neo-mycin base and 10,000 units polymyxin B sulfate	In 5 and 10 ml.
Dexacidin Suspension (*Ciba Vision*)			In 5 ml.[11]
AK-Trol Suspension (*Akorn*)			In 5 ml.[12]
Maxitrol Suspension (*Alcon*)			In 5 ml Drop-Tainers.[13]

[1] As a prepared solution.
[2] Cholesterol, methylcellulose, 0.01% benzethonium chloride, boric acid,

[3] 0.001% thimerosal, cetyl alcohol, glyceryl monostearate, polyoxyl 40 stearate, propylene glycol, mineral oil, NaCl.
[4] Mineral oil and aluminum tristearate
[5] 1.4% polyvinyl alcohol, 0.001% thimerosal, polysorbate 80, propylene glycol.
[6] 1.4% polyvinyl alcohol, 0.005% benzalkonium chloride, EDTA, hydroxypropyl methylcellulose, polysorbate 80, NaCl.
[7] Polysorbate 80, EDTA, 0.2% benzalkonium Cl, 0.1% sodium bisulfite.
[8] 0.01% benzalkonium Cl, EDTA, polysorbate 80, sodium bisulfite.
[9] 0.02% benzalkonium Cl, polysorbate 80, EDTA, 0.1% sodium bisulfite.
[10] 0.01% benzalkonium Cl, tyloxapol, EDTA, hydroxyethylcellulose, sodium sulfate, NaCl.
[11] Hydroxypropyl methylcellulose, polysorbate 20, 0.04% benzalkonium chloride, NaCl.
[12] 0.004% benzalkonium chloride, polysorbate 20, 0.5% hydroxypropyl methylcellulose, NaCl.
[13] 0.5% hydroxypropyl methylcellulose, polysorbate 20, 0.004% benzalkonium chloride.

Anti-infective Agents		
Generic Name Trade Name	**Dose form/ Strength**	**How Supplied**
Silver Nitrate Silver Nitrate (*Lilly*)	Solution: 1%	With acetic acid and sodium acetate. In 100s (wax ampules).
Zinc Sulfate Solution Eye-Sed (*Scherer*)	Solution: 0.25%	In 15 ml.[1]
Natamycin Natacyn (*Alcon*)	Suspension: 5%	With 0.02% benzalkonium. In 15 ml.
Vidarabine (Adenine Arabinoside; Ara-A) Vira-A (*Parke-Davis*)	Ointment: 3% vidarabine monohydrate (equivalent to 2.8% vidarabine)	In a liquid petrolatum base. In 3.5 g.
Trifluridine (Trifluorothymidine) Trifluridine (*Schein*)	Solution: 1%	In aqueous solution with NaCl and 0.001% thimerosal. In 7.5 ml Drop-Dose.
Viroptic (*Monarch*)	1%	In aqueous solution with NaCl and 0.001% thimerosal. In 7.5 ml Drop-Dose.
Ganciclovir (DHPG) Capsules and Powder for Injection Cytovene (*Syntex*)	Capsules: 250 mg	In 180s.
Cytovene (*Syntex*)	Powder for Injection, lyophilized: 500 mg/ vial ganciclovir (as sodium)	In 10 ml vials.
Ganciclovir Intravitreal Implant Vitrasert (*Chiron Vision*)	Implant: Minimum 4.5 mg	In individual unit boxes in a sterile Tyvek package.
Foscarnet Sodium (Phosphonoformic acid) Foscavir (*Astra*)	Injection: 24 mg/ml	In 250 and 500 ml bottles.
Cidofovir Vistide (*Gilead Sciences*)	Injection: 75 mg/ml	5 ml amp.

[1] With 0.05% tetrahydrozoline HCl, EDTA, benzalkonium Cl and NaCl.

Epinephrines		
Generic Name Trade Name	**Dose form/ Strength**	**How Supplied**
Epinephrine HCl		
Epinephrine HCl (*Ciba Vision*)	Solution: 0.1%	In 1 ml Dropperettes (12s).[1]
Epifrin (*Allergan*)	0.5% (as base)	In 15 ml dropper bottles.[2]
Epifrin (*Allergan*)	1% (as base)	In 15 ml dropper bottles.[2]
Glaucon (*Alcon*)	1%	In 10 ml Drop-Tainers.[3]
Epifrin (*Allergan*)	2% (as base)	In 15 ml dropper bottles.[2]
Glaucon (*Alcon*)	2%	In 10 ml Drop-Tainers.[3]
Epinephryl Borate		
Epinal (*Alcon*)	Solution: 0.5%	In 7.5 ml.[4]
Epinal (*Alcon*)	1%	In 7.5 ml.[4]
Dipivefrin HCl (Dipivalyl epinephrine)		
Dipivefrin HCl (*Various, eg, Falcon, Schein*)	Solution: 0.1%	In 5, 10 and 15 ml.
Propine (*Allergan*)	0.1%	In 5, 10 & 15 ml C Cap Compliance Cap B.I.D.[5]
AKPro (*Akorn*)	0.1%	In 2, 5, 10 and 15 ml dropper bottles.[5]

[1] With 0.5% chlorobutanol and sodium bisulfite.
[2] With benzalkonium chloride, sodium metabisulfite, EDTA and hydrochloric acid.
[3] With 0.01% benzalkonium chloride, sodium metabisulfite, EDTA, sodium chloride, hydrochloric acid and sodium hydroxide.
[4] With 0.01% benzalkonium chloride, ascorbic acid, acetylcysteine, boric acid and sodium carbonate.
[5] With 0.005% benzalkonium chloride, sodium chloride, EDTA and hydrochloric acid.

Alpha$_2$ Adrenergic Agonists		
Generic Name Trade Name	**Dose form/ Strength**	**How Supplied**
Apraclonidine HCl		
Iopidine (*Alcon*)	Solution: 0.5%	With 0.01% benzalkonium chloride. In 5 ml and 10 ml Drop-Tainers.
Iopidine (*Alcon*)	Solution: 1%	With 0.01% benzalkonium chloride. In 0.1 ml (2s).
Brimonidine Tartrate		
Alphagan (*Allergan*)	Solution: 0.2% brimonidine tartrate, 0.05 mg benzalkonium chloride	In 5 and 10 ml dropper bottles.

Beta-Adrenergic Blocking Agents		
Generic Name Trade Name	**Dose form/ Strength**	**How Supplied**
Betaxolol HCl		
Betoptic (*Alcon*)	Solution: 5.6 mg (equiv. to 5 mg base) per ml (0.5%)	In 2.5, 5, 10 and 15 ml Drop-Tainer bottles.[1]
Betoptic S (*Alcon*)	Suspension: 2.8 mg (equiv. to 2.5 mg base) per ml (0.25%)	In 2.5, 5, 10 and 15 ml Drop-Tainer bottles.[2]
Carteolol HCl		
Ocupress (*Otsuka America*)	Solution: 1%	In 5 and 10 ml dropper bottles.[3]
Levobunolol HCl		
Levobunolol (*Various, eg, Bausch & Lomb*)	Solution: 0.25%	In 5 and 10 ml.
AKBeta (*Akorn*)	0.25%	In 5 and 10 ml.
Betagan Liquifilm (*Allergan*)	0.25%	In 5 and 10 ml dropper bottles with B.I.D. *C Cap*.[4]
Levobunolol (*Various, eg, Bausch & Lomb*)	0.5%	In 5, 10 and 15 ml.
AKBeta (*Akorn*)	0.5%	In 5, 10 and 15 ml.
Betagan Liquifilm (*Allergan*)	0.5%	In 2 ml bottles with B.I.D. and Q.D. *C Cap*.[4]
Metipranolol HCl		
OptiPranolol (*Bausch & Lomb*)	Solution: 0.3%	In 5 or 10 ml dropper bottles.[5]
Timolol Maleate		
Timolol Maleate (*Various, eg, Alcon*)	Solution: 0.25%	In 5, 10 and 15 ml.
Betimol (*Ciba Vision*)	0.25%	In 2.5, 5, 10 and 15 ml.[6]
Timoptic (*Merck*)	0.25%	In 2.5, 5, 10 & 15 ml Ocumeters[6] & UD 60s Ocudose.[7]
Timolol (*Various, eg, Alcon*)	0.5%	In 5, 10 and 15 ml.
Betimol (*Ciba Vision*)	0.5%	In 2.5, 5, 10 and 15 ml.[6]
Timoptic (*Merck*)	0.5%	In 2.5, 5, 10 & 15 ml Ocumeters[6] & UD 60s Ocudose.[7]
Timoptic-XE (*Merck*)	Solution, gel-forming: 0.25%	In 2.5 and 5 ml.[8]
Timoptic-XE (*Merck*)	0.5%	In 2.5 and 5 ml.[8]

[1] With 0.01% benzalkonium chloride and EDTA.
[2] With 0.01% benzalkonium chloride, mannitol, poly sulfonic acid, carbomer 934P and EDTA.
[3] With 0.005% benzalkonium chloride.
[4] With 1.4% polyvinyl alcohol, 0.004% benzalkonium chloride, sodium metabislufite and EDTA.
[5] With 0.004% benzalkonium chloride and EDTA.
[6] With 0.01% benzalkonium chloride.
[7] Preservative free; use immediately after opening; discard remaining contents.
[8] With 0.012% benzododecinium bromide.

Miotics, Direct-Acting		
Generic Name Trade Name	**Dose form/ Strength**	**How Supplied**
Acetylcholine Chloride, Intraocular		
Miochol-E (*Ciba Vision*)	Solution: 1:100 acetylcholine chloride when reconstituted	In 2 ml dual chamber univial (lower chamber 20 mg lyophilized acetylcholine chloride and 56 mg mannitol; upper chamber 2 ml electrolyte diluent[1] and sterile water for injection).
Carbachol, Intraocular		
Carbastat (*Ciba Vision*)	Solution: 0.01%	In 1.5 ml vials.[2]
Miostat (*Alcon*)	0.01%	In 1.5 ml vials.[2]
Carbachol, Topical		
Isopto Carbachol (*Alcon*)	Solution: 0.75%	In 15 and 30 ml Drop-Tainers.[3]
Isopto Carbachol (*Alcon*)	1.5%	In 15 and 30 ml Drop-Tainers.[3]
Isopto Carbachol (*Alcon*)	2.25%	In 15 ml Drop-Tainers.[3]
Isopto Carbachol (*Alcon*)	3%	In 15 and 30 ml Drop-Tainers.[3]
Carboptic (*Optopics*)	3%	In 15 ml.[4]
Pilocarpine HCl		
Isopto Carpine (*Alcon*)	Solution: 0.25%	In 15 ml.[5]
Pilocarpine HCl (*Various, eg, Rugby*)	0.5%	In 15 and 30 ml.
Isopto Carpine (*Alcon*)	0.5%	In 15 and 30 ml.
Pilocar (*Ciba Vision*)	0.5%	In 15 ml and twin-pack (2 × 15 ml).[6]
Piloptic - ½ (*Optopics*)	0.5%	In 15 ml.[7]
Pilostat (*Bausch & Lomb*)	0.5%	In 15 ml.[9]
Pilocarpine HCl (*Various, eg, Alcon, Goldline, Rugby*)	1%	In 2, 15 and 30 ml and UD 1 ml.
Adsorbocarpine (*Alcon*)	1%	In 15 ml.[8]
Akarpine (*Akorn*)	1%	In 15 ml.
Isopto Carpine (*Alcon*)	1%	In 15 and 30 ml.[5]
Pilocar (*Ciba Vision*)	1%	In 15 ml, twin-pack (2 × 15 ml) and 1 ml dropperettes.[6]
Piloptic-1 (*Optopics*)	1%	In 15 ml.[7]
Pilostat (*Bausch & Lomb*)	1%	In 15 ml and twin-pack (2 × 15 ml).[9]
Pilocarpine HCl (*Various, eg, Alcon, Zenith-Goldline*)	2%	In 2, 15 and 30 ml.

Adsorbocarpine (*Alcon*)	2%	In 15 ml dropper bottles.[8]
Akarpine (*Akorn*)	2%	In 15 ml dropper bottles.
Isopto Carpine (*Alcon*)	2%	In 15 and 30 ml.[5]
Pilocar (*Ciba Vision*)	2%	In 15 ml, twin-pack (2 × 15 ml) and 1 ml dropperettes.[6]
Piloptic-2 (*Optopics*)	2%	In 15 ml.[7]
Pilostat (*Bausch & Lomb*)	2%	In 15 ml and twin-pack (2 × 15 ml).[9]
Isopto Carpine (*Alcon*)	3%	In 15 and 30 ml.[5]
Pilocar (*Ciba Vision*)	3%	In 15 ml, twin-pack (2 × 15 ml).[6]
Piloptic-3 (*Optopics*)	3%	In 15 ml.[7]
Pilostat (*Bausch & Lomb*)	3%	In 15 ml and twin-pack (2 × 15 ml).[9]
Pilocarpine HCl (*Various, eg, Alcon, Zenith-Goldline*)	4%	In 2, 15 and 30 ml.
Adsorbocarpine (*Alcon*)	4%	In 15 ml dropper bottles.[8]
Akarpine (*Akorn*)	4%	In 15 ml dropper bottles.
Isopto Carpine (*Alcon*)	4%	In 15 and 30 ml.[5]
Pilocar (*Ciba Vision*)	4%	In 15 ml, twin-pack (2 × 15 ml) and 1 ml dropperettes.[6]
Piloptic-4 (*Optopics*)	4%	In 15 ml.[8]
Pilopto-Carpine (*Lebeh Pharmacal*)	4%	In 15 ml.
Pilostat (*Bausch & Lomb*)	4%	In 15 ml and twin-pack (2 × 15 ml).[9]
Isopto Carpine (*Alcon*)	5%	In 15 and 30 ml.[5]
Pilocarpine HCl (*Various, eg, Rugby*)	6%	In 15 ml.
Isopto Carpine (*Alcon*)	6%	In 15 ml.[5]
Pilocar (*Ciba Vision*)	6%	In 15 ml and twin-pack (2 × 15 ml).[7]
Piloptic-6 (*Optopics*)	6%	In 15 ml.[7]
Pilostat (*Bausch & Lomb*)	6%	In 15 ml.[7]
Isopto Carpine (*Alcon*)	8%	In 15 ml.
Pilocarpine HCl (*Alcon*)	8%	In 2 ml.
Isopto Carpine (*Alcon*)	10%	In 15 ml.[5]

Pilopine HS (*Alcon*)	Gel: 4%	In 3.5 g.[10]
Pilocarpine Nitrate Pilagan (*Allergan*)	Solution: 1%	In 15 ml.[11]
Pilagan (*Allergan*)	2%	In 15 ml.[11]
Pilagan (*Allergan*)	4%	In 15 ml.[11]
Pilocarpine Ocular Therapeutic System Ocusert Pilo-20 (*Alza*)	Ocular Therapeutic System: Releases 20 mcg pilocarpine per hour for 1 week	In packs of 8 individ. sterile systems
Ocusert Pilo-40 (*Alza*)	Releases 40 mcg pilocarpine per hour for 1 week	In packs of 8 individ. sterile systems

[1] Sodium chloride, potassium chloride, magnesium chloride hexahydrate, calcium chloride dihydrate.
[2] With 0.64% sodium chloride, 0.075% potassium chloride, 0.048% calcium chloride dihydrate, 0.03% magnesium chloride hexahydrate, 0.39% sodium acetate trihydrate, 0.17% sodium citrate dihydrate, sodium hydroxide, hydrochloric acid.
[3] With 0.005% benzalkonium chloride, 1% hydroxypropyl methylcellulose, sodium chloride, boric acid and sodium borate.
[4] With benzalkonium chloride, polyvinyl alcohol and sodium phosphate dibasic and monobasic.
[5] With 0.5% hydroxypropyl methylcellulose and 0.01% benzalkonium chloride.
[6] With hydroxypropyl methylcellulose, benzalkonium chloride and EDTA.
[7] With polyvinyl alcohol, benzalkonium chloride and EDTA.
[8] With 0.004% benzalkonium chloride, EDTA, povidone, PEG and hydroxyethyl cellulose.
[9] With hydroxypropyl methylcellulose, 0.01% benzalkonium chloride and EDTA.
[10] With 0.008% benzalkonium chloride, carbopol 940 and EDTA.
[11] With 1.4% polyvinyl alcohol, 0.5% chlorobutanol, menthol, camphor, phenol and eucalyptol.

Cholinesterase Inhibitors

Generic Name Trade Name	Dose form/ Strength	How Supplied
Physostigmine Eserine Sulfate (*Ciba Vision*)	Ointment: 0.25% (as sulfate)	In 3.5 g.
Demecarium Bromide Humorsol (*Merck*)	Solution: 0.125%	In 5 ml Ocumeters.[1]
Humorsol (*Merck*)	0.25%	In 5 ml Ocumeters.[1]
Echothiophate Iodide Phospholine Iodide (*Wyeth-Ayerst*)	Powder for Reconstitution: 1.5 mg to make 0.03%	With 5 ml diluent.[2]
Phospholine Iodide (*Wyeth-Ayerst*)	3 mg to make 0.06%	With 5 ml diluent.[2]
Phospholine Iodide (*Wyeth-Ayerst*)	6.25 mg to make 0.125%	With 5 ml diluent.[2]
Phospholine Iodide (*Wyeth-Ayerst*)	12.5 mg to make 0.25%	With 5 ml diluent.[2]
Pilocarpine and Epinephrine E-Pilo-1 (*Ciba Vision*)	Solution: 1% pilocarpine HCl, 1% epinephrine bitartrate	In 10 ml dropper bottles.[3]
P_1E_1 (*Alcon*)	1% pilocarpine HCl, 1% epinephrine bitartrate	In 15 ml Drop-Tainers.[4]
E-Pilo-2 (*Ciba Vision*)	2% pilocarpine HCl, 1% epinephrine bitartrate	In 10 ml dropper bottles.[3]
P_2E_1 (*Alcon*)	2% pilocarpine HCl, 1% epinephrine bitartrate	In 15 ml Drop-Tainers.[4]
P_3E_1 (*Alcon*)	3% pilocarpine HCl, 1% epinephrine bitartrate	In 15 ml Drop-Tainers.[4]
E-Pilo-4 (*Ciba Vision*)	4% pilocarpine HCl, 1% epinephrine bitartrate	In 10 ml dropper bottles.[3]
P_4E_1 (*Alcon*)	4% pilocarpine HCl, 1% epinephrine bitartrate	In 15 ml Drop-Tainers.[4]
E-Pilo-6 (*Ciba Vision*)	6% pilocarpine HCl, 1% epinephrine bitartrate	In 10 ml dropper bottles.[3]

P_6E_1 (*Alcon*)	6% pilocarpine HCl, 1% epinephrine bitartrate	In 15 ml Drop-Tainers.[4]

[1] With 1:5000 benzalkonium chloride and sodium chloride.
[2] With potassium acetate, 0.55% chlorobutanol and 1.2% mannitol.
[3] With benzalkonium chloride, EDTA, mannitol and sodium bisulfite.
[4] With 0.01% benzalkonium chloride, methylcellulose, EDTA, chlorobutanol, polyethylene glycol and sodium bisulfite.

Carbonic Anhydrase Inhibitors

Generic Name Trade Name	**Dose form/ Strength**	**How Supplied**
Acetazolamide		
Acetazolamide (*Various, eg, Mutual, URL*)	Tablets: 125 mg	In 50s, 100s, 250s, 500s and 1000s.
Diamox (*Lederle*)	125 mg	In 100s.
Acetazolamide (*Various, eg, Qualitest, Schein, URL*)	250 mg	In 100s, 500s, 1000s and UD 100s.
Dazamide (*Major*)	250 mg	In 100s, 250s, 1000s and UD 100s.
Diamox (*Lederle*)	250 mg	In 100s, 1000s and UD 100s.
Diamox Sequels (*Lederle*)	Capsules, sustained release: 500 mg	In 30s and 100s.
Acetazolamide (*Various, eg, Bedford Labs*)	Powder for injection, lyophilized: 500 mg (as sodium)	In vials.
Dichlorphenamide		
Daranide (*Merck*)	Tablets: 50 mg	Lactose. In 100s.
Methazolamide		
Methazolamide (*Various, eg, Mikart*)	Tablets: 25 mg	In 100s.
Methazolamide (*Various, eg, Mikart*)	50 mg	In 100s.
Neptazane (*Lederle*)	25 mg	In 100s.
Neptazane (*Lederle*)	50 mg	In 100s.
GlaucTabs (*Akorn*)	25 mg	In 100s.
GlaucTabs (*Akorn*)	50 mg	In 100s.
MZM Tablets (*Ciba Vision*)	25 mg	Lactose. In 100s.
MZM Tablets (*Ciba Vision*)	50 mg	Lactose. In 100s.
Dorzolamide HCl		
Trusopt (*Merck*)	Solution: 2%	In 5 and 10 ml.

Prostaglandins		
Generic Name Trade Name	**Dose form/ Strength**	**How Supplied**
Latanoprost Xalatan (*Pharmacia & Upjohn*)	Solution: 0.005%	In 2.5 ml plastic ophthalmic dispenser bottle with dropper tip.[1]

[1] With 0.02% benzalkonium chloride, sodium chloride, sodium dihydrogen phosphate monohydrate, disodium hydrogen phosphate anhydrous.

Hyperosmotic Agents

Generic Name Trade Name	Dose form/ Strength	How Supplied
Glucose, Topical		
Glucose-40 (*Ciba Vision*)	Ointment: 40%	White petrolatum, anhydrous lanolin, parabens. In 3.5 g.
Glycerin, Topical		
Ophthalgan (*Wyeth-Ayerst*)	Solution: Glycerin	0.55% chlorobutanol. In 7.5 ml.
Sodium Chloride, Hypertonic		
Adsorbonac (*Alcon*)	Solution: 2%	In 15 ml.[1]
Muro 128 (*Bausch & Lomb*)	Solution: 2%	In 15 ml.[2]
Adsorbonac (*Alcon*)	Solution: 5%	In 15 ml.[1]
AK-NaCl (*Akorn*)	Solution: 5%	In 15 ml.[3]
Muro 128 (*Bausch & Lomb*)	Solution: 5%	In 15 and 30 ml.[4]
Muroptic-5 (*Optopics*)	Solution: 5%	In 15 ml.[5]
AK-NaCl (*Akorn*)	Ointment: 5%	Preservative free. In 3.5 g.[6]
Muro 128 (*Bausch & Lomb*)	Ointment: 5%	In 3.5 g single and twin packs.[7]
Glycerin (Glycerol)		
Osmōglyn (*Alcon*)	Solution: 50% (0.6 g glycerin/ml)	Lime flavor. In 220 ml.
Isosorbide		
Ismotic (*Alcon*)	Solution: 45% (100 g per 220 ml)	With 4.6 mEq sodium and 0.9 mEq potassium per 220 ml. Alcohol, saccharin, sorbitol. Vanilla-mint flavor. In 220 ml.
Mannitol		
Osmitrol (*Baxter*)	Injection: 5%	In 1000 ml.
Osmitrol (*Baxter*)	Injection: 10%	In 500 and 1000 ml.
Osmitrol (*Baxter*)	Injection: 15%	In 500 ml.
Osmitrol (*Baxter*)	Injection: 20%	In 250 and 500 ml.
Mannitol (*Various, eg, American Regent, Astra, IMS, Taylor Pharmaceuticals*)	Injection: 25%	In 50 ml.

[1] With povidone, hydroxyethylcellulose 2910, PEG-90M, poloxamer 188, 0.004% thimerosal, EDTA.
[2] With hydroxypropyl methylcellulose 2906, 0.046% methylparaben, 0.02% propylparaben, propylene glycol, boric acid.
[3] With hydroxypropyl methylcellulose, propylene glycol, 0.023% methylparaben, 0.01% propylparaben, boric acid.
[4] Boric acid, hydroxypropyl methylcellulose 2910, propylene glycol, 0.023% methylparaben, 0.01% propylparaben.
[5] With benzalkonium chloride, EDTA, polyvinyl alcohol, propylene.
[6] With mineral oil, white petrolatum, lanolin oil.
[7] With mineral oil, white petrolatum, lanolin.

Surgical Adjuncts

Generic Name Trade Name	Dose form/ Strength	How Supplied
Intraocular Irrigating Solutions		
Balanced Salt Solution (*Various, eg, Akorn*)	Solution: 0.64% NaCl, 0.075% KCl, 0.03% magnesium chloride, 0.048% calcium chloride, 0.39% sodium acetate, 0.17% sodium citrate and hydrochloric acid or hydrochloric acid	In 18 and 500 ml.
AMO Endosol (*Allergan*)	0.64% NaCl, 0.075% KCl, 0.03% magnesium chloride, 0.048% calcium chloride, 0.39% sodium acetate, 0.17% sodium citrate and hydrochloric acid or hydrochloric acid	Preservative free. In 500 ml.
BSS (*Alcon*)	0.64% NaCl, 0.075% KCl, 0.03% magnesium chloride, 0.048% calcium chloride, 0.39% sodium acetate, 0.17% sodium citrate and hydrochloric acid or hydrochloric acid	Preservative free. In 15, 30, 250 and 500 ml.
Iocare Balanced Salt (*Ciba Vision*)	0.64% NaCl, 0.075% KCl, 0.03% magnesium chloride, 0.048% calcium chloride, 0.39% sodium acetate, 0.17% sodium citrate and hydrochloric acid or hydrochloric acid	Preservative free. In 15 ml.
AMO Endosol Extra (*Allergan*)	Mix aseptically just prior to use. **Part I:** 7.14 mg NaCl, 0.38 mg KCl, 0.154 mg calcium chloride dihydrate, 0.2 mg magnesium chloride hexahydrate, 0.92 mg dextrose, hydrochloric acid or sodium hydroxide/ml	Preservative free. In 515 ml.
	Part II: 1081 mg sodium bicarbonate, 216 mg dibasic sodium phosphate (anhydrous) and 95 mg glutathione disulfide (oxidized glutathione)/vial	Preservative free. In 60 ml.
BSS Plus (*Alcon*)	Mix aseptically just prior to use. **Part I:** 7.44 mg NaCl, 0.395 mg KCl, 0.433 mg dibasic sodium phosphate, 2.19 mg sodium bicarbonate, hydrochloric acid or sodium hydroxide/ml	Preservative free. In 240 ml.
	Part II: 3.85 mg calcium chloride dihydrate, 5 mg magnesium chloride hexahydrate, 23 mg dextrose, 4.6 mg glutathione disulfide/ml	Preservative free. In 10 ml.

B-Salt Forte (*Akorn*)	Mix aseptically just prior to use. **Part I:** 7.14 mg NaCl, 0.38 mg KCl, 0.154 mg calcium chloride dihydrate, 0.2 mg magnesium chloride hexahydrate, 0.92 mg dextrose, hydrochloric acid or sodium hydroxide/ml	Preservative free. In 515 ml.
	Part II: 1081 mg sodium bicarbonate, 216 mg dibasic sodium phosphate (anhydrous) and 95 mg glutathione disulfide (oxidized glutathione)/vial	Preservative free. In 60 ml.
Povidone Iodine Betadine 5% Sterile Ophthalmic Prep Solution (*Akorn*)	Solution: 5% povidone iodine	In 50 ml.[1]
Sodium Hyaluronate Healon (*Kabi Pharmacia*)	Injection: 10 mg/ml[2]	In 0.4, 0.55, 0.85 and 2 ml disp. syringes.
ProVisc (*Alcon*)		In 0.4, 0.55 and 0.85 ml disposable glass syringes.
Amvisc (*Chiron*)	12 mg/ml[3]	In 0.5 or 0.8 ml disp. syringes.
Healon GV (*Kabi Pharmacia*)	14 mg/ml[2]	In 0.55 and 0.85 ml disp. syringes.
Amvisc Plus (*Chiron*)	16 mg/ml[3]	In 0.5 or 8 ml disp. syringes.
AMO Vitrax (*Allergan*)	30 mg/ml[4]	In 0.65 ml disp. syringe.
Sodium Hyaluronate and Chondroitin Sulfate Viscoat (*Alcon*)	Solution: ≤ 40 mg sodium chondroitin sulfate, 30 mg sodium hyaluronate per ml	0.45 mg sodium dihydrogen phosphate hydrate, 2 mg disodium hydrogen phosphate, 4.3 mg sodium chloride per ml. In 0.5 ml disposable syringes.
Sodium Hyaluronate and Fluorescein Sodium Healon Yellow (*Pharmacia & Upjohn*)	Solution: 10 mg sodium hyaluronate, 0.005 mg fluorescein sodium per ml	8.5 mg NaCl, 0.28 mg disodium hydrogen phosphate dihydrate, 0.04 mg sodium dihydrogen phosphate hydrate per ml. In 0.55 or 0.85 ml disposable syringes with cannula.
Hydroxypropyl Methylcellulose OcuCoat (*Storz*)	Solution: 2%	In a balanced salt solution. In 1 ml syringe with cannula.
Gonak (*Akorn*)	Solution: 2.5%	In 15 ml.[5]
Goniosol (*Ciba Vision*)	Solution: 2.5%	In 15 ml.[5]

Hydroxyethyl-cellulose Gonioscopic (*Alcon*)	Solution: Hydroxyethylcellulose	0.004% thimerosal, 0.1% EDTA. In 15 ml Drop-Tainers.
Absorbable Gelatin Film, Sterile Gelfilm (*Pharmacia & Upjohn*) Gelfilm Ophthalmic (*Pharmacia & Upjohn*)	100 mm x 125 mm 25 mm x 50 mm	In 1s. In 6s.
Miotics, Direct-Acting Acetylcholine Chloride, Intraocular Miochol-E (*Ciba Vision*)	Solution: 1:100 acetylcholine chloride when reconstituted	In 2 ml dual chamber univial (lower chamber 20 mg lyophilized acetylcholine chloride and 56 mg mannitol; upper chamber 2 ml electrolyte diluent[6] and sterile water for injection).
Miotics, Direct-Acting Carbachol, Intraocular Carbastat (*Ciba Vision*) Miostat (*Alcon*)	Solution: 0.01% 0.01%	In 1.5 ml vials.[7] In 1.5 ml vials.[7]
Polydimethylsilox-ane (Silicone Oil) AdatoSil 5000 (*Escalon Ophthalmics*)	Injection: Polydimethylsiloxane oil	In single-use 10 and 15 ml vials.
Botulinum Toxin Type A Botox (*Allergan*)	Powder for Injection (lyophilized): 100 units of lyophilized *Clostridium botulinum* toxin type A[8]	Preservative free. 0.05 mg albumin (human), 0.9 mg sodium chloride. In vials.

[1] Glycerin, sodium chloride, sodium hydroxide and sodium phosphate.
[2] With 8.5 mg NaCl per ml.
[3] With 9 mg NaCl per ml.
[4] With 3.2 mg NaCl, 0.75 mg KCl, 0.48 mg calcium chloride, 0.3 mg magnesium chloride, 3.9 mg sodium acetate and 1.7 mg sodium citrate per ml.
[5] With 0.01% benzalkonium chloride and EDTA.
[6] Sodium chloride, potassium chloride, magnesium chloride hexahydrate, calcium chloride dihydrate.
[7] With 0.64% sodium chloride, 0.075% potassium chloride, 0.048% calcium chloride dihydrate, 0.03% magnesium chloride hexahydrate, 0.39% sodium acetate trihydrate, 0.17% sodium citrate dihydrate, sodium hydroxide, hydrochloric acid.
[8] One unit corresponds to the calculated median lethal intraperitoneal dose (LD/50) in mice of the reconstituted drug injected.

Nonsurgical Adjuncts

Generic Name Trade Name	**Dose form/ Strength**	**How Supplied**
Dapiprazole HCl		
Rēv-Eyes (*Storz/Lederle*)	Powder, lyophilized: 25 mg (0.5% solution when reconstituted)	In vial with 5 ml diluent and dropper.[1]
Extraocular Irrigating Solutions		
AK-Rinse (*Akorn*)	Solution: Sodium carbonate, KCl, boric acid, EDTA, 0.01% benzalkonium Cl	In 30 and 118 ml.
Blinx (*Akorn*)	Solution: NaCl, KCl, sodium phosphate, 0.005% benzalkonium Cl, 0.02% EDTA	In 120 ml.
Collyrium for Fresh Eyes Wash (*Wyeth-Ayerst*)	Solution: Boric acid, sodium borate, benzalkonium chloride	In 120 ml.
Dacriose (*Ciba Vision*)	Solution: NaCl, KCl, sodium phosphate, sodium hydroxide, 0.01% benzalkonium Cl, EDTA	In 15 and 120 ml.
Eye Stream (*Alcon*)	Solution: 0.64% NaCl, 0.075% KCl, 0.03% magnesium Cl hexahydrate, 0.048% calcium Cl dihydrate, 0.39% sodium acetate trihydrate, 0.17% sodium citrate dihydrate, 0.013% benzalkonium Cl	In 30 and 118 ml.
Eye Wash (*Bausch & Lomb*)	Solution: Boric acid, KCl, EDTA, sodium carbonate, 0.01% benzalkonium Cl	In 118 ml.
Eye Wash (*Zenith-Goldline*)	Solution: Boric acid, KCl, EDTA, anhydrous sodium carbonate, 0.01% benzalkonium Cl	In 118 ml.
Eye Wash (*Lavoptik*)	Solution: 0.49% NaCl, 0.4% sodium biphosphate, 0.45% sodium phosphate, 0.005% benzalkonium Cl	In 180 ml with eyecup.
Eye Irrigating Wash (*Roberts Hauck*)	Solution: Boric acid, KCl, sodium carbonate, EDTA, 0.01% benzalkonium Cl	In 120 ml.
Eye Irrigating Solution (*Rugby*)	Solution: NaCl, mono- and dibasic sodium phosphate, benzalkonium Cl, EDTA	In 118 ml.
Irrigate Eye Wash (*Optopics*)	Solution: NaCl, mono- and dibasic sodium phosphate, benzalkonium Cl, EDTA	In 118 ml.
Optigene (*Pfeiffer*)	Solution: NaCl, mono- and dibasic sodium phosphate, EDTA, benzalkonium Cl	In 118 ml.

Visual-Eyes (*Optopics*)	Solution: NaCl, mono- and dibasic sodium phosphate, benzalkonium Cl, EDTA	In 120 ml.
Lid Scrubs		
Eye-Scrub (*Ciba Vision*)	Solution: PEG-200 glyceryl tallowate, disodium laureth sulfosuccinate, cocoamidopropyl-amine oxide, PEG-78 glyceryl cocoate, benzyl alcohol, EDTA	In UD 30s (pads) and kit (120 ml and 60 pads).
Lid Wipes-SPF (*Akorn*)	Solution: PEG-200 glyceryl tallowate, PEG-80 glyceryl cocoate, laureth-23, cocoamidopropylamine oxide, NaCl, glycerin, sodium phosphate, sodium hydroxide	Preservative free. In UD 30s (pads).
OCuSOFT (*OCuSOFT*)	Solution: PEG-80 sorbitan laurate, sodium trideceth sulfate, PEG-150 distearate, cocoamidopropyl hydroxysultaine, lauroampha-carboxyglycinate, sodium laureth-13 carboxylate, PEG-15 tallow polyamine, quarternium-15	Alcohol and dye free. In UD 30s (pads), 30, 120 and 240 ml and compliance kit (120 ml and 100 pads).
Tear Test Strips		
Sno-Strips (*Akorn*)	Strips: Sterile tear flow test strips	In 100s.
Schirmer Tear Test (*Various, eg, Alcon*)	Strips: Sterile test strips	In 250s.
Zone-Quick (*Menicon USA*)	Threads: Phenol red threads (PRT)	In 50 Aluminum pkg sets (100 threads).
Hamamelis Water		
Succus Cineraria Maritima (*Walker Pharm*)	Solution: Aqueous and glycerin solution of senecio compositae, hamamelis water, boric acid	In 7 ml.
Zinc Sulfate Solution		
Eye-Sed (*Scherer*)	Solution: 0.25%	In 15 ml.[2]
Vitamins and Minerals		
Vitamin A Palmitate (*Freeda*)	Tablets: 10,000 IU	In 100s and 250s.
Vitamin A Palmitate (*Freeda*)	Tablets: 15,000 IU	In 100s and 250s.
Vitamin A Palmitate (*Freeda*)	Tablets: 25,000 IU	In 100s and 250s.
Beta Carotene (*Freeda*)	Tablets: 10,000 IU	In 100s, 250s and 500s.
Palmitate-A (*Akorn*)	Tablets: 15,000 IU vitamin A palmitate	In 100s.
Palmitate-A 5000 (*Akorn*)	Tablets: 5000 IU vitamin A palmitate	In 100s.

Icaps Plus (*Ciba Vision*)	Tablets: 6000 IU vitamin A[3], 200 mg C, 20 mg B_2, 60 IU E, 40 mg Zn[4], 2 mg Cu, 5 mg Mn, 20 mcg Se	In 60s, 120s and 180s.
Icaps Time Release (*Ciba Vision*)	Tablets: 7000 IU vitamin A[3], 200 mg C, 20 mg B_2, 100 IU E, 40 mg Zn[4], 2 mg Cu, 20 mcg Se	In 60s and 120s.
AntiOxidants (*Akorn*)	Caplets: 5000 IU vitamin A[3], 400 mg C[5], 200 IU E[6], 40 mg Zn[7], 5 mg L-glutathione, 3 mg sodium pyruvate, 2 mg Cu[8], 40 mcg Se[9]	In 60s.
Oxi-Freeda (*Freeda*)	Tablets: 5000 IU beta carotene, 150 IU E, 20 mg B_1, 20 mg B_2, 20 mg B_6, 10 mcg B_{12}, 15 mg elemental Zn, 50 mcg Se, 20 mg calcium pantothenate, 40 mg glutathione, 40 mg B_3, 100 mg C, 75 mg L-cysteine	In 100s and 250s.
One-A-Day Extras Antioxidant (*Bayer*)	Capsules, softgel: 5000 IU vitamin A[3], 200 IU E, 250 mg C, 7.5 mg Zn, 1 mg Cu, 15 mcg Se, 1.5 mg Mn	Tartrazine. In 50s.
OCuSoft VMS (*OCuSoft*)	Tablets: 5000 IU vitamin A, 30 IU E, 60 mg C, 40 mg Zn, 2 mg Cu, 40 mcg Se	Film coated. In 60s.
Ocuvite (*Storz/Lederle*)	Tablets: 40 mg elemental Zn[10], 2 mg elemental Cu[11], 40 mcg elemental Se[12], 5000 IU vitamin A[3], 30 IU E[5] and 60 mg C[6]	In 60s and 120s.
Ocuvite Extra (*Storz/ Lederle*)	Tablets: 40 mg elemental Zn[10], 2 mg elemental Cu[11], 200 mg C, 50 IU E, 6000 IU vitamin A[3], 40 mcg elemental Se, 3 mg B_2, 40 mg B_3, 5 mg elemental Mn, 5 mg L-glutathione	In 50s.

[1] With 2% mannitol, 0.4% hydroxypropyl methylcellulose, 0.01% EDTA, 0.01% benzalkonium chloride and sodium chloride.
[2] With 0.05% tetrahydrozoline HCl, EDTA, benzalkonium Cl and NaCl.
[3] As beta carotene.
[4] As zinc acetate.
[5] As ascorbic acid.
[6] As dl-alpha tocopheryl acetate.
[7] As zinc ascorbate.
[8] As copper ascorbate.
[9] As L-selenomethionine.
[10] As zinc oxide.
[11] As cupric oxide.
[12] As sodium selenate.

INDEX

This **Index** lists all generic names, brand names *(italics)* and group names included in *Ophthalmic Drug Facts*. Additionally, many drug tables, synonyms, pharmacological actions and therapeutic uses for the agents listed are included.

Index entries may refer to more than one form of a product (eg, tablets, solutions, suspensions, ointments) when all forms are included on the single page. Separate index entries are included when multiple forms of a product appear on different pages or when products are listed in more than one therapeutic group.